Dedicated to John S. Thompson, MD

A Department Chairman
A Mentor and Friend

From the Chief Residents at the
University of Kentucky
Department of Medicine
1980–1990

Contents

Associate Editors

James Barker, MD
Pulmonary and Critical Care Medicine
Nebraska Methodist Hospital
Medical Director
Nebraska Methodist School of Respiratory Care
Omaha, Nebraska

Marianne Billeter, PharmD
Assistant Professor of Clinical Pharmacy
College of Pharmacy
Xavier University of Louisiana
New Orleans, Louisiana

David P. Haynie, MD
Staff Cardiologist
The Medical and Surgical Clinic
Wichita Falls, Texas

Monty S. Metcalfe, MD
Assistant Professor
Division of Hematology-Oncology
Markey Cancer Center
Department of Medicine
University of Kentucky Medical Center
Lexington, Kentucky

Benjamin Stahr, MD, FCAP
Associate Pathologist
Atlanta Dermatopathology and Pathology Associates
Atlanta, Georgia

Contributors

James Barker, MD
Pulmonary and Critical Care Medicine
Nebraska Methodist Hospital
Medical Director
Nebraska Methodist School of Respiratory Care
Omaha, Nebraska

David J. Bensema, MD
General Internist
Private Practice
Lexington, Kentucky

Marianne Billeter, PharmD
Assistant Professor of Clinical Pharmacy
College of Pharmacy
Xavier University of Louisiana
New Orleans, Louisiana

David W. Dozer, MD
Chief Resident
Department of Medicine
University of Kentucky Medical Center
Lexington, Kentucky

D. Randolph Drosick, MD
Fellow, Division of Hematology-Oncology
Department of Medicine
University of Kentucky Medical Center
Lexington, Kentucky

Rita M. Egan, MD, PhD
Assistant Professor of Medicine
Division of Rheumatology
Department of Medicine
University of Kentucky Medical Center
Lexington, Kentucky

G. Paul Eleazer, MD
Assistant Professor of Medicine
Division of General Internal Medicine
Department of Medicine
University of South Carolina
Columbia, South Carolina

Douglas L. Fraker, MD
Senior Resident
Department of Surgery
University of California, San Francisco
San Francisco, California

David K. Goebel, MD
Fellow, Division of Hematology-Oncology
Department of Medicine
University of Kentucky Medical Center
Lexington, Kentucky

John J. Gohmann, MD
Medical Oncologist
Private Practice
Lexington, Kentucky

Tricia L. Gomella, MD
Neonatal Consultant
Department of Pediatrics
Division of Neonatology
Francis Scott Key Medical Center
Baltimore, Maryland

C. Gary Grigsby, Jr, MD
Fellow, Cardiology
Department of Medicine
University of Kentucky Medical Center
Lexington, Kentucky

Steven A. Haist, MD
Assistant Professor of Medicine
Division of General Internal Medicine and Geriatrics
Department of Medicine
University of Kentucky Medical Center
Lexington, Kentucky

David P. Haynie, MD
Staff Cardiologist
The Medical and Surgical Clinic
Wichita Falls, Texas

William J. John, MD
Assistant Professor of Medicine
Division of Digestive Diseases and Nutrition
Department of Medicine
University of Kentucky Medical Center
Lexington, Kentucky

Craig B. Kaplan, MD
Associate Professor of Medicine
Division of General Internal Medicine
Department of Internal Medicine
Medical College of Virginia
Richmond, Virginia

Gale G. Kerns, MD, FACC
Cardiologist
The Duluth Clinic
Duluth, Minnesota

Ross E. Kerns, MD
Hematologist-Oncologist
Private Practice
Knoxville, Tennessee

Alan T. Lefor, MD
Assistant Professor of Surgery and Oncology
Department of Surgery
University of Maryland
Baltimore, Maryland

Jerry J. Lierl, MD
Cardiologist
Cardiology Associates
Crestview Hill, Kentucky

Ralph A. Manchester, MD
Medical Chief
University Health Service
Assistant Professor of Medicine
General Medicine Unit
Department of Medicine
University of Rochester School of Medicine and Dentistry
Rochester, New York

Rick R. McClure, MD
Fellow and Clinical Scholar
Division of Cardiovascular Medicine
Department of Medicine
University of Kentucky Medical Center
Lexington, Kentucky

Monty S. Metcalfe, MD
Assistant Professor
Division of Hematology-Oncology
Markey Cancer Center
Department of Medicine
University of Kentucky Medical Center
Lexington, Kentucky

Thomas B. Montgomery, MD
Assistant Professor of Medicine
Division of General Internal Medicine and Geriatrics
Department of Medicine
University of Kentucky Medical Center
Lexington, Kentucky

Rita K. Munn, MD
Fellow, Division of Hematology-Oncology
Department of Medicine
University of Kentucky Medical Center
Lexington, Kentucky

Mark V. Paciotti, MD
Cardiologist
Harrison Memorial Hospital
Bremerton, Washington

Carol B. Peddicord, MD
Chief Resident
Department of Medicine
University of Kentucky Medical Center
Lexington, Kentucky

John B. Robbins, MD
Assistant Professor of Medicine
Division of General Internal Medicine and Geriatrics
Department of Medicine
University of Kentucky Medical Center
Lexington, Kentucky

Benjamin Stahr, MD, FCAP
Associate Pathologist
Atlanta Dermatopathology and Pathology Associates
Atlanta, Georgia

R. Douglas Strickland, MD
Chief Resident
Department of Medicine
University of Kentucky Medical Center
Lexington, Kentucky

Michael N. Tate, MD
Medical Oncologist
Hickory Oncology and Hematology Clinic
Hickory, North Carolina

Eric C. Westman, MD
Fellow, Division of General Medicine
Department of Medicine
Duke University
Durham, North Carolina

Eric A. Wiebke, MD
Chief Resident
Department of Surgery
The Johns Hopkins Hospital
Baltimore, Maryland

Timothy A. Winchester, MD
General Internist
Private Practice
Lexington, Kentucky

Preface

Internal Medicine On Call provides a readily available reference that will assist in the initial evaluation and treatment of frequently encountered problems in internal medicine. It will aid houseofficers and medical students when they are called about potentially life-threatening as well as common problems. The following pages will provide a concise, practical approach to these problems and will serve to bridge the gap between classroom, textbook, and patient care. We have not attempted to provide a comprehensive discussion of each topic, but rather the essential elements in the initial assessment and management that will aid the houseofficer and student when they are called to evaluate these problems.

The on-call problems are introduced with a case scenario. This is followed by the questions the clinician must initially ask. A differential diagnosis for the problem is given with key points to help the physician arrive at the final diagnosis. Evaluation and treatment are then outlined. Recommendations for treatment are specific with regard to dosage and dosing intervals, but it is emphasized that hepatic and renal disease as well as other factors (eg, age) can greatly affect the metabolism of drugs. In addition, variations in institutional practices exist. For these reasons, treatment may need to be individualized.

Houseofficers and medical students often have questions regarding appropriate use of laboratory tests, proper procedural technique, and frequently used medications. These areas as well as blood component therapy and ventilator management have been incorporated into this manual.

We are grateful to Tricia Gomella, MD, for providing the "on-call" concept originally used in her book *Neonatology: Basic Management, On Call Problems, Diseases, and Drugs,* published by Appleton & Lange in 1988. We are also grateful to Leonard Gomella, MD, and Alan T. Lefor, MD, since many of the problems as well as other sections from their *Surgery On Call,* published by Appleton & Lange in 1990, have been modified in this manual for the houseofficer and student in internal medicine. We thank Appleton & Lange for providing us the forum to present unique approaches for medical student and houseofficer education.

Finally, we extend to Beverly Jones our sincerest appreciation for the dedicated secretarial support that she provided. Without her assistance, completion of this text would not have been possible.

We hope this manual will enhance your training and help you provide the best care for your patients.

Steven A. Haist, MD
John B. Robbins, MD

1 On Call Problems

■ ABDOMINAL PAIN

I. **Problem.** A 34-year-old woman admitted for control of her diabetes develops acute abdominal pain that increases in severity over several hours.

II. **Immediate Questions**

A. **What are the patient's vital signs?** Acute abdominal pain in this woman could signify a condition as benign as gastroenteritis or as catastrophic as an infarcted bowel or perforated viscus. The significant morbidity and mortality of the acute surgical abdomen can be obviated by early diagnosis. **Tachycardia** and **hypotension** would suggest circulatory or septic shock from perforation, hemorrhage, or fluid loss into the intestinal lumen or peritoneal cavity. Orthostatic blood pressure and pulse changes would also be helpful in ascertaining the presence of volume loss. **Fever** occurs in inflammatory conditions such as cholecystitis and appendicitis. When the temperature exceeds 102°F, gangrene or perforation of a viscus should be suspected. Fever may not be present in elderly patients, patients on corticosteroids, or patients who are immunocompromised.

B. **Where is the pain located?** Abdominal pain is produced by three mechanisms: (1) tension within the walls of the alimentary tract (biliary or intestinal obstruction); (2) ischemia (strangulated bowel, mesenteric vascular occlusion); and (3) peritoneal irritation. The first two causes result in visceral pain, a dull pain perceived in the midline and **poorly localized.** Generally, **midepigastric pain** is caused by disorders of the stomach, duodenum, pancreas, liver, and biliary tract. Disease of the small intestine, appendix, upper ureters, testes, and ovaries results in **periumbilical pain. Lower abdominal pain** is caused by processes in the colon, bladder, lower ureters, and uterus. Inflammation of the parietal peritoneum results in more severe pain that is **well localized** to the area of inflammation.

C. **Does the pain radiate?** Pain that becomes generalized rapidly implies perforation and leakage of fluid into the peritoneal cavity. Biliary pain can radiate from the right upper quadrant to the right inferior scapula. Pancreatic and abdominal aneurysmal pain may radiate to the back. Ureteral colic may be referred to the groin and thigh.

D. When did the pain begin? Sudden onset suggests perforated ulcer, mesenteric occlusion, ruptured aneurysm, or ruptured ectopic pregnancy. A more gradual onset over 1 hour or longer implies an inflammatory condition such as appendicitis or cholecystitis or an obstructed viscus such as bowel obstruction.

E. What is the quality of pain? Intestinal colic occurs as cramping abdominal pain interspersed with pain-free intervals. Biliary colic is not a true colicky pain in that it usually presents as sustained, persistent pain. Unfortunately, the terms *sharp, dull, burning,* and *tearing,* although used by the patient to describe pain, seldom assist in distinguishing the etiology.

F. What makes the pain better or worse? Pain with deep inspiration is associated with diaphragmatic irritation, such as with pleurisy or upper abdominal inflammation. Patients with intestinal or ureteral colic tend to be restless and active, whereas patients with peritonitis attempt to avoid all motion. Coughing frequently exacerbates abdominal pain with peritonitis.

G. Are there any associated symptoms? Vomiting may result from intestinal obstruction or could result from a visceral reflex caused by pain. In conditions causing an acute surgical abdomen, the vomiting usually follows rather than precedes the onset of pain. **Hematemesis** suggests gastritis or peptic ulcer disease. **Diarrhea** could result from gastroenteritis, but could also result from ischemic colitis or inflammatory disease. **Obstipation** (absence of passage of stool or flatus) suggests mechanical bowel obstruction. **Hematuria** would suggest genitourinary disease. **Cough** and **sputum production** might occur if lower lobe pneumonia is present.

H. If female, what is her menstrual history? A missed period in a sexually active woman would suggest ectopic pregnancy. A foul vaginal discharge might indicate pelvic inflammatory disease.

I. What is the patient's past medical history? Does the patient have a history of peptic ulcer disease, gallstones, alcohol abuse, abdominal operations resulting in adhesions, or abdominal aortic aneurysm? Is there any known history of cardiac arrhythmias or other cardiac disease that could result in embolization to a mesenteric artery?

III. Differential Diagnosis. There are several potential causes of acute abdominal pain, some of which are listed in Table 1–1. Many of these diseases can be managed medically; others require urgent surgery. Abdominal pain can result from extra-abdominal processes as well as intra-abdominal disease.

A. Intra-abdominal disease

1. Hollow viscera. Perforation of a hollow viscus represents a surgical emergency.

a. Upper abdomen: Esophagitis, gastritis, peptic ulcer disease, cholecystitis.

TABLE 1–1. COMMON CAUSES OF ACUTE ABDOMEN[a]

- **Gastrointestinal tract disorders**
  - *Appendicitis*
  - *Small and large bowel obstruction*
  - *Strangulated hernia*
  - *Perforated peptic ulcer*
  - *Bowel perforation*
  - *Meckel's diverticulitis*
  - *Boerhaave's syndrome*
  - Diverticulitis
  - Inflammatory bowel disorders
  - Mallory-Weiss syndrome
  - Gastroenteritis
  - Acute gastritis
  - Mesenteric adenitis
- **Liver, spleen, and biliary traet disorders**
  - *Acute cholecystitis*
  - *Acute cholangitis*
  - *Hepatic abscess*
  - *Ruptured hepatic tumor*
  - *Spontaneous rupture of the spleen*
  - Splenic infarct
  - Biliary colic
  - Acute hepatitis
- **Pancreatic disorders**
  - Acute pancreatitis
- **Urinary tract disorders**
  - Ureteral or renal colic
  - Acute pyelonephritis
  - Acute cystitis
  - Renal infarct
- **Gynecologic disorders**
  - *Ruptured ectopic pregnancy*
  - *Twisted ovarian tumor*
  - *Ruptured ovarian follicle cyst*
  - Acute salpingitis
  - Dysmenorrhea
  - Endometriosis
- **Vascular disorders**
  - *Ruptured aortic and visceral aneurysms*
  - *Acute ischemic colitis*
  - *Mesenteric thrombosis*
- **Peritoneal disorders**
  - *Intra-abdomonal abscesses*
  - Primary peritonitis
  - Tuberculous peritonitis
- **Retroperitoneal disorders**
  - Retroperitoneal hemorrhage

[a] Conditions in italic often require urgent operation.
From Boey JH. Acute abdomen. In: Way LW, ed. Current Surgical Diagnosis and Treatment. *8th ed. Norwalk, Conn: Appleton & Lange; 1988. Used with permission.*

  b. **Midgut:** Small bowel obstruction or infarction.
  c. **Lower abdomen:** Inflammatory bowel disease, appendicitis, obstruction, diverticulitis.

2. Solid organ
  a. Hepatitis
  b. Pancreatitis
  c. Splenic infarction
  d. Pyelonephritis

3. Pelvis
  a. Pelvic inflammatory disease
  b. Ruptured ectopic pregnancy

4. Vascular system
  a. Ruptured aneurysm

b. **Dissecting aneurysm**
c. **Mesenteric thrombosis or embolism**

B. **Extra-abdominal disease.** These causes of acute abdominal pain should be considered to spare the patient unnecessary surgery.
1. **Diabetic ketoacidosis**
2. **Acute adrenal insufficiency**
3. **Acute porphyria**
4. **Lower lobe pneumonia**
5. **Pulmonary embolism**
6. **Pneumothorax**
7. **Sickle cell crisis**

IV. Database

A. **Physical examination key points** (See Table 1–2.)
1. **Vital signs** (See Section II.A.)
2. **Lungs.** Percuss for dullness at the bases which would suggest a pleural effusion or consolidation. In addition to dullness, the presence of crackles or bronchial breath sounds would suggest a pneumonia or infarction.
3. **Heart.** Look for jugular venous distension, S_3 gallop, or a displaced point of maximal impulse indicative of congestive heart failure that might predispose to passive congestion of the liver or mesenteric ischemia. An irregular pulse could indicate atrial fibrillation which might result in mesenteric artery embolism.
4. **Abdomen**
   a. **Inspection.** Examine for the presence of distension (obstruction, ileus, ascites), ecchymoses (hemorrhagic

TABLE 1–2. PHYSICAL FINDINGS WITH VARIOUS CAUSES OF ACUTE ABDOMEN

Condition	Helpful Signs
Perforated viscus	Scaphoid, tense abdomen; diminished bowel sounds (late); loss of liver dullness; guarding or rigidity
Peritonitis	Motionless; absent bowel sounds (late); cough and rebound tenderness; guarding or rigidity
Inflamed mass or abscess	Tender mass (abdominal, rectal, or pelvic); punch tenderness; special signs (Murphy's, psoas, or obturator)
Intestinal obstruction	Distension; visible peristalsis (late); hyperperistalsis (early) or quiet abdomen (late); diffuse pain without rebound tenderness; hernia or rectal mass (some)
Paralytic ileus	Distension; minimal bowel sounds; no localized tenderness
Ischemic or stangulated bowel	Not distended (until late); bowel sounds variable; severe pain but little tenderness; rectal bleeding (some)
Bleeding	Pallor, shock; distension; pulsatile (aneurysm) or tender (eg, ectopic pregnancy) mass; rectal bleeding (some)

From Boey JH. Acute abdomen. In Way LW, ed. Current Surgical Diagnosis and Treatment. *8th ed. Norwalk, Conn: Appleton & Lange; 1988. Used with permission.*

pancreatitis), caput medusae (portal hypertension), and surgical scars.

b. **Auscultation.** Listen for bowel sounds (absent or occasional tinkle with ileus, hyperperistaltic with gastroenteritis, high-pitched rushes with small bowel obstruction).

c. **Percussion.** Tympany is associated with distended loops of bowel. Shifting dullness and a fluid wave suggest the presence of ascites. Loss of liver dullness may occur if a viscus has ruptured and free air has entered the abdominal cavity.

d. **Palpation.** Involuntary guarding, rigidity, and rebound tenderness are hallmarks of peritonitis. Localized tenderness and guarding suggest perforation with spillage of gastrointestinal contents into the peritoneal cavity. Costovertebral angle tenderness is common with pyelonephritis. Murphy's sign is inspiratory arrest on palpation of the gall bladder and is seen with acute cholecystitis. Pain with active hip flexion or with extension of the patient's right thigh while lying on the left side (psoas sign) could result from an inflamed retrocecal appendix. The obturator sign (pain on internal rotation of the flexed thigh) can occur with retrocecal or pelvic appendicitis.

5. **Rectum.** Evaluation of acute abdominal pain is not complete until a rectal exam has been performed. A mass could suggest the presence of rectal carcinoma. Lateral rectal tenderness occurs with pelvic appendicitis, a condition in which examination of the abdomen may not reveal localized findings. If stool is present, evaluate for occult blood.

6. **Female genitalia.** Examine for pain with cervical motion and cervical discharge that may suggest pelvic inflammatory disease. Also palpate for adnexal masses that would indicate an ectopic pregnancy, ovarian abscess, cyst, or neoplasm.

B. **Laboratory data.** The decision to operate on a patient with acute abdominal pain is seldom made solely on the basis of laboratory data. This information serves mainly as an adjunct in those cases in which the etiology of the pain is not clear, or to assist preoperative resuscitation in those individuals for whom the diagnosis is certain and the decision to perform surgery has already been made.

1. **Hematology.** An increased hematocrit suggests hemoconcentration from volume loss. A low hematocrit could suggest a process that has resulted in chronic blood loss, or possibly acute intra-abdominal hemorrhage; however, with acute blood loss, the hematocrit may not decrease for several hours. An elevated white blood cell count suggests an inflammatory process such as appendicitis or cholecystitis.

2. **Electrolytes, blood urea nitrogen (BUN), creatinine.** Bowel

obstruction with vomiting can result in hypokalemia, azotemia, and volume contraction alkalosis. A strangulated bowel or sepsis may result in a metabolic gap acidosis.

3. **Liver function tests including bilirubin, transaminases, and alkaline phosphatase.** These may be elevated in acute hepatitis, cholecystitis, and other liver diseases.
4. **Amylase.** Markedly elevated levels are associated with pancreatitis; however, amylase may be normal initially in up to 30% of patients with acute pancreatitis, especially in patients with lipemic serum. Conversely, amylase can also be elevated in conditions other than pancreatitis such as acute cholecystitis, perforated ulcer, small bowel obstruction with strangulation, and ruptured ectopic pregnancy.
5. **Arterial blood gases (ABG).** Hypoxemia is often an early sign of sepsis and may occur with pancreatitis. As mentioned, acidosis may result from ischemic bowel or sepsis.
6. **Pregnancy test.** All premenopausal women with acute right or left lower abdominal pain should be tested for human chorionic gonadotropin (HCG) to rule out ectopic pregnancy whether or not they missed their last period.
7. **Urinalysis.** Hematuria may indicate nephrolithiasis; pyuria and hematuria can be present in urinary tract infections and, occasionally, appendicitis.
8. **Cervical culture.** Obtain a cervical culture for chlamydia and gonorrhea when pelvic inflammatory disease is suspected.

C. **Radiology and other studies**

1. **Flat and upright abdominal films.** These films can be readily obtained and may provide important information. Observe for the following: gas pattern, evidence of bowel dilation, air-fluid levels, presence or absence of air in the rectum, pancreatic calcifications, biliary and renal calcifications, aortic calcifications, loss of psoas margin (suggesting retroperitoneal bleeding), and presence or absence of air in the biliary tract.
2. **Chest film.** This may reveal lower lobe pneumonia, pleural effusion, or elevation of a hemidiaphragm indicating a subdiaphragmatic inflammatory process. Free air under the diaphragm suggests a perforated viscus and is most often seen on the upright chest film. Up to 15% to 20% of cases of perforation do not manifest this sign.
3. **Ultrasound.** This readily obtainable and noninvasive test may reveal the presence or absence of gallstones, biliary tract dilation, or ectopic pregnancy.
4. **Electrocardiogram (ECG).** An ECG is needed to rule out an acute myocardial infarction or pericarditis which may present with acute upper abdominal pain.
5. **Paracentesis.** (See Chapter 3, Paracentesis, p 334.) In a patient with known ascites presenting with acute abdominal pain, this test is required to rule out the possibility of spontaneous

bacterial peritonitis. If ascites is suspected but has not been documented then an ultrasound should be performed prior to an attempted paracentesis.

6. **Other studies** may be obtained in a more leisurely fashion to determine the nature of the pain provided the patient does not appear to have a case of acute abdominal pain requiring surgery. These tests can include the following:
   a. **Intravenous pyelogram (IVP)**
   b. **Abdominal CT scan**
   c. **Hepato-iminodiacetic acid (HIDA) scan** to rule out acute cholecystitis
   d. **Contrast bowel study,** such as an upper GI and small bowel series, to look for evidence of occult perforation or mechanical obstruction. A barium enema may be helpful in evaluation for sigmoid or cecal volvulus.
   e. **Endoscopic studies,** such as esophagogastroduodenoscopy (EGD), colonoscopy, or endoscopic retrograde cholangiopancreatography (ERCP).
   e. **Arteriography.** This may be necessary in those patients in whom mesenteric artery ischemia is suspected.

V. **Plan.** As mentioned previously, the initial goal in evaluating a patient with acute abdominal pain is to determine whether or not surgical treatment is indicated to prevent further morbidity. When pain has been present 6 or more hours and has not improved, there is an increased likelihood that the patient will require surgical exploration to determine the cause of pain. Often the specific etiology of the patient's abdominal pain is not determined until laparotomy. The use of analgesics remains controversial, but many surgeons now favor the use of moderate doses of pain medication to make the patient more comfortable and facilitate further examination.

A. **Observation.** With the exception of those conditions that require urgent surgical exploration (see Table 1–1), most cases of abdominal pain can be initially managed with close observation, correction of any fluid or electrolyte disturbances, and judicious use of analgesics.

1. Any patient on a medical service developing acute abdominal pain should receive an evaluation by a general surgeon as expediently as possible.
2. In those cases in which mechanical obstruction is suspected or vomiting is present, nasogastric decompression should be initiated. (See Chapter 3, Gastrointestinal Tubes, p 336.)
3. Patients who appear in septic or circulatory shock should receive vigorous intravenous volume replacement. If hypotension persists, they may require a vasopressor such as dopamine. (See Hypotension, Section V, p 178.)
4. Meperidine (Demerol) 50–75 mg IM every 3 to 4 hours may be used to provide patient comfort; however, avoid oversedation which could obscure patient evaluation.

TABLE 1–3. INDICATIONS FOR URGENT OPERATION IN PATIENTS WITH ACUTE ABDOMEN

- **Physical findings**
  - Involuntary guarding or rigidity, especially if spreading
  - Increasing or severe localized tenderness
  - Tense or progressive distension
  - Tender abdominal or rectal mass with high fever or hypotension
  - Rectal bleeding with shock or acidosis
  - Equivocal abdominal findings along with
    - Septicemia (high fever, marked or rising leukocytosis, mental changes, or increasing glucose intolerance in a diabetic patient)
    - Bleeding (unexplained shock or acidosis, falling hematocrit)
    - Supsended ischemia (acidosis, fever, tachycardia)
    - Deterioration on conservative treatment
- **Radiologic findings**
  - Pneumoperitoneum
  - Gross or progressive bowel distension
  - Free extravasation of contrast material
  - Space-occupying lesion on scan, with fever
  - Mesenteric occlusion on angiography
- **Endoscopic findings**
  - Perforated or uncontrollably bleeding lesion
- **Paracentesis findings**
  - Blood, bile, pus, bowel contents, or urine

From Boey JH. Acute abdomen. In Way LW, ed. Current Surgical Diagnosis and Treatment. *8th ed. Norwalk, Conn: Appleton & Lange; 1988. Used with permission.*

5. Serial physical examinations by the same examiner are very helpful in determining the patient's symptoms and establishing the diagnosis or need for surgery.

B. Surgery. Those indications that mandate urgent operation without a period of observation or establishment of a specific preoperative diagnosis are outlined in Table 1–3.

REFERENCES

Hendrix TR, Bulkley GB, Schuster MM. Abdominal Pain. In: Harvey AM, Johns RJ, McKusick VA et al, eds. *The Principles and Practice of Medicine,* 22nd ed. Norwalk, Conn: Appleton & Lange; 1988:787–797.

Jung PJ, Merrell PC. Acute abdomen. *Gastroenterol Clin North Am* 1988;17:227–245.

Way LW. Abdominal pain. In: Sleisinger MH, Fortran JS, eds. *Gastrointestinal Disease.* 4th ed. Philadelphia: WB Saunders; 1989:238–250.

ACIDOSIS

I. Problem. A 30-year-old male is brought into the emergency room unconscious. He was found at home by a friend. No other history is available. Physical examination is unremarkable except for rapid, shallow breathing. An arterial blood gas reveals a pH of 7.10.

II. Immediate Questions

A. Is the acidosis metabolic, respiratory, or mixed? A quick look at the pCO_2 on the arterial blood gas slip will reveal whether the disturbance is a primary metabolic or respiratory acidosis. If the pCO_2 is less than 40 mm Hg, then the primary disturbance is a metabolic acidosis. If the pCO_2 is greater than 40 mm Hg, the disturbance may be a primary respiratory acidosis or may be a mixed disturbance. Many arterial blood gas slips list the base excess (BE). The BE may help determine the etiology of the acidosis. If the BE is positive, the acidosis is respiratory; if the BE is negative, the acidosis is at least partially metabolic. Remember, the BE is calculated from the pH and assumes that both the pH and pCO_2 are correct.

B. What are the patient's vital signs? A common cause of metabolic acidosis is lactic acidosis from hypoperfusion. If there is hypotension or if the patient is orthostatic, immediate fluid resuscitation is indicated. Vasopressor agents may also be needed. (See Hypotension, p 174.) Bradypnea may suggest a narcotics overdose. Tachypnea may arise from hyperventilation as respiratory compensation for a metabolic acidosis or increased respiratory effort but hypoventilation resulting in a respiratory acidosis.

C. Are there any arrhythmias or ectopy? With a profound acidosis of any cause, there may be disturbances of the cardiac rhythm or ventricular ectopy. Obtain an ECG and monitor the patient.

D. What is the serum bicarbonate? To fully understand an acid-base problem, it is imperative to obtain the serum bicarbonate from an electrolyte panel. A high serum bicarbonate is evidence for a primary respiratory acidosis. A low serum bicarbonate is evidence for either a primary metabolic acidosis or a mixed metabolic and respiratory acidosis.

E. Does the serum bicarbonate, pH, and pCO_2 fit? Once you have the serum bicarbonate, you should make sure the pH, pCO_2, and HCO_3^- fit:

$$pH = pK_a + \log\frac{[HCO_3^-]}{[H_2CO_3]}$$

which can be simplified to

$$[H^+] = 24 \times \frac{pCO_2}{HCO_3^-}$$

In this patient with a pH of 7.10, if the pCO_2 was 20 mm Hg and the serum bicarbonate was 6 mmol/L, then

$$[H^+] = 24 \times \frac{20}{6}$$
$$[H^+] = 80$$

Does a pH of 7.10 equal a $[H^+]$ of 80 nmol/L? There are some simple rules to help convert pH to $[H^+]$. At a pH of 7.40, the $[H^+]$ = 40 nmol/L. pH is a log scale and for every 0.3 change in pH, the $[H^+]$ doubles or is halved. For instance, if pH = 7.70, $[H^+]$ = 20 nmol/L and at pH = 8.00, $[H^+]$ = 10 nmol/L. In this patient, if pH = 7.10, then $[H^+]$ = 80 nmol/L. Also around a pH of 7.40, the $[H^+]$ changes 1 nmol/L for every 0.01 change in pH. Lastly, on the back of many arterial blood gas slips, there may be a scale showing the relationship between pH and $[H^+]$. If when given the pH, pCO_2 and HCO_3^-, the numbers do not fit reasonably well into the equation

$$pH = 24 \times \frac{pCO_2}{HCO_3^-}$$

then it is difficult to determine the acid-base disturbance and the blood gas and serum bicarbonate should be repeated. For insance, if pH = 7.30, pCO_2 = 45 mm Hg, and HCO_3^- = 30 mmol/L, a superficial interpretation might be respiratory acidosis; however, closer scrutiny is necessary.

pH of 7.30 corresponds to a $[H^+]$ of 50 mmol/L

$$50 = 24 \times \frac{45}{30}$$
$$50 = 36$$

Either the pH, the pCO_2, or the HCO_3^- is in error. For instance, if there was too much heparin in the syringe, the pH could be falsely low. You must also check the compensation to see if it is appropriate.

F. **Is the compensation appropriate?** Checking to see whether the compensation is appropriate may unmask mixed disturbances.

1. For respiratory acidosis, immediate compensation is through buffers. In the short term, you expect the HCO_3^- to increase by 1 mmol/L for every 10 mm Hg increase in pCO_2 over normal (40 mm Hg). Renal compensation is not present for up to 24 hours. For chronic respiratory acidosis, expect an increase in the HCO_3^- of 3.5 to 4.0 mmol/L for every 10 mm Hg increase in pCO_2. For instance, in a 25-year-old with an acute episode of asthma, the ABG revealed a pCO_2 of 90. You would expect the bicarbonate to increase by 5 mmol/L from the calculation 1

mmol/L × (90 mm Hg − 40 mm Hg)/10 mm Hg. You would expect the HCO_3^- to be 31 mmol/L from the calculation 26 mmol/L (normal bicarbonate range 23–29) + 5 mmol/L. If the bicarbonate were 25 mmol/L, then a relative metabolic acidosis would be present along with the primary respiratory acidosis. If the bicarbonate were 36 mmol/L, then a metabolic alkalosis would also be present along with the primary respiratory acidosis.

2. For metabolic acidosis, compensation begins immediately through buffers and hyperventilation; however, steady state may not be reached for up to 24 hours. The expected change in pCO_2 is 1 to 1.5 times the change in HCO_3^-. For instance, in a 40-year-old with renal failure, the serum bicarbonate was found to be 15 mmol/L. The change in bicarbonate from normal should be 11 mmol/L or 26 mmol/L − 15 mmol/L. The expected change in pCO_2 would be between 11 and 16 mm Hg (11 × 1 and 11 × 1.5). The pCO_2 would be expected to be between 24 and 29 mm Hg (40 − 16 and 40 − 11).

If the actual pCO_2 were 19 mm Hg, then a respiratory alkalosis would also be present along with the primary metabolic acidosis. If the actual pCO_2 were 36 mm Hg, then a relative respiratory acidosis would be present along with the primary metabolic acidosis.

III. Differential Diagnosis. An acidosis is either metabolic or respiratory. There are many causes for both and sometimes a patient may have more than one cause of an acidosis.

A. Respiratory acidosis. By definition respiratory acidosis occurs secondary to hypoventilation. Hypoventilation can be caused by central nervous system, lung, or chest disorders.

1. Lungs

a. Asthma. May progress from a respiratory alkalosis to respiratory acidosis. A normal or elevated pCO_2 indicates impending respiratory failure and may require prompt intubation.

b. Pulmonary edema. Mild pulmonary edema usually causes a respiratory alkalosis. Severe pulmonary edema may cause a respiratory acidosis and intubation will probably be required.

c. Pneumonia. Again, usually causes respiratory alkalosis. But if more than one lobe is involved or if there is underlying chronic obstructive disease, pneumonia may cause a respiratory acidosis.

d. Upper airway obstruction. Foreign body, tumor, or laryngospasm.

e. Pneumothorax. Usually causes respiratory alkalosis; can cause a respiratory acidosis.

f. Large pleural effusion. Usually causes a respiratory alkalosis; can cause a respiratory acidosis.

2. **Chest abnormalities**
   a. **Kyphoscoliosis.** Resulting in a restrictive defect.
   b. **Scleroderma.** Resulting in a restrictive defect.
   c. **Marked obesity (Pickwickian syndrome)**
   d. **Muscular disorders.** Muscular dystrophy, severe hypophosphatemia, or myasthenia gravis.
   e. **Peripheral neurologic disorders,** such as Guillain-Barré syndrome.
3. **Central nervous system disorders**
   a. **Drugs or toxins** causing depression of respiratory drive
      (1) **Ethanol intoxication** at levels of 400–500 mg%
      (2) **Barbiturates,** especially overdoses
      (3) **Narcotics**
      (4) **Benzodiazepines,** especially when taken with alcohol
   b. **Cerebrovascular accident**
   c. **Brainstem bleed or cervical spinal cord injuries**

B. **Metabolic acidosis.** Can be divided into gap and nongap acidosis.

$$\text{Anion gap} = [Na^+] - ([Cl^-] + [HCO_3^-])$$

The normal anion gap is 8–12 mmol/L. An increase in anion gap may result from an increase in an unmeasured anion. Other causes of an elevated anion gap include dehydration, alkalosis, use of penicillin antibiotics that contain large amounts of sodium such as carbenicillin, and therapy with sodium salts or organic acids such as sodium lactate, acetate, and citrate. Sodium citrate is used in whole blood and packed red cells as an anticoagulant. With massive transfusion, the anion gap may increase.

1. **Normal anion gap (metabolic nongap acidosis)**
   a. **Loss of bicarbonate through gastrointestinal tract**
      (1) **Diarrhea**
      (2) **Small bowel fistula**
      (3) **Pancreatocutaneous fistula**
      (4) **Ureterosigmoidostomy**
      (5) **Chloride-containing exchange resins,** such as cholestyramine or with calcium chloride or magnesium chloride.
   b. **Loss of bicarbonate through kidney**
      (1) **Renal tubular acidosis.** Distal and proximal.
      (2) **Carbonic anhydrase inhibitors**
   c. **Other causes not from gastrointestinal or renal loss of HCO_3^-**
      (1) **Early renal failure**
      (2) **Hydrochloric acid**
      (3) **Hyperalimentation**
      (4) **Dilutional**
2. **Elevated anion gap (metabolic gap acidosis)**
   a. **Lactic acidosis.** Results from overproduction or impair-

ment of lactate utilization by the liver. Often from tissue hypoperfusion.

(1) **Shock.** Cardiogenic, hypovolemic, septic.
(2) **Severe anemia**
(3) **Hypoxia**
(4) **Malignancy**
(5) **Seizures**
(6) **Ethanol**
(7) **Crush injury**

b. **Renal failure.** Loss of secretion of acid and failure to filter anions.

c. **Ketoacidosis**
(1) **Diabetic ketoacidosis**
(2) **Alcoholic ketoacidosis**
(3) **Starvation ketoacidosis**

d. **Toxins**
(1) **Salicylates.** Cause an isolated metabolic gap acidosis (10%), an isolated respiratory alkalosis (30%), and most commonly a mixed metabolic gap acidosis and respiratory alkalosis (57%).
(2) **Methanol.** Metabolized to formic acid and formaldehyde. May cause blindness, abdominal pain, and headache.
(3) **Ethylene glycol.** Metabolized to oxalate, glycoaldehyde, and hippurate. Renal failure, neurologic disturbances, hypertension, and cardiovascular collapse may occur.

Note: Isopropyl alcohol ingestion does not cause an acidosis. Isopropyl alcohol is metabolized to acetone. It may cause a positive nitroprusside test for ketones.

e. The anion gap is also helpful in differentiating a pure metabolic acidosis, a mixed metabolic gap acidosis and metabolic nongap acidosis, and a mixed metabolic gap acidosis and metabolic alkalosis. For instance, if the HCO_3^- were 14 with a gap of 23, this would most likely represent a **pure metabolic gap acidosis** as calculated by:

23 mmol/L	Actual gap
− 10 mmol/L	Normal gap
13 mmol/L	Expected change in HCO_3^- from normal

26 mmol/L	Normal HCO_3^- (range 23–29)
− 13 mmol/L	Expected change
13 mmol/L	Expected HCO_3^-

Actual HCO_3^- 14 mmol/L ≅ expected gap of 13 mmol/L

An HCO_3^- of 19 with a gap of 25 would most likely represent a **mixed metabolic gap acidosis and metabolic alkalosis** as calculated by:

25 mmol/L	Actual gap
− 10 mmol/L	Normal gap
15 mmol/L	Expected change in HCO_3^- from normal

26 mmol/L	Normal HCO_3^- (range 23–29)
− 15 mmol/L	Expected change in HCO_3^-
11 mmol/L	Expected HCO_3^-

The actual HCO_3^-, however, is 19 mmol/L, 8 mmol/L higher than expected. Thus, there must also be a metabolic alkalosis in addition to the metabolic gap acidosis.

An HCO_3^- of 8 mmol/L with a gap of 22 mmol/L would most likely represent a **mixed metabolic gap acidosis and metabolic nongap acidosis** as calculated by:

22 mmol/L	Actual gap
− 10 mmol/L	Normal gap
12 mmol/L	Expected change in HCO_3^- from normal

26 mmol/L	Normal HCO_3^- (range 23–29)
− 12 mmol/L	Expected change in HCO_3^-
14 mmol/L	Expected HCO_3^-

The actual HCO_3^-, however, is 8 mmol/L or 6 mmol/L lower than expected. Thus, there must also be a metabolic nongap acidosis in addition to the metabolic gap acidosis.

IV. Database

A. Physical exam key points

1. **Vital signs.** A low respiratory rate suggests hypoventilation; a high rate points toward respiratory failure or compensation for a metabolic acidosis. Fever suggests sepsis. Hypotension suggests hypoperfusion.
2. **Skin.** Changes of scleroderma indicate a restrictive defect. Cool, clammy, and mottled skin on extremities suggests shock.
3. **HEENT.** Ketosis or fruity odor on breath suggests diabetic ketoacidosis. Look for tracheal shift from a space-occupying lesion or venous distension (congestive heart failure or tension pneumothorax). Pinpoint pupils are consistent with overdose.
4. **Lungs.** Evaluate for absent or decreased breath sounds, stridor in upper airway obstruction, wheezes, and rales.
5. **Abdomen.** Peritoneal signs indicate an acute abdomen; marked distension may inhibit respiration.
6. **Neuromuscular exam.** Generalized weakness or focal neurologic signs, depressed level of consciousness, obtundation, and coma should be noted.

B. Laboratory data

1. **Hemograms.** Anemia may be associated with renal failure. Anemia may cause ischemia resulting in lactic acidosis. Leukocytosis may suggest sepsis.

2. **Electrolytes** Serum chloride is elevated in metabolic nongap acidosis. Serum potassium is increased with acidosis and decreased with alkalosis. The serum potassium may be especially helpful in determining the acid-base status given the serum bicarbonate prior to the arterial blood gas. For instance, a serum bicarbonate of 34 mmol/L could indicate a primary metabolic alkalosis or compensation for a chronic respiratory acidosis. If the potassium were 5.6 mmol/L, this would argue that the bicarbonate of 34 mmol/L was from compensation for a chronic respiratory acidosis. If the potassium were 3.1 mmol/L, this would argue that the bicarbonate of 34 mmol/L was from a metabolic alkalosis. The potassium, BUN, and creatinine may be elevated with renal failure. The creatinine may be falsely elevated with ketoacidosis.
3. **Metabolic gap acidosis.** The following **must** be ordered:
   a. **Glucose.** If elevated, may indicate diabetic ketoacidosis.
   b. **Ketone levels.** May indicate alcoholic, starvation, or diabetic ketoacidosis.
   c. **Lactate.** Lactic acidosis may be seen with alcohol use, severe anemia, sepsis, hypoperfusion (either generalized or local), hypoxemia, end-stage liver disease, and postictally.
   d. **Salicylate level**
   e. **Ethanol**
   f. **Methanol**
   g. **Ethylene glycol**
   h. **Paraldehyde.** Very rare cause of metabolic acidosis.
   i. **BUN and creatinine**
4. **Metabolic nongap acidosis.** If the history does not reveal an obvious cause such as diarrhea, then renal tubular acidosis needs to be considered.
   a. **Distal renal tubular acidosis.** Inability to lower urine pH below 5.5 with NH_4Cl (ammonium chloride).
   b. **Proximal renal tubular acidosis.** Urine pH will decrease to less than 5.5; however, the excretion of HCO_3^- is increased to greater than 15% when serum HCO_3^- is raised to the normal range.
5. **Respiratory acidosis.** Order a serum and urine drug screen. If hypoventilation with decreased respirations, need to rule out overdose. Also, with an intentional salicylate overdose, ingestion of other substances must be ruled out as intentional overdoses often involve multiple substances.

C. **Radiologic and other studies**
1. If respiratory acidosis:
   a. **Chest x-ray (CXR).** Rule out pneumothorax, pulmonary edema, infiltrative processes.
   b. **CT scan of head.** Consider with hypoventilation and altered mental status or focal neurologic exam.

c. **Electromyography (EMG).** May be helpful to assess for neuromuscular disorders.

V. Plan. In general for both respiratory and metabolic acidosis, treatment of the underlying cause of the acidosis is the primary goal. In emergent situations, the two methods to reverse metabolic and respiratory acidosis in the short term are to administer sodium bicarbonate intravenously and to hyperventilate the patient. Be sure to check serial pH values to monitor the progress of therapy.

A. Severe acidosis (pH < 7.20). Use continuous cardiac monitoring for potential arrhythmia.

B. Metabolic acidosis

1. **Bicarbonate therapy.** Although controversial, the present recommendation is to administer IV bicarbonate if the pH < 7.20.
   a. Calculate the total body bicarbonate deficit:

      Patient's weight (in kg) $\times$ 0.50 $\times$ (26$-$[HCO_3^-]) = total mmol of HCO_3^- needed

   b. Give 50% of this amount over the first 12 hours as a mixture of bicarbonate with D5W. A normal bicarbonate drip is made by adding 3 ampoules of $NaHCO_3$ (50 mmol/ampoule) to 1 L of D5W.
   c. Complications of bicarbonate therapy include:
      (1) **Hypernatremia**
      (2) **Volume overload**
      (3) **Hypokalemia.** Caused by intracellular shifts of potassium as the pH increases.
2. **Treatment of underlying causes**
   a. Volume resuscitation with normal saline for sepsis and hemorrhagic shock. Vasopressors may be needed.
   b. Dialysis as needed for renal failure.
   c. Normal saline and insulin for diabetic ketoacidosis. (See Hyperglycemia, Section V, page 139.)
   d. Normal saline and dextrose for alcoholic ketoacidosis along with replacement of other electrolytes and vitamins such as thiamine and folate as needed.
   e. Starvation ketosis is treated with normal saline and dextrose.
   f. Salicylate intoxication is treated with alkalinization of urine. Intravenous fluids containing $NaHCO_3$ (3 ampoules 50 mEq in 1 L of D5W or 2 ampoules in 1 L D5 1/4NS) to run at 100–250 mL/h. Check urine pH every 1 to 2 hours. Urine pH should be maintained at or above 7.5–8.0. ABG and serum bicarbonate should be followed closely and severe alkalemia (pH > 7.55) avoided. Hemodialysis may be required.
   g. Methanol and ethylene glycol ingestion is treated with eth-

anol infusion, which decreases the accumulation of toxic metabolites. Hemodialysis may be required.

C. Respiratory acidosis. The main goal is to treat the underlying cause.

1. If necessary, intubate the patient and treat with mechanical ventilation. If a patient is already intubated and has a significant respiratory acidosis, then increase alveolar ventilation either by increasing tidal volume (up to 10–15 mL/kg), while following peak inspiratory pressures, or by increasing the respiratory rate.
2. In an emergent situation, disconnect the patient from the ventilator and hyperventilate by hand. The importance of good pulmonary toilet, ie, suctioning of secretions, cannot be overemphasized. Sedation is often a necessary adjunct to mechanical ventilation (See Chapter 6, Ventilator Management, p 354.)

REFERENCES

Davenport H. *The ABC of Acid-Base Chemistry.* 6th ed. Chicago: University of Chicago Press; 1984.

Emmett M, Narins RG. Clinical use of the anion gap. *Medicine* 1977;56:38–54.

Kaehny WD. Pathogenesis and management of respiratory and mixed acid-base disorders. In: Schrier RW, ed. *Renal and Electrolyte Disorders.* 3rd ed. Boston: Little, Brown; 1986.

Kaehny WD, Gabow PA. Pathogenesis and management of metabolic acidosis and alkalosis. In: Schrier RW, ed. *Renal and Electrolyte Disorders.* 3rd ed. Boston: Little, Brown; 1986.

Narins RG, Emmett M. Simple and mixed acid-base disorders: A practical approach. *Medicine* 1980;59:161–187.

■ ALKALOSIS

I. Problem. You are consulted to see a 60-year-old male with a pH of 7.65 who is 3 days status post cholecystectomy.

II. Immediate Questions

A. Is the alkalosis metabolic, respiratory, or mixed? A quick look at the pCO_2 on the ABG slip will reveal whether the disturbance is a primary metabolic or respiratory alkalosis. If the pCO_2 is greater than 40 mm Hg, the primary disturbance is a metabolic alkalosis with at least partial respiratory compensation. If the pCO_2 is less than 40 mm Hg, the disturbance may be a primary respiratory alkalosis or a mixed disturbance. Many arterial blood gas slips list the base excess (BE). The BE may help determine the etiology of the alkalosis. If the BE is negative, the alkalosis is respiratory; if the BE is positive, the alkalosis is at least partially metabolic. Remember, the BE is calculated from the pH and assumes that both the pH and pCO_2 are correct.

B. **What are the patient's vital signs?** An elevated respiratory rate, fever, hypotension, or all three may indicate sepsis. Respiratory alkalosis is associated with sepsis. Tachypnea may also indicate anxiety, central nervous system disease, or pulmonary disease.

C. **What medications is the patient taking?** Thiazide diuretics can cause a contraction alkalosis. Acetate in hyperalimentation solutions, antacids, exogenous steroids, or large doses of penicillin or carbenicillin may cause an alkalosis. Salicylate overdose and progesterone can cause respiratory alkalosis.

D. **Is a nasogastric tube in place or is there vomiting?** Loss of HCl from the stomach is a common cause of metabolic alkalosis.

E. **Is there any history of mental status changes, seizures, paresthesias, or tetany?** Alkalemia may cause the above and if so, prompt action is indicated.

F. **Is there any ventricular ectopy?** Severe alkalemia may cause ventricular arrhythmias unresponsive to the usual pharmacologic treatments.

Note: Mortality in critically ill surgical patients is associated with a rise in serum pH. Mortality was 69% with a pH greater than 7.60 and was 44% with a pH between 7.55 and 7.59 in a study by R. F. Wilson.

G. **What is the serum bicarbonate?** To fully understand an acid-base problem, it is imperative to obtain the serum bicarbonate from an electrolyte panel. A low serum bicarbonate is evidence for a primary respiratory alkalosis with at least partial metabolic compensation. A high serum bicarbonate is evidence for either a primary metabolic alkalosis or a mixed metabolic and respiratory alkalosis.

H. **Does the serum bicarbonate fit the pH and pCO_2?** (See Acidosis, Section II.F.)

I. **Is the compensation appropriate?** Checking to see if the compensation is appropriate may unmask mixed disturbances.

1. For a respiratory alkalosis, immediate compensation is through buffers. The compensation for acute respiratory alkalosis is a decrease of 2 mmol of HCO_3^- (range 1–3 mmol) for each 10 mm Hg decrease in pCO_2. Renal compensation is complete between 24 and 48 hours. The compensation for chronic respiratory alkalosis is a decrease of about 5 mmol of HCO_3^- for each 10 mm Hg decrease in pCO_2. For instance, in a 35-year-old woman who is 36 weeks pregnant, the ABG revealed a pCO_2 of 25. You would expect the HCO_3^- to decrease by 7.5 mmol from the calculation 5 mmol/L × (40 mm Hg − 25 mm Hg)/10 mm Hg. You would expect the HCO_3^- to be 18.5 or 26 mmol/L (normal HCO_3^-) − 7.5 mmol (expected change in HCO_3^-). If the HCO_3^- were 23 mmol, a relative metabolic alkalosis would be present along with the primary respiratory alkalosis. If the HCO_3^- were 12 mmol, there would be a metabolic acidosis along with the primary respiratory alkalosis.

2. For metabolic alkalosis, compensation begins immediately through buffers and hypoventilation. Hypoventilation as a means of compensation is limited by resulting hypoxemia. Seldom will the pCO_2 be greater than 55 mm Hg secondary to compensation. The expected increase in pCO_2 is 0.6 mm Hg (range 0.25–1.0 mm Hg) for each 1-mmol increase in HCO_3^-. For instance, in a 60-year-old status post cholecytectomy, the HCO_3^- was 36 mmol/L. The expected pCO_2 is 46 mm Hg (36 mmol/L − 26 mmol/L) × 0.6 mm Hg per 1 mmol/L change in HCO_3^-. If the pCO_2 were 40 mm Hg, there would be a relative respiratory alkalosis along with the primary metabolic alkalosis. If the pCO_2 were 55 mm Hg, there would be a respiratory acidosis along with a primary metabolic alkalosis.

III. Differential Diagnosis. An alkalosis is either metabolic or respiratory. There may be many causes for both and sometimes a patient may have more than one cause of an alkalosis.

A. Respiratory alkalosis. By definition, respiratory alkalosis occurs secondary to hyperventilation. Hyperventilation can result from either central or peripheral stimulation of respiration. Common causes include medications, central nervous system disease, pulmonary disease, anxiety, and systemic disorders.

1. **Medications**
   a. **Salicylate overdose.** Causes an isolated respiratory alkalosis (30%), isolated metabolic gap acidosis (10%), and most commonly a mixed metabolic gap acidosis and respiratory alkalosis (57%).
   b. **Progesterone**
2. **Central nervous system disease** (See Coma, Acute Mental Status Changes, p 65.)
   a. **Cerebrovascular accident**
   b. **Infection**
   c. **Tumor.** Primary or metastatic.
   d. **Trauma**
3. **Pulmonary disease** (See Dyspnea, p 91.)
   a. **Interstitial lung disease**
   b. **Pneumonia.** If multiple lobes, may cause respiratory acidosis.
   c. **Asthma.** If mild to moderate, will cause a respiratory alkalosis; if severe, respiratory acidosis may result.
   d. **Pulmonary emboli**
   e. **Pneumothorax**
4. **Anxiety**
5. **Pulmonary edema.** If mild, causes a respiratory alkalosis; if severe, may cause a respiratory acidosis.
6. **Pain**
7. **Pregnancy.** Secondary to progesterone.
8. **Liver disease.** Cirrhosis.
9. **Fever**

10. **Gram-negative sepsis**
11. **Hyperthyroidism**
12. **Iatrogenic**
13. **Hypoxemia**

B. **Metabolic alkalosis.** Can be divided into chloride responsive and chloride unresponsive. The urine Cl^- is less than 10 to 20 mmol/L with the chloride-responsive causes and greater than 20 to 30 mmol/L with the chloride-unresponsive causes.

1. **Chloride responsive causes**
   a. **Gastric losses.** Vomiting or nasogastric tube.
   b. **Diarrhea.** Chloride wasting.
   c. **Diuretics**
   d. **Correction of chronic hypercapnia**
   e. **Sulfates, phosphates, or high-dose penicillins**
   f. **Massive blood transfusion.** Citrate is used as an anticoagulant and is metabolized to HCO_3^-. One unit of whole blood and one unit of packed red cells contain 17 and 5 mEq of citrate, respectively.
2. **Chloride-unresponsive causes**
   a. **Cushing's syndrome.** Elevated glucocorticoids from a variety of causes including pituitary adenoma, adrenal adenoma, and ectopic production. Results in hypertension, glucose intolerance, fluid retention, and osteoporosis.
   b. **Hyperaldosteronism.** Rare cause of hypertension. Also associated with hypokalemia and hypernatremia.
   c. **Exogenous steroid ingestion**
   d. **Bartter's syndrome.** Also hypokalemia. Hyperreninemia and hyperaldosteronemia secondary to hyperplasia of the juxtaglomerular apparatus. Patients are normotensive.
   e. **Potassium or magnesium deficiency**
   f. **Calcium carbonate–containing antacids**
   g. **Milk-alkali syndrome**
   h. **Refeeding with glucose after starvation**

IV. **Database**

A. **Physical exam key points**

1. **Vital signs.** Respiratory rate. Tachypnea may indicate pulmonary disease, pulmonary edema, or CNS respiratory stimulation. An elevated temperature may indicate an infection or sepsis.
2. **Chest.** Must be thorough. Look for evidence of pneumothorax, pleural effusion, bronchospastic disease, and pulmonary edema.
3. **Abdomen.** Look for evidence of chronic liver disease such as ascites and caput medusae.
4. **Skin.** Look for evidence of chronic liver disease such as palmar erythema, Dupuytren's contractures, and spider angiomas. Also look for changes associated with Cushing's syndrome such as buffalo hump, purple striae, and easy bruisability.

5. **Neurologic exam.** Look for focal abnormalities as evidence for tumor, cerebrovascular accident, and infection. Tremor and hyperreflexia may suggest hyperthyroidism.

B. **Laboratory data**
1. **Anion gap.** May unmask a mixed metabolic gap acidosis and metabolic alkalosis. (See Acidosis, p 12.)
2. **Serum electrolytes.** Hypokalemia and hypomagnesemia may cause a metabolic alkalosis. Hypokalemia may also result from alkalosis as potassium ions shift intracellularly in exchange for hydrogen ions.
3. **Respiratory alkalosis**
   a. **Salicylate level.** If elevated, check serum and urine drug screen for other ingested substances.
   b. **Liver function tests**
   c. **Thyroid function studies**
   d. **Blood cultures**
4. **Metabolic alkalosis.** Need spot urine for chloride. A urine chloride below 10–20 mmol/L represents a "chloride-responsive" alkalosis. A urine chloride above 20 mmol/L represents a "chloride-unresponsive" alkalosis.
5. **Chloride-unresponsive metabolic alkalosis.** May need to rule out Cushing's syndrome and primary aldosteronism.

C. **Radiological and other studies.** If respiratory alkalosis, consider the following:
1. **Chest x-ray.** To look for pulmonary disease and pulmonary edema.
2. **CT scan of head.** Rule out central nervous system disease.

V. **Plan.** It is essential to identify the cause of alkalosis and treat it.

A. **Respiratory alkalosis**
1. If hypoxic, give supplemental oxygen.
2. If anxious, give sedative such as diazepam 1–5 mg PO or 1–2 mg IV or lorazepam 1–2 mg PO or 0.5 mg IV.
3. If nonintubated, increase $FiCO_2$ (fraction of inspired carbon dioxide) by use of a rebreathing mask. Would consider for a pH greater than 7.55.
4. If intubated, will need to decrease minute ventilation by decreasing the rate or tidal volume. Be sure the tidal volume is set for 10–15 mL/kg. The respirator may need to be changed from assist control to intermittent mandatory ventilation.
5. If salicylate overdose, consider alkalinization of urine. Alkalinization of urine should be done cautiously in a patient who is already alkalotic for other reasons. Follow serum pH and serum bicarbonate closely. See Acidosis, Section V, p 16, for instructions on alkalinization of urine. Hemodialysis may be required.

B. **Metabolic alkalosis**
1. In the presence of severe alkalemia with seizures or ventricular arrhythmias, prompt, immediate action is needed. Treatment

would include increasing the pCO_2 or administering an acid such as hydrochloric acid. Hydrochloric acid must be given slowly through a central line.

2. Bicarbonate precursors such as acetate salts (amino acids) found in hyperalimentation solutions or solutions containing lactate should be eliminated if possible.
3. If chloride responsive, give normal saline.
4. If chloride unresponsive, treat underlying disorder.
   a. If potassium or magnesium deficient, will often need massive replacement.
   b. Evaluation and specific treatment of endogenous mineralocorticoid disorders.

REFERENCES

Davenport H. *The ABC of Acid-Base Chemistry.* 6th ed. Chicago: University of Chicago Press; 1984.

Kaehny WD. Pathogenesis and management of respiratory and mixed acid-base disorders. In: Schrier RW, ed. *Renal and Electrolyte Disorders.* 3rd ed. Boston: Little, Brown; 1986.

Kaehny WD, Gabow PA. Pathogenesis and management of metabolic acidosis and alkalosis. In: Schrier RW, ed. *Renal and Electrolyte Disorders.* 3rd ed. Boston: Little, Brown; 1986.

Narins RG, Emmett M. Simple and mixed acid-base disorders: A practical approach. *Medicine* 1980;59:161–187.

Wilson RF, Gibson D, Percinel AK, et al. Severe alkalosis in critically ill surgical patients. *Arch Surg* 1972;105:197–203.

■ ANAPHYLACTIC REACTION

I. **Problem.** Within 10 minutes of receiving an intramuscular injection, a patient develops respiratory distress and becomes unresponsive.

II. **Immediate Questions.** Anaphylaxis can be a life-threatening situation and requires immediate evaluation and treatment.

   A. **What are the patient's vital signs?** Tachycardia is a common finding and could result from an arrhythmia or as a response to hypoxia, fear, or hypotension. Hypotensive shock, which can occur with or without other symptoms, poses the greatest danger from anaphylaxis and must be recognized and treated promptly.

   B. **Can the patient still communicate?** The ability to provide appropriate answers to simple questions implies adequate cerebral oxygenation. Inability to speak or stridor could indicate upper airway obstruction from laryngospasm or laryngeal edema.

   C. **What medication did the patient receive?** Anaphylaxis can result from a variety of agents including medications, foods, venoms, pollens, and serum. The most common medications causing anaphylaxis are penicillins, cephalosporins, tetracycline, amphotericin, and local anesthetics. Anaphylactoid reactions nonimmunologically mediated result from aspirin, indomethacin, other nonsteroidal anti-inflammatory drugs, and radiopaque contrast material.

III. Differential Diagnosis. Signs and symptoms of anaphylaxis are produced by the release of biologically active mediators such as histamine from basophils and mast cells. This release can either be mediated immunologically through the interaction of antigen with IgE residing on the basophils and mast cells or can occur as the result of a nonimmunologic release of mediators. These mediators affect several organ systems including the skin, upper and lower airways, vascular system, and gastrointestinal tract. Anaphylaxis may involve only one or all of the preceding organ systems, and thus must be distinguished from other disease processes occurring at those sites.

- **A. Upper airway obstruction.** This could result from aspiration of a foreign body such as a food bolus, or may occur with other causes of laryngeal edema such as hereditary angioneurotic edema.
- **B. Acute asthmatic attack.** There is a known history of previous asthma.
- **C. Wheezing, from other causes** (See p 257.)
- **D. Pulmonary embolus.** This diagnosis must be considered in any patient developing sudden acute shortness of breath.
- **E. Dyspnea** (See p 91.)
- **F. Vasovagal reaction.** This can also cause acute cardiovascular collapse but is usually associated with bradycardia and resolves quickly with recumbency.
- **G. Urticaria.** This condition can be produced by a wide variety of causes other than anaphylaxis.

IV. Database. Knowledge of the patient's prior history of allergies and current medications is essential. The temporal relationship between the medication administration and the onset of symptoms is also important since anaphylaxis usually occurs within minutes of administration.

- **A. Physical examination key points**
  1. **Vital signs.** Hypotension must be recognized immediately.
  2. **Lungs.** Listen for wheezing (suggests bronchospasm) and stridor (suggests upper airway obstruction).
  3. **Skin.** Generalized flushing, urticaria, and angioedema may occur.
  4. **Extremities.** Look for cyanosis.
  5. **Mental status.** Impaired mentation may indicate significant respiratory compromise and would suggest the need for immediate respiratory support.
- **B. Laboratory data—Arterial blood gases.** Hypoxia and hypercapnia occur with respiratory compromise; however, most often the problem must be addressed before results of this test are available.
- **C. Radiologic and other studies.**
  1. **Chest x-ray.** Can be obtained after the patient is stabilized to

exclude other causes of respiratory distress such as pneumonia and congestive heart failure.

2. **Electrocardiogram.** Acute myocardial infarction can present with severe dyspnea and also can occur as a result of anaphylaxis.

V. Plan. Treatment should be initiated quickly without waiting for the results of laboratory testing. If the patient is pulseless, external cardiac compressions must be initiated.

A. Oxygen. Oxygen by face mask should be instituted if the patient appears dyspneic. Intubation may be required if the patient is severely somnolent or becomes hypoxemic. Tracheostomy may be necessary if upper airway edema precludes intubation.

B. Epinephrine. Epinephrine 1:1000 solution 0.3–0.5 mL intramuscularly should be given immediately for laryngospasm or vascular collapse. It may be given every 15 to 30 minutes as needed; however, it must be used with caution in patients exceeding 40 years of age. Intravenous administration of epinephrine 2–4 mL in 1:10,000 solution should be given only if there is severe hypotension.

C. Diphenhydramine (Benadryl). Diphenhydramine 25–50 mg IM should follow epinephrine to reduce the effects of histamine release. This may alleviate hypotension as well as lessen the symptoms associated with mild urticaria.

D. High-dose glucocorticosteroids. Steroids are of questionable benefit in anaphylactic shock, but hydrocortisone 100 mg IV should be given for episodes of anaphylactic bronchospasm. They may also help prevent the late phase response that sometimes occurs several hours after the initial presentation.

E. Aminophylline. For patients whose bronchospasm does not respond to epinephrine, aminophylline 6 mg/kg over 20 to 30 minutes should be given (see Wheezing, Section V, page 259).

F. Blood pressure support. Hypotension usually responds to administration of epinephrine; however, normal saline may be necessary for those patients failing to respond. Occasionally, vasopressors such as dopamine are needed if the patient fails to respond to volume repletion and epinephrine. (See Hypotension, Section V, p 178.)

G. Monitoring. Relapse of anaphylaxis can occur hours after the initial presentation. Close monitoring for the first 24 hours is essential.

REFERENCES

Fisher M. Anaphylaxis. *Disease-A-Month* 1987;(33):435–475.

Wasserman SI. Anaphylaxis. In: Middleton E, Reed CE, Ellis EF, eds. *Allergy: Principles and Practice.* 3rd ed. St. Louis, Mo: CV Mosby; 1988:1365–1376.

■ ANEMIA

I. **Problem.** A patient is admitted for pneumonia. The hematocrit (HCT) is noted to be 25%.

II. **Immediate Questions**

A. **What are the patient's vital signs?** If the patient is not hypotensive or severely tachycardic, transfusion therapy is probably not emergently indicated.

B. **Is the patient symptomatic?** With angina or hemodynamic compromise, transfusion therapy is not emergently indicated. Lack of symptoms indicates chronicity of the anemia.

C. **Is there evidence of acute or recent blood loss such as melena, hematochezia, bright red blood per rectum, or menorrhagia?** Gastrointestinal (GI) blood loss can be divided into acute or chronic, upper GI (see Hematemesis, Melena, p 117) and lower GI (see Hematochezia, p 121). Patients more frequently succumb from acute upper GI blood loss; however, lower GI blood loss, though not seen as frequently by internists, can still be lethal.

D. **What medications does the patient take?** Aspirin and nonsteroidal anti-inflammatory drugs (NSAIDs) may lead to GI blood loss. Alkylating agents (melphalan, *cis*-platinum), folate antagonists (Bactrim, pentamidine), anticonvulsants (Dilantin), and anti-inflammatory drugs (phenylbutazone) may cause marrow suppression or aplasia. Penicillin, sulfonamides, and methyldopa (Aldomet) may cause hemolysis. Alcohol, isoniazid, and trimethoprim may cause maturation defects.

E. **Is there significant organ dysfunction or a current inflammatory disease?** Severe liver, kidney, adrenal, and thyroid dysfunction may lead to anemia. Rheumatoid arthritis, systemic lupus erythematosus (SLE), and vasculitides are associated with anemia of chronic or inflammatory disease.

F. **Does the patient have other medical problems associated with excess total body water that may lead to a pseudoanemia, such as congestive heart failure, cirrhosis, and pregnancy?** In settings with increased plasma volume relative to the red cell mass, an apparent anemia may be manifest or an existing anemia may be made more apparent.

G. **Does the patient have a history or a family history of anemia, thalassemia, sickle cell anemia, or glucose 6-phosphatase deficiency?** Hereditary disorders of hemoglobin usually present nonacutely and a family history may be suggestive of an inherited cause of the anemia.

III. **Differential Diagnosis.** There are well over 100 causes of anemia. A look at the peripheral smear with careful attention to the red cell indices is of particular importance when evaluating a patient with anemia.

TABLE 1–4. CAUSES OF MICROCYTIC ANEMIA

	Iron Deficiency	β-Thalassemia	Chronic Disease	Sideroblastic Anemia
Iron	Low	Normal/increased	Low	Increased
TIBC	Increased	Normal	Low	Normal
Ferritin	Low	Normal/increased	Normal/increased	Increased
Hemoglobin A_2[a]	Normal	Increased	Normal	Normal

[a] A type of hemoglobin detected by hemoglobin electrophoresis.

A. **Pancytopenia.** The platelet and white blood cell (WBC) counts are decreased along with the hemoglobin (HGB) and HCT. Usually caused by either marrow invasion, failure, or suppression. Most commonly caused by drugs, solid tumors, hematologic malignancies, and inflammatory diseases. May be idiopathic.

B. **Anemia with a low mean corpuscular volume (MCV).** Associated with microcytic red cells on the peripheral smear. Iron deficiency is the most common etiology and is seen in approximately 20% of menstruating females. Thalassemias are also in this category. Hypochromic, microcytic red blood cells (RBCs), target cells, basophilic stippling, marked anisocytosis, and poikilocytosis are noted. Sideroblastic anemia and anemia of chronic disease may also be associated with low MCV. The MCV should never be less than 70 if it is due to chronic disease. Microcytic anemias can easily be differentiated by looking at the peripheral smear and various laboratory studies. Serum iron, total iron-binding capacity or transferrin, ferritin, and hemoglobin electrophoresis may be helpful. (See Table 1–4.)

C. **Normal-MCV anemias.** Many anemias are associated with a normal MCV. Anemia of chronic disease is probably the most common normocytic anemia. Chronic infections (tuberculosis, osteomylitis), collagen vascular disease, and malignancies may produce an anemia with a normal MCV. Kidney, liver, thyroid, and adrenal dysfunction may also lead to a normal-MCV anemia. Correction of the underlying disorder should correct the anemia.

D. **High-MCV anemias.** Many anemias are macrocytic, but only a few are megaloblastic. Folate and vitamin B_{12} deficiencies are the most common megaloblastic anemias. Vitamin B_{12} deficiency can be secondary to pernicious anemia (lack of intrinsic factor), bacterial overgrowth, ileal disease, and dietary deficiency which is rare. Vitamin B_{12} stores last 3 to 4 years. Folate deficiency is often caused by dietary deficiency but may be secondary to increased needs such as with pregnancy or hyperthyroidism. If there is not an obvious cause of folate deficiency, then the possibility of malabsorption must be considered. Along with macrocytic RBCs, the peripheral smear of folate or vitamin B_{12} deficiency may demonstrate hypersegmented neutrophils and nucleated RBCs. Other anemias that may be associated with macrocytes are myelodysplasias, aplastic anemias, acquired sideroblastic anemias, anemias induced by chemotherapy (antimetabolites), and anemia associated with hypothyroidism and with chronic liver disease. An increased MCV may be seen in the presence of a markedly increased reticulocyte count, as reticulocytes are large cells that increase the mean RBC size.

E. **Anemias with increased reticulocytosis.** Many anemias listed earlier are associated with an increased reticulocyte count. A reticulocyte is a very young red cell approximately 1 day old. As the RBC life span is approximately 100 days (actually 120), the normal reticulocyte count is approximately 1/100 or 1%. An increased reticulocyte count indicates that the bone marrow is making red cells faster than normal. This is usually due to red cells having a shortened life span or to blood loss. The peripheral smear may reveal large polychromatophilic RBCs which are reticulocytes; however, a reticulocyte stain is needed to definitively do a reticulocyte count. Examples of anemias with an increased reticulocyte count are acquired or autoimmune hemolytic anemias and congenital hemolytic anemias (sickle cell anemia, thalassemias). Correction of a particular deficit such as B_{12} deficiency by the administration of B_{12} will also lead to a reticulocytosis.

IV. Database

A. Physical examination key points

1. **Vital signs.** Make sure the patient is not hypotensive. The patient may be **orthostatic.** Look for an increase in heart rate of 20 beats per minute and/or a decrease in systolic blood pressure of 10 mm Hg on movement from a supine to a standing position after 1 minute.
2. **Skin.** Telangiectasia, palmar erythema, and jaundice may indicate liver disease. Isolated jaundice may point toward hemolysis.
3. **Oropharynx.** Glossitis commonly seen in iron and B_{12} deficiency.
4. **Heart.** Murmurs may be indicative of hemolysis from valvular disease or merely a flow murmur resulting from anemia.
5. **Abdomen.** Check for splenomegaly. Associated with hemolysis, thalassemias, chronic leukemias, lymphomas, and occasionally acute leukemias. Could also indicate portal hypertension secondary to cirrhosis. Also look for ascites and hepatomegaly.
6. **Rectum.** Stool hemoccult to look for GI blood loss.
7. **Neurologic exam.** Loss of vibration and position sense and dementia are associated with B_{12} deficiency but could also represent effects of alcohol and hypothyroidism.

B. Laboratory data

1. **Peripheral smear.** Review on all patients with anemia. Note the size and shape of the RBCs and the presence or absence of platelets. Nucleated RBCs, reticulocytes, schistocytes, sickle cells, and target cells may aid in the diagnosis. Examine WBC morphology for hypersegmented neutrophils.
2. **Reticulocyte count.** The most important laboratory test after reviewing the peripheral smear. An increased count indicates an appropriate response to anemia or that the RBC survival through blood loss or hemolysis is shortened. A low reticulocyte count indicates that the marrow is inappropriately responding to the anemia.
3. **Iron and total iron binding capacity (TIBC) or transferrin.** And occasionally a ferritin should be obtained if the anemia is microcytic. Will aid in the diagnosis of iron deficiency anemia. Iron deficiency anemia results in a low iron and a normal or elevated TIBC or transferrin. The ferritin is also low. If the patient has a very low MCV (<70) and a normal iron and TIBC, the likelihood of thalassemia is high. It is important to realize that many acute and chronic illnesses can dramatically affect the iron and TIBC, making their utility in the diagnosis of anemia low. If the question of iron deficiency requires a definite answer, a bone marrow exam with iron stains is indicated.
4. **B_{12} and folate.** Order on any patient suspected of having B_{12} and folate deficiency prior to transfusion. If folate deficiency is secondary to malnutrition, a serum folate may be normal after one or two well-balanced meals. If folate deficiency is suspected and the patient has recently eaten, then consider checking a red blood cell folate.
5. **Haptoglobin and urine hemosiderin.** A low haptoglobin and a positive urine hemosiderin are indicative of hemolysis.
6. **Direct and indirect Coombs' test.** May indicate that the hemolysis is immunologic. A direct Coombs' measures the presence of antibody and/or complement on the RBC; an indirect Coombs' detects antibody in the plasma that has dissociated from the RBC but is directed at the RBC. The direct Coombs' is the most valuable test in evaluating the possibility of immunohemolytic disease, whereas the indirect Coombs' is primarily of value as a blood banking procedure. Detection of an antibody in the plasma but not on the RBC indicates it is an alloantibody and not an autoantibody. Most immunohemolytic anemias are due to warm-reacting antibodies, usually IgG. These are manifest by a direct Coombs' that is positive for IgG with or without complement.
7. **Platelet count.** May be elevated in early iron deficiency. Decreased in folate and vitamin B_{12} deficiency and with marrow replacement.

C. Radiologic and other studies. Not usually needed unless gastrointestinal blood loss is suspected and then order as clinically indicated.

V. Plan

A. Anemia with hemodynamic compromise or complications

1. If the patient is hemodynamically unstable or having angina, an urgent transfusion is indicated. When this is the case, the source of blood loss is usually obvious. For specifics on transfusion, see Chapter 5.
2. Be sure the patient has adequate intravenous access if there is evidence of acute bleeding.

B. Anemia without hemodynamic compromise or complications. If the patient is not hemodynamically compromised, the workup may proceed in an orderly fashion. In many cases, the cause of the anemia is not obvious. Furthermore, laboratory testing is not always diagnostic. If the patient has an unremarkable history and physical, ambivalent laboratory testing, and no obvious underlying infectious, malignant, or inflammatory disease, a bone marrow biopsy is indicated.

C. Iron deficiency anemia. A source of blood loss must be found. This usually entails a flexible sigmoidoscopy and air-contrast barium enema, or a colonoscopy and either an upper endoscopy or a barium study of the upper gastrointestinal tract. Remember, heavy menstrual losses are the most common cause of an iron deficiency anemia in a young woman. Once the source of blood loss is determined, the iron stores need to be repleted. Most patients tolerate oral iron as ferrous sulfate 325 mg orally TID. Tolerance to oral iron may be improved by gradually increasing the dose from 325 mg QD to TID.

D. Folate deficiency. Generally, this is due to dietary insufficiency (pregnancy, chronic alcoholism). In this setting, daily folate supplementation at 1 mg PO is indicated.

E. Vitamin B_{12} deficiency. Inadequate dietary intake is a rare cause of B_{12} deficiency. True pernicious anemia can be diagnosed by the use of Schilling's test. This test involves the administration of a loading dose of 1000 mg vitamin B_{12} to saturate receptor sites, followed by the administration of radiolabeled B_{12} and measurement of the radioactivity in a 24-hour urine. If the amount of radioactive vitamin B_{12} in the urine is small, oral intrinsic factor can be given along with a second dose of radioactive B_{12} and a 24-hour urine recollected. An abnormal first step and a normal second step help differentiate between pernicious anemia and other causes of vitamin B_{12} deficiency such as bacterial overgrowth and ileal diseases. The history may also give an obvious etiology for B_{12} deficiency (status post gastrectomy or ileal resection). Vitamin B_{12} is replaced by administration of 100 μg IM daily for a week, then 100 μg IM twice a week for a month, and thereafter 100 μg IM monthly for life.

F. **Hemolytic anemia.** In the face of an elevated reticulocyte count and no obvious source of blood loss, a destructive process must be considered. Immune-mediated processes can be diagnosed by use of the Coombs' test. In the setting of Coombs' negative hemolytic anemia, other processes must be considered such as disseminated intravascular coagulation and microangiopathic hemolytic anemia. A review of the peripheral smear will be helpful. A concomitant low platelet count, low fibrinogen, and elevated prothrombin time, partial thromboplastin time, and fibrin degradation products point toward disseminated intravascular coagulation. The possibility of an inherited disorder such as thalassemia, sickle cell anemia, or an enzymopathy must be ruled out. Hemoglobin electrophoresis and review of the peripheral smear are indicated. If an enzymopathy is considered, specific assays are indicated (glucose-6-phosphate dehydrogenase, pyruvate kinase, and so on). The possibility of paroxysmal nocturnal hemoglobinuria must be considered in cases where etiology is unclear. Ham's test is indicated in this instance. Discussion of specific treatments for hemolytic anemia is beyond the scope of this book.

G. **Anemia of chronic disease.** This is usually a diagnosis of exclusion. The etiology may be obvious as in a patient with advanced malignancy. There is no specific diagnostic test for this disorder. Treatment is of the underlying disease. It is generally manifest by a low reticulocyte count, a low iron and TIBC, and normal bone marrow morphology. These are not specific findings, however.

REFERENCES

Jandl JH. The anemias. In: Jandl JH, ed. *Blood: Textbook of Hematology.* Boston/Toronto: Little, Brown; 1987:111–432.

■ ARTERIAL LINE PROBLEMS

(See also Chapter 3, Arterial Line Placement, p 305.)

I. **Problem.** You are called to the intensive care unit to see a patient in whom a low, dampened arterial line pressure is being obtained.

II. **Immediate Questions**

A. **Does the pressure accurately reflect the patient's status?** Mental status changes (See Coma, Acute Mental Status Changes, p 65), tachycardia, and a decreased urine output would be expected with hypotension.

B. **Is the problem with the catheter itself or with the monitoring apparatus (tubing, transducer, electronic equipment)?** If the patient's clinical status does not reflect the low blood pressure obtained by the arterial line, the problem may be in the equipment.

C. **Is an extremity at risk?** Thrombosis secondary to the arterial line can cause ischemia and tissue loss.

D. Has the tracing changed recently? Find out if the tracing was satisfactory earlier. A good tracing followed by a poor tracing suggests either deterioration in clinical status or a new problem with the catheter.

III. Differential Diagnosis. A low and/or dampened blood pressure results from problems with the monitoring equipment, problems with the arterial line catheter, or actual hemodynamic deterioration of the patient.

A. Patient status. If the patient's hemodynamic status has deteriorated, the decrease in blood pressure/dampening of the waveform is actually indicative of the patient's status. Often, other clinical indicators of the patient's status such as mental status changes, tachycardia, decreased urine output, and electrocardiographic changes suggesting ischemia are apparent.

B. Monitoring apparatus problems

1. Air is present in the tubing/transducer.
2. The tubing is kinked.
3. Electrical equipment is faulty.

C. Catheter problems

1. There are kinks in the catheter.
2. A thrombus is present in the catheter or in the vessel.
3. The catheter tip is resting against the wall of the artery because of the way the catheter was anchored (by suture and/or taping).
4. The catheter has punctured the arterial wall causing bleeding and compression of the catheter.

IV. Database

A. Physical examination: Key points.

1. **Blood pressure.** If the arterial line pressure is low, perform a cuff pressure. If this confirms hypotension, prompt action is indicated. The manual blood pressure is usually within 10–15 mm Hg of the arterial line pressure.
2. **Pulses.** Check immediately for distal pulses and for swelling and/or tenderness in the area of the catheter insertion. Failure to find a pulse or a decrease in pulse with significant swelling at the catheter site represents a potentially serious vascular compromise.
3. **Inspection of the equipment**
   - **a.** Check for air in the lines or the transducer. The search must be thorough and almost certainly will require the assistance of the nursing staff.
   - **b.** Have nursing staff confirm that the electrical equipment is working properly.
   - **c.** Attempt to withdraw blood through the catheter. Inability to do so suggests the catheter tip is in poor position, there is a kink or a thrombus in the catheter, at the catheter tip, or in the artery. ***Caution:*** Do not attempt to flush a catheter through which blood cannot be drawn!

V. **Plan**

A. **Maintaining perfusion to the extremity.** A potentially ischemic extremity often results from hypotension, a large catheter-to-vessel ratio, bleeding into surrounding tissues, inadequate flushing techniques, or prolonged catheter indwelling time.

1. Failure of the pulse to return will probably necessitate a cutdown attempt at thrombus removal and/or repair of the artery. Consult a vascular surgeon immediately.
2. If bleeding from the artery into the surrounding tissue seems probable, watch carefully for compartmental syndrome (pain, pain with extension of the digits, pallor, hypesthesia, and loss of motor function). Surgical evacuation of the blood may be necessary. Consult a vascular surgeon immediately if compartmental syndrome is suspected.
3. Search for evidence of infection. If infection is present, culture and treat appropriately and remove the catheter.

B. **Monitoring apparatus problems**

1. Flush the transducer and tubing thoroughly.
2. Retape the tubing to eliminate kinks.
3. Replace faulty electrical equipment.
4. An armboard may prevent the catheter or tubing from kinking extra-arterially.

C. **Catheter problems**

1. Loosen sutures or tape to reposition catheter tip away from the wall.
2. If a thrombus or kink in the intra-arterial catheter is suspected, the line will probably have to be removed and placed elsewhere.
3. In general, one should not attempt to place a new arterial line over a guide wire. Remove the old catheter and replace it with a new one preferably at a different site. Perforation of the kink with the guide wire (possibly causing a foreign body embolus), damage to the arterial wall, and/or dislodgement of a thrombus in or at the tip of the catheter all serve to make the risks outweigh potential benefits.

■ ASPIRATION

I. **Problem.** After a generalized seizure, a patient is observed to vomit and subsequently develops acute respiratory distress.

II. **Immediate Questions**

A. **What are the vital signs?** On the basis of the history, it must be assumed that the patient has aspirated gastric contents. This can result in acute respiratory compromise either through lodging of particulate matter in the larynx or trachea or through the rapid onset of pulmonary edema. In either case, both **tachycardia** and

tachypnea may result. In severe episodes of respiratory compromise, **apnea** and **shock** may also occur.

B. Is the patient able to communicate? Aphonia may result from lodging of particulate matter in the larynx or trachea and requires immediate endotracheal suctioning.

C. Is the patient cyanotic? Cyanosis would indicate severe respiratory compromise and probable need for emergent intubation.

D. Does the patient need to be repositioned? To prevent further aspiration of gastric contents, the patient should be placed in a lateral decubitus position with the head down.

III. Differential Diagnosis. Three distinct aspiration syndromes are recognized depending on the nature of the aspirated contents: (1) acidic gastric contents; (2) nonacid and/or particulate material; and (3) oropharyngeal bacterial pathogens. These syndromes should be distinguished from each other as well as from other causes of acute respiratory distress because the complications and treatment differ for each.

A. Acid aspiration. Aspiration of gastric contents with a pH less than 2.5 results in immediate alveolar injury and chemical pneumonitis. Noncardiogenic pulmonary edema and shock may occur. Clinically, there is the abrupt onset of dyspnea, fever, wheezing, rales, and hypoxemia.

B. Particulate aspiration. This can result in mechanical obstruction and bronchospasm. It must be distinguished from aspiration of a foreign body and asthma. Pneumonia can ensue if particulate material remains lodged in peripheral airways.

C. Oropharyngeal bacteria. Saliva contains 10^8 organisms per milliliter. Aspiration of saliva into the lower airway can cause an early pneumonitis followed by necrotizing pneumonia or abscess in 7 to 14 days.

D. Asthma (See Wheezing, p 257.)

E. Pneumonia. Pneumonia can be very difficult to distinguish from acute aspiration of gastric contents as both can result in tachypnea, tachycardia, rales, fever, sputum production, and radiographic infiltrates.

F. Pulmonary embolism. This diagnosis must be considered in the differential of any patient developing acute respiratory distress.

G. Foreign body aspiration. This occurs mainly in younger children and occasionally in debilitated elderly people who aspirate a food bolus.

IV. Database. Attempt to identify those conditions that predispose to aspiration. Disorders resulting in **impairment of consciousness** include anesthesia, alcohol abuse, seizure disorder, cerebrovascular accident, cardiopulmonary arrest, and drug overdose. **Esophageal dysfunction** predisposes to aspiration and includes esophageal stricture, hiatal hernia, and nasogastric intubation. **Impaired swallowing** may result from a cerebrovascular accident, polymyositis, myasthenia gravis, Parkinson's disease, a tracheostomy, or cancer involving the head and neck.

A. Physical examination key points

1. **Vital signs** (See Section II.A.)
2. **HEENT.** Check dentition for loose or missing teeth and evidence of gingivitis.
3. **Neck.** Examine for evidence of tumor involving of the oropharynx. Also look for any evidence of prior surgical procedures or radiation of the head and neck.
4. **Lungs.** Wheezing and crackles can occur after aspiration of gastric contents. Wheezing and diminished breath sounds may result from aspiration of particulate material.
5. **Skin.** Examine for presence of cyanosis.
6. **Neurologic exam.** Determine the patient's degree of consciousness and also the presence or absence of a gag reflex.

B. Laboratory data

1. **Arterial blood gases.** Hypoxemia and hypercapnia may occur and, if present, intubation may be required.
2. **Hemogram.** Aspiration of acid contents and pneumonia can cause a leukocytosis and left shift.
3. **Sputum gram stain and culture.** If the patient manifests fever, leukocytosis, and sputum production 2 to 3 days after aspiration, sputum gram stain and culture may be helpful in confirming pneumonia and directing subsequent antibiotic therapy.

C. Radiologic and other studies

1. **Chest x-ray** may show:
   - **a.** Hyperaeration from air trapping on side of foreign body aspiration.
   - **b.** Infiltrate in dependent segments of the lungs. Infiltrates may not be seen immediately after aspiration; therefore, if the initial CXR is normal but there is a strong clinical suspicion of aspiration, repeat the CXR in 4 to 5 hours.
   - **c.** Wedge-shaped pleural-based density suggests pulmonary infarction.
   - **d.** Clear fields in uncomplicated asthma.
   - **e.** Lung abscess formation does not generally occur until 7 to 14 days following aspiration and will not be observed on initial films.
2. **Other studies.** Ventilation/perfusion ($\dot{V}/\dot{Q}$) scan if a pulmonary embolism is suspected.

V. Plan. Aspiration should be suspected in any patient with a predisposing factor who develops sudden respiratory distress. Early treatment is important as death from respiratory failure can occur if the condition is not recognized early. Ideally, the best treatment is prevention.

A. Prevention

1. For patients being administered tube feedings, gastric emptying should be confirmed and the head of the bed elevated.

2. Unconscious patients should be placed in a lateral, slightly head-down position whenever possible.
3. When not being used for enteral feedings, nasogastric tubes should be placed only when continuous suction is required.
4. Patients with recent strokes should not be fed by mouth until they have demonstrated an intact gag reflex.

B. Oxygenation. Supplemental oxygen should be given in an amount sufficient to ensure oxygen saturation greater than 90%.

C. Intubation and positive pressure breathing. Will be required in the patient in whom supplemental oxygen therapy is not able to maintain adequate oxygenation or in the patient who is obtunded and unable to protect her or his airway.

D. Endotracheal suction. Should be attempted in any patient who is observed to aspirate.

E. Medications

1. Bronchodilators such as aminophylline (6 mg/kg IV loading dose over 30 minutes, then 0.3–0.6 mg/kg/h continuous infusion) and nebulized beta agonists such as Alupent (0.3 mL in 3 mL of normal saline) may be necessary if bronchospasm is present.
2. Prophylactic corticosteroids have not been shown to decrease subsequent morbidity and mortality from aspiration and are not indicated.
3. Prophylactic antibiotics likewise have not been shown to diminish morbidity and mortality. Antibiotics should be administered only if the patient continues to manifest fever, leukocytosis, purulent sputum, and infiltrates 2 to 3 days after the initial aspiration. For those patients with in-hospital aspiration, a regimen that provides coverage for gram-negative aerobes as well as *Staphylococcus aureus* should be used. A combination including ticarcillin and tobramycin is generally recommended.

F. Rigid bronchoscopy. This should be performed only when large particulate aspiration is suspected and atelectasis persists.

REFERENCE

Wynne JW, Modell H. Respiratory aspiration of stomach contents. *Ann Intern Med* 1977;87:466–474.

■ BRADYCARDIA

I. Problem. A nurse on the telemetry unit calls to notify you that a 30-year-old woman admitted last night has a heart rate of 42 beats per minute. The woman has mitral stenosis and was admitted to undergo percutaneous mitral balloon valvotomy.

II. Immediate Questions

A. What are the patient's other vital signs? A given heart rate must always be considered in relation to the patient's blood pressure (BP) and other signs of peripheral perfusion. A BP below 90 mm Hg in a bradycardic patient requires more rapid action than in a patient with bradycardia and a normal BP. Cerebrovascular accident and myocardial ischemia or infarction may result from prolonged untreated hypotension.

B. **What has the patient's heart rate been since admission?** The range of normal heart rates is wide and depends on activity, age, conditioning, and medications.

C. **Does the patient have any symptoms associated with the bradycardia?** Fatigue, dizziness, nausea, dyspnea, chest pain, or neurologic alterations.

III. Differential Diagnosis

A. Sinus bradycardia

1. **High vagal tone.** May be precipitated by sudden stressful or painful experience.
2. **Sinus node disease.** Associated with hypothyroidism, hypothermia, certain infiltrating diseases, drug effects, or as part of sick-sinus syndrome.
3. **Myocardial infarction.** Usually with inferior infarction.
4. **Cushing's reflex.** This reflex results from an increase in intracranial pressure secondary to a variety of causes such as hemorrhagic stroke, meningitis, or intracranial tumor. Hypertension occurs in addition to bradycardia.
5. **Drug effect.** Beta blockers such as propranolol (Inderal), metoprolol (Lopressor), and atenolol (Tenormin); calcium channel blockers such as verapamil (Calan, Isoptin), diltiazem (Cardiazem), and clonidine; and certain antiarrhythmic drugs such as amiodarone (Cordarone).

B. Atrioventricular (AV) block

1. **Second-degree AV block, Mobitz type I (Wenckebach).** Characterized by progressive, cyclical prolongation of the PR interval until a ventricular complex is dropped. This results in intermittent AV block.
   a. **Acute myocardial infarction.** Mostly inferior.
   b. **Drug toxicity.** Digoxin (Lanoxin), beta blockers, calcium channel blockers, and amiodarone.
   c. **Infectious.** Acute rheumatic fever, Lyme disease.
   d. **Other.** Can be seen in normal people and relates to vagal tone.
2. **Second-degree AV block, Mobitz type II.** Cyclical AV block without progressive prolongation of PR interval. The QRS complex of conducted beats is often wide because of a bundle branch block.
   a. **Acute myocardial infarction.** Anterior more common than inferior.
   b. **Degenerative disease** of the conduction system of the bundle of His.

c. **Infectious diseases** such as viral myocarditis, acute rheumatic fever, and Lyme disease.

3. **Third-degree AV block.** Associated with the same conditions as type II second-degree heart block. Occurs when there is no conduction through the AV node. This results in the P waves and QRS complexes being totally independent of one another.

IV. Database

A. Physical examination: Key points

1. **Vital signs** (See Section II.A.)
2. **Neck veins.** Intermittent cannon "A" waves suggest AV dissociation. A cannon "A" wave is an exaggerated A wave in the jugular veins that results from simultaneous right atrial contraction and a closed tricuspid valve (AV dissociation) causing increased backward pressure to be transmitted into the superior vena cava and jugular veins.
3. **Lungs.** Rales suggest decompensated heart failure which can occur as a result of bradycardia.
4. **Heart.** Listen for murmurs and gallops. An S_4 may point toward an acute myocardial infarction as the etiology of the bradycardia. A murmur (see Heart Murmur, p 112) may be seen in myocardial infarction, acute rheumatic fever, and myocarditis.
5. **Skin.** Cool, pale extremities suggest decreased peripheral perfusion.
6. **Mental status.** Inadequate perfusion may result in altered mental status.

B. Laboratory data

1. **Electrolytes.** Look for hypokalemia if the patient is on digoxin.
2. **Digoxin level.** A must if patient is on digoxin.
3. **Thyroid hormone levels.** Rule out hypothyroidism.

C. Radiologic and other studies. Electrocardiogram and rhythm strip.

1. Look for presence of P waves. Leads I, aVR, and aVL and inferior leads demonstrate the morphology of P waves the best. The absence of P waves suggests a nodal rhythm.
2. A varying PR interval with a dropped QRS complex is Mobitz type I second-degree heart block.
3. P waves that occur intermittently without an associated QRS complex and an otherwise constant PR interval suggest second-degree heart block Mobitz type II. Third-degree heart block is present when the P waves and QRS complexes are independent.
4. Look for evidence of myocardial infarction or ischemia. ST elevation or depression, T wave inversion, or Q waves.
5. Pacemaker spikes if appropriate.

V. Plan. Therapy is dictated by the clinical setting and symptoms associated with the bradycardic rhythm. Try not to overreact.

A. Drugs

1. Consider stopping or holding doses of drugs associated with bradycardic rhythms. If the patient is asymptomatic, discontinuing a medication such as propranolol is all that needs to be done.
2. Atropine 0.5–1.0 mg IV should be used to increase the heart rate in sinus bradycardia, second-degree AV block, or third-degree AV block if the patient is symptomatic.
3. As atropine is usually only a temporary measure, isoproterenol 1–3 μg/min infusion can be given following atropine if a heart rate is not maintained to sustain hemodynamic stability.

B. Treatment of bradycardia secondary to a CNS event. Decrease intracranial pressure in patients with CNS disturbances. Hyperventilation, furosemide, and dexamethasone should be given if there is an increase in intracranial pressure resulting in bradycardia. (See Coma, Acute Mental Status Changes, Section V, p 71.)

C. Pacemakers. Permanent or temporary. Temporary pacemakers include external and transvenous pacemakers. External pacemakers can be applied quickly in an emergent situation such as severe bradycardia with hypotension. Transvenous pacemakers can be placed with central venous access at the bedside when the patient is hemodynamically stable for any of the following indications.

1. **Temporary**
   - **a.** Mobitz type II second-degree or third-degree AV block associated with myocardial infarction.
   - **b.** Symptomatic AV block associated with drug toxicity such as with digoxin.
   - **c.** Sinus bradycardia with congestive heart failure complicated by chronotropic incompetence.
   - **d.** Prolonged sinus pauses (>3.5 seconds) associated with syncope.
2. **Permanent**
   - **a.** Sick-sinus syndrome **with** symptoms as a result of bradycardia or sinus pauses.
   - **b.** Mobitz type II second-degree or third-degree AV block.

REFERENCES

Marriott H. *Practical Electrocardiography.* 7th ed. Baltimore: Williams and Wilkins; 1983.

Zipes DP. Management of cardiac arrhythmias. In: Braumwald E, ed. *Heart Disease: A Textbook of Cardiovascular Medicine.* 3rd ed. Philadelphia: WB Saunders; 1988:621–657.

Zipes DP. Specific arrhythmias: Diagnosis and treatment. In: Braumwald E, ed. *Heart Disease: A Textbook of Cardiovascular Medicine.* 3rd ed. Philadelphia: WB Saunders; 1988:658–716.

■ CARDIOPULMONARY ARREST

I. **Problem.** You are the first member of a code team to arrive at the bedside of a patient found unresponsive by the nurse.

II. **Immediate Questions**

   A. **Is the patient unresponsive?** Cardiopulmonary resuscitation (CPR) begins with an attempt to arouse the patient. Call the patient and gently shake him or her by the shoulders. If the patient is unresponsive, begin CPR.

   B. **Is the patient in optimal position for CPR?** The patient must be supine and on a firm, flat surface to provide effective external chest compression. The head must be at the same level as the thorax for optimal cerebral perfusion.

   C. **Is the airway obstructed?** In the unconscious patient, the tongue and epiglottis may fall backward and occlude the airway. A head tilt/chin lift maneuver will lift these structures and open the airway. Vomitus or foreign material should be removed from the mouth by either a finger sweep or suction.

   D. **After establishment of a patent airway, is the patient breathing?** This can be assessed within 3 to 5 seconds by looking for chest movement, listening for air movement, and feeling for breath on the rescuer's face. If breathing is not present, then institute rescue breathing with two full breaths.

   E. **Is there evidence of adequate circulation?** Establish whether a carotid pulse is present. If no pulse is felt after 10 seconds of palpation, begin external chest compressions. After basic and then advanced cardiac life support has been instituted, other questions may help elucidate the cause of the patient's arrest.

   F. **What medications is the patient taking?** Cardiac medications are particularly important. Drugs that prolong the QT interval such as quinidine and procainamide may predispose to torsades de pointes, characterized by recurrent ventricular tachycardia and ventricular fibrillation. Phenothiazines and tricyclic antidepressants may also cause this condition. Digoxin (Lanoxin) is a frequent cause of a variety of cardiac arryhthmias.

   G. **Has the patient received any administered medications that could have resulted in an anaphylactic reaction?** (See Anaphylactic Reaction, p 22.)

   H. **Is there any history of electrolyte disturbance or conditions that could predispose to electrolyte disturbance?** Hypokalemia and hypomagnesemia can predispose to arrhythmias. Hyperkalemia can cause complete heart block and cardiac arrest.

   I. **What are the patient's other medical problems?** Inquire specifically regarding a prior history of coronary artery disease or other cardiac disease. Is there any recent history to suggest the possibility of acute stroke or any conditions that might predispose to acute pulmonary embolism such as recent surgery? The aggressiveness of CPR can also be determined by ascertaining if the patient has any associated medical problems such as malignancy which carries an extremely poor prognosis with resuscitation.

III. Differential Diagnosis. Cardiopulmonary arrest can result either from a primary cardiac disturbance or from primary respiratory arrest. Cardiac rhythms that may result in arrest include ventricular fibrillation, ventricular tachycardia, asystole, and electromechanical dissociation. There are a wide variety of causes of cardiopulmonary arrest; some of the more common are listed here:

- **A. Cardiac**
  1. **Acute myocardial infarction**
  2. **Acute pulmonary edema**
  3. **Ventricular arrhythmias**
  4. **Cardiac tamponade**
- **B. Pulmonary**
  1. **Pulmonary embolus**
  2. **Acute respiratory failure**
  3. **Aspiration**
  4. **Tension pneumothorax**
- **C. Hemorrhagic.** Acute massive hemorrhage such as from a ruptured aortic aneurysm.
- **D. Metabolic**
  1. **Electrolyte disturbances.** Hypokalemia, hyperkalemia, and hypomagnesemia can induce arrhythmias.
  2. **Acidosis and alkalosis**
  3. **Rewarming** during the treatment of acute hypothermia may induce ventricular fibrillation or arrhythmias.
- **E. Neurologic.** Acute subarachnoid hemorrhage.

IV. Database

- **A. Physical examination key points.** The initial assessment of airway, breathing, and circulation is described in Section II, p 39. Resuscitation should obviously be initiated before a detailed physical examination is performed. Other signs to be looked for:
  1. **Tracheal deviation.** Would indicate the possibility of tension pneumothorax.
  2. **Distended neck veins.** May also indicate a tension pneumothorax or pericardial tamponade.
- **B. Laboratory data.** These should be obtained early in resuscitation but should not result in delaying the start of therapy.
  1. **Arterial blood gases.** Acidosis could be the cause of an arrhythmia or result from prolonged hypoperfusion. A low pO_2 can result from a variety of causes including pulmonary edema and pulmonary embolus, or again it may result from prolonged hypoperfusion.
  2. **Serum electrolytes.** Including serum magnesium.
  3. **Complete blood count.** Realize that with massive hemor-

rhage the hematocrit may not have had sufficient time to equilibrate and therefore may not indicate the severity of bleeding.

C. Radiologic and other studies

1. **Continuous cardiac monitoring.** Preferably with a 12-lead electrocardiogram. Should be obtained as early as possible.
2. **Chest x-ray.** Should be obtained to determine the position of the endotracheal tube or any central venous lines.

V. Plan. A full description of definitive therapy for each of the causes of cardiopulmonary arrest is beyond the scope of this text. The reader is referred to the excellent references at the end of this section. In general, the best success in performing CPR has been achieved in those patients in whom basic life support has been initiated within 4 minutes of the time of arrest and advanced cardiac life support within 8 minutes of arrest. Fairly early recognition of unresponsiveness and initiation of CPR are crucial. Once basic life support has been instituted, the next goal should be to obtain endotracheal intubation and venous access, either via the antecubital vein or through a central vein. Once a 12-lead ECG has been obtained, the physician can establish a specific cause of the arrest and direct treatment accordingly. Listed here are brief summaries of the management of the major cardiac causes of arrest.

A. Ventricular fibrillation (See Figure 1–1) Immediate defibrillation is the most important element in the treatment of ventricular fibrillation. In fact, defibrillation should be attempted prior to attempts at intubating or establishing intravenous access. This is facilitated by the use of quick-look paddles now available on most defibrillators.

1. The first attempt should be with 200 joules. If the patient remains in ventricular fibrillation, the second attempt should be increased to 300 joules and administered immediately. If fibrillation still persists, a third countershock with 360 joules should be delivered.
2. If the patient remains in ventricular fibrillation after three countershocks, CPR should be resumed, the patient should be intubated, intravenous access should be established, and the patient should be connected to a 12-lead ECG. Epinephrine 1 mg of a 1:10,000 solution should be administered every 5 minutes. This drug is probably the most important pharmacologic agent used during CPR.
3. After 4 to 5 minutes, defibrillation should be attempted again with 360 joules. If the patient remains in ventricular fibrillation, a 50- to 100-mg IV bolus of lidocaine should be administered followed by a continuous infusion of 2 mg/min.
4. After administration of this drug, defibrillation should again be attempted. If fibrillation persists, a second 50– to 100-mg IV bolus of lidocaine can be administered followed by defibrillation.

Witnessed Arrest	Unwitnessed Arrest
↓	↓
Check Pulse—If No Pulse	Check Pulse—If No Pulse
↓	↓
Precordial Thump	
↓	
Check Pulse—If No Pulse	↓

↓

CPR Until a Defibrillator Is Available

↓

Check Monitor for Rhythm—if VF of VT[a]

↓

Defibrillate 200 Joules[b]

↓

Defibrillate, 200–300 Joules[b]

↓

Defibrillate With up to 360 Joules[b]

↓

CPR If No Pulse

↓

Establish IV Access

↓

Epinephrine, 1:10,000, 0.5–1.0 mg IV Push[c]

↓

Intubate If Possible[d]

↓

Defibrillate With up to 360 Joules[b]

↓

Lidocaine, 1 mg/kg IV Push

↓

Defibrillate With up to 360 Joules[b]

↓

Bretylium, 5 mg/kg IV Push[c]

↓

(Consider Bicarbonate)[f]

↓

Defibrillate With up to 360 Joules[b]

↓

Bretylium, 10 mg/kg IV Push[c]

↓

Defibrillate With up to 360 Joules[b]

↓

Repeat Lidocaine or Bretylium

↓

Defibrillate With up to 360 Joules[b]

5. Finally, if ventricular fibrillation still persists, bretylium 500 mg IV bolus can be administered and followed by another attempt at defibrillation.

B. Sustained ventricular tachycardia with no palpable pulse. This should be managed identically to ventricular fibrillation.

C. Ventricular tachycardia with a palpable pulse (See Figure 1–2.)

1. Ventricular tachycardia that is stable

a. The initial drug of choice is lidocaine with an initial loading dose of 50–100 mg followed by an IV infusion of 2 mg/min. An additional 50–75 mg of lidocaine can be administered every 5–10 minutes as necessary until a loading dose of 225 mg has been given.

b. If this fails to convert the patient, procainamide can be administered IV in 100-mg increments every 5 minutes until either the arrhythmia is suppressed or the QRS complex is widened more than 50% or until a loading dose of 1 g is given.

c. Finally, if both lidocaine and procainamide have been unsuccessful, bretylium 500 mg infused over 10 minutes can be administered followed by continuous infusion of 2 mg/min.

d. If none of the preceding agents is successful in converting the patient, synchronized cardioversion with an initial ener

---

Figure 1-1. Ventricular fibrillation (and pulseless ventricular tachycardia). *(From "Standards and Guidelines for Cardiopulmonary Resuscitation and Emergency Cardiac Care,"* Journal of the American Medical Association, *Volume 255, Number 21, June 6, 1986. Copyright 1986, American Medical Association.)*

—Ventricular fibrillation (and pulseless ventricular tachycardia). This sequence was developed to assist in teaching how to treat a broad range of patients with ventricular fibrillation (VF) or pulseless ventricular tachycardia (VT). Some patients may require care not specified herein. This algorithm should not be construed as prohibiting such flexibility. Flow of algorithm presumes that VF is continuing. CPR indicates cardiopulmonary resuscitation.

[a]Pulseless VT should be treated identically to VF.

[b]Check pulse and rhythm after each shock. If VF recurs after transiently converting (rather than persists without ever converting), use whatever energy level has previously been successful for defibrillation.

[c]Epinephrine should be repeated every five minutes.

[d]Intubation is preferable. If it can be accomplished simultaneously with other techniques, then the earlier the better. However, defibrillation and epinephrine are more important initially if the patient can be ventilated without intubation.

[e]Some may prefer repeated doses of lidocaine, which may be given in 0.5-mg/kg boluses every eight minutes to a total dose of 3 mg/kg.

[f]Value of sodium bicarbonate is questionable during cardiac arrest, and it is not recommended for routine cardiac arrest sequence. Consideration of its use in a dose of 1 mEq/kg is appropriate at this point. Half of original dose may be repeated every ten minutes if it is used.

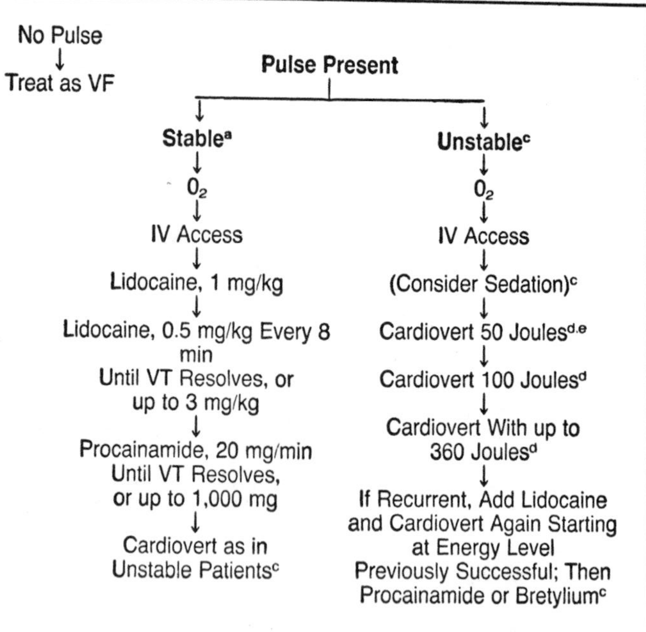

Figure 1-2. Sustained ventricular tachycardia. *(From "Standards and Guidelines for Cardiopulmonary Resuscitation and Emergency Cardiac Care,"* Journal of the American Medical Association, *Volume 255, Number 21, June 6, 1986. Copyright 1986, American Medical Association.)*

—Sustained ventricular tachycardia (VT). This sequence was developed to assist in teaching how to treat a broad range of patients with sustained VT. Some patients may require care not specified herein. This algorithm should not be construed as prohibiting such flexibility. Flow of algorithm presumes that VT is continuing. VF indicates ventricular fibrillation.

[a]If patient becomes unstable (see footnote b for definition) at any time, move to "Unstable" arm of algorithm.

[b]Unstable indicates symptoms (eg, chest pain or dyspnea), hypotension (systolic blood pressure <90 mm Hg), congestive heart failure, ischemia, or infarction.

[c]Sedation should be considered for all patients, including those defined in footnote b as unstable, except those who are hemodynamically unstable (eg, hypotensive, in pulmonary edema, or unconscious).

[d]If hypotension, pulmonary edema, or unconsciousness is present, unsynchronized cardioversion should be done to avoid delay associated with synchronization.

[e]In the absence of hypotension, pulmonary edema, or unconsciousness, a precordial thump may be employed prior to cardioversion.

[f]Once VT has resolved, begin intravenous (IV) infusion of antiarrhythmic agent that has aided resolution of VT. If hypotension, pulmonary edema, or unconsciousness is present, use lidocaine if cardioversion alone is unsuccessful, followed by bretylium. In all other patients, recommended order of therapy is lidocaine, procainamide, and then bretylium.

gy level of 50 joules may be attempted. If this is unsuccessful, 100 joules and then 200 joules can be administered.

2. **Ventricular tachycardia that is unstable**
   - **a.** If the patient has a pulse but is hemodynamically unstable (hypotension, unconsciousness, pulmonary edema), antiarrhythmic therapy should be deferred; instead, immediate unsynchronized cardioversion with 100 joules should be administered.
   - **b.** After cardioversion, a continuous infusion of lidocaine should be administered to prevent a recurrence of arrhythmia.

D. Asystole (See Figure 1–3.) This rhythm has an extremely poor prognosis.

1. Epinephrine 1 mg should be administered IV and repeated every 5 minutes.
2. As massive parasympathetic discharge can occasionally result in asystole, an initial dose of atropine 1 mg may be administered if there is no response to the epinephrine. This dose may be repeated after 5 minutes if there is no response.
3. Sodium bicarbonate and calcium chloride are no longer recommended for routine administration in asystole.
4. In general, pacemaker therapy will not be successful if the heart fails to respond to either of the preceding measures.
5. Be aware that occasionally fine ventricular fibrillation may be mistaken as asystole. This problem can be avoided by evaluating the ECG in several leads; however, if only one lead is available and there is a question of fine ventricular fibrillation, then defibrillation can be attempted.

E. Electromechanical dissociation (See Figure 1–4.) This condition is characterized by the presence of electrical activity on the ECG but no associated effective myocardial contraction. It is associated with a grave prognosis.

1. Electromechanical dissociation is caused by a variety of conditions including hypoxemia, severe acidosis, pericardial tamponade, tension pneumothorax, hypovolemia, and pulmonary embolus. It is therefore important to evaluate for potentially reversible causes such as tamponade and pneumothorax.
2. If tamponade is suspected, pericardiocentesis should be performed.
3. If tension pneumothorax is suspected, insertion of a 14- or 16-gauge Intracath (Jelco) in the second intercostal space midclavicular line should be attempted.
4. Otherwise, treatment consists of epinephrine 1 mg IV every 5 minutes along with CPR.
5. Fluid challenge should also be considered.
6. The administration of calcium chloride for this condition is no longer recommended.

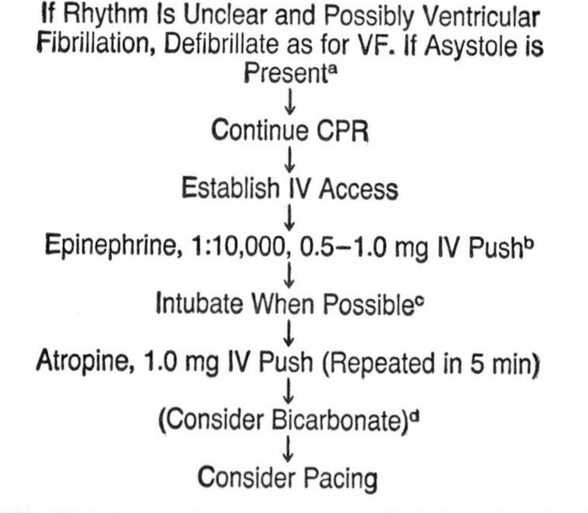

If Rhythm Is Unclear and Possibly Ventricular Fibrillation, Defibrillate as for VF. If Asystole is Present[a]
↓
Continue CPR
↓
Establish IV Access
↓
Epinephrine, 1:10,000, 0.5–1.0 mg IV Push[b]
↓
Intubate When Possible[c]
↓
Atropine, 1.0 mg IV Push (Repeated in 5 min)
↓
(Consider Bicarbonate)[d]
↓
Consider Pacing

Figure 1-3. Asystole (Cardiac Standstill). *(From "Standards and Guidelines for Cardiopulmonary Resuscitation and Emergency Cardiac Care,"* Journal of the American Medical Association, *Volume 255, Number 21, June 6, 1986. Copyright 1986, American Medical Association.)*

—Asystole (cardiac standstill). This sequence was developed to assist in teaching how to treat a broad range of patients with asystole. Some patients may require care not specified herein. This algorithm should not be construed to prohibit such flexibility. Flow of algorithm presumes asystole is continuing. VF indicates ventricular fibrillation; IV, intravenous.

[a]Asystole should be confirmed in two leads.

[b]Epinephrine should be repeated every five minutes.

[c]Intubation is preferable; if it can be accomplished simultaneously with other techniques, then the earlier the better. However, cardiopulmonary resuscitation (CPR) and use of epinephrine are more important initially if patient can be ventilated without intubation. (Endotracheal epinephrine may be used.)

[d]Value of sodium bicarbonate is questionable during cardiac arrest, and it is not recommended for the routine cardiac arrest sequence. Consideration of its use in a dose of 1 mEq/kg is appropriate at this point. Half of original dose may be repeated every ten minutes if it is used.

REFERENCES

Grauer K, Cavallaro D. Overall approach to management of cardiopulmonary arrest: Algorithms for treatment. In *ACLS Certification Preparation and a Comprehensive Review.* 2nd ed. St. Louis, Mo: CV Mosby; 1987:3–22.

1985 National Conference on Cardiopulmonary Resuscitation and Emergency Cardiac Care: Standards and guidelines for cardiopulmonary resuscitation and emergency cardiac care. *JAMA* 1986;255:2905–2954.

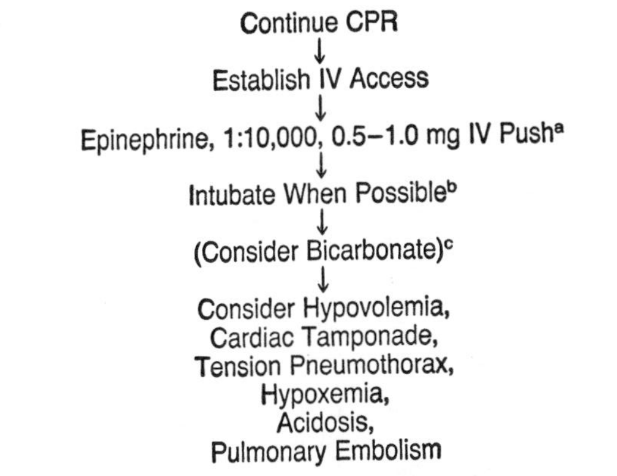

Continue CPR
↓
Establish IV Access
↓
Epinephrine, 1:10,000, 0.5–1.0 mg IV Push[a]
↓
Intubate When Possible[b]
↓
(Consider Bicarbonate)[c]
↓
Consider Hypovolemia,
Cardiac Tamponade,
Tension Pneumothorax,
Hypoxemia,
Acidosis,
Pulmonary Embolism

Figure 1-4. Electromechanical dissociation. *(From "Standards and Guidelines for Cardiopulmonary Resuscitation and Emergency Cardiac Care,"* Journal of the American Medical Association, *Volume 255, Number 21, June 6, 1986. Copyright 1986, American Medical Association.)*

—Electromechanical dissociation. This sequence was developed to assist in teaching how to treat a broad range of patients with electromechanical dissociation. Some patients may require care not specified herein. This algorithm should not be construed to prohibit such flexibility. Flow of algorithm presumes that electromechanical dissociation is continuing. CPR indicates cardiopulmonary resuscitation; IV, intravenous.

[a]Epinephrine should be repeated every five minutes.

[b]Intubation is preferable. If it can be accomplished simultaneously with other techniques, then the earlier the better. However, epinephrine is more important initially if the patient can be ventilated without intubation.

[c]Value of sodium bicarbonate is questionable during cardiac arrest, and it is not recommended for routine cardiac arrest sequence. Consideration of its use in a dose of 1mEq/kg is appropriate at this point. Half of original dose may be repeated every ten minutes if it is used.

■ CENTRAL VENOUS LINE PROBLEMS

(See also Pulmonary Artery Catheter Problems, p 228.)

I. Problem. The nursing staff calls to report a subclavian line has stopped functioning.

II. Immediate Questions

A. If the central line is used for central venous pressure (CVP) monitoring, what does the waveform look like? The CVP waveform drops on inspiration, raises with expiration, and should show monophasic to triphasic fluctuations with each cardiac cycle. If there is no waveform, the catheter may not be patent or there may be a thrombus in the vein or catheter.

B. **Do intravenous fluids easily flow into the catheter or does fluid leak from around the insertion site?** Again, this could be evidence for a thrombosed central vein or possibly a kinked catheter.

C. **Is the patient febrile?** A temperature in conjunction with a malfunctioning catheter suggests either a central line infection, associated deep vein thrombosis, or both. If any suspicion of associated infection or thrombosis exists, malfunctioning lines should be removed immediately and cultured.

D. **Are there any arrhythmias?** A central line catheter that extends into the right atrium or right ventricle can cause atrial or ventricular ectopy and arrhythmias.

E. **What is the line being used for? What is its relative necessity?** If drugs are being administered centrally that should not be given peripherally (vincristine or adriamycin as a continuous infusion), the situation is different than if the line has outlived its usefulness and could be replaced by peripheral lines.

III. Differential Diagnosis

A. **Clotted catheter.** This can occur when central lines are allowed to run dry or are running very slowly. Blood backs up into the catheter lumen and clots.

B. **Misdirected catheter.** Subclavian catheters from either the right or the left side may be inadvertently placed retrograde into the ipsilateral internal jugular vein. This results in a line that cannot really be used to measure central venous pressure. Much more rarely, subclavian or internal jugular attempts end up in the long thoracic vein and fail to function correctly. The catheter may also extend into the right atrium or right ventricular rather than the proximal venous circulation.

C. **Kinked catheter.** Catheters can kink at the skin line or more deeply. From the right subclavian insertion site, it is not uncommon for catheters within relatively stiff sheaths to kink at the turn from the subclavian vein to the brachiocephalic vein as it joins the superior vena cava. Kinking at this bend is uncommon for single-lumen catheters or triple-lumen catheters not inside a sheath. Internal jugular lines and left subclavian lines are not generally subject to this problem. It should be stressed that any line can be misdirected and kink. The catheters are easily seen fluoroscopically and radiographically; a chest x-ray will usually diagnose the problem.

D. **Infected catheter.** Central line sepsis will usually not result in any apparent malfunction of the catheter. Fever, sepsis, and positive blood cultures may all result from the spread of skin flora to the intravascular segment of the catheter.

E. **Thrombosis of the vein of insertion.** All the deep veins accessed for central line insertion can thrombose as a result of the trauma associated with the procedure as well as the presence of a foreign body within the vein. Clinically, these events resemble natural deep vein thrombosis and can result in associated bland or septic pulmonary emboli.

IV. Database

A. Physical examination key points

1. **Vital signs.** An elevated temperature suggests an infection. If the catheter has been in place more than 3 days, you must consider the central venous catheter as the source of the fever.
2. **Extremities.** Look for evidence of deep vein thrombosis. Unilateral edema and venous engorgement suggest deep vein thrombosis.
3. **Skin.** Examine insertion site for evidence of tissue infiltration, bleeding, catheter kinking, or leakage. Also, erythema around the insertion site can be from a localized infection.

B. Laboratory data

1. **Complete blood count with differential.** An elevated white count with an increase in banded neutrophils is often present with catheter-related sepsis.
2. **Prothrombin time (PT), partial thromboplastin time (PTT), platelet count.** Should be obtained if a central line needs to be changed and a coagulopathy is possible, such as in patients with severe liver disease or malnutrition.
3. **Blood culture.** Should be obtained as part of routine evaluation of a fever. Remember, if a central venous catheter has been in place more than 3 days, there is a significant risk of catheter-related sepsis.

C. Radiologic and other studies

1. **Chest x-ray.** Useful in determining whether a catheter is in the correct position or kinked.
2. **Culture of catheter tip.** If catheter-related sepsis or infection is suspected, the catheter must be removed and the catheter tip sent for culture.
3. **Impedance plethysmography and Doppler ultrasound.** Noninvasive tests for suspected lower extremity venous thrombosis.
4. **Venography.** The gold standard for diagnosing venous thrombosis. If there is a history of allergy to contrast, venography should be preceded by treatment with corticosteroids and diphenhydramine.
5. **Nuclear venogram.** Can diagnose venous thrombosis and pulmonary embolism simultaneously with lower extremity injection.

V. Plan.

(For replacement of central venous catheters, see Chapter 3, Central Venous Catheterization, p 314.)

A. **Clotted catheter.** A line can sometimes be salvaged by aspirating the catheter while it is slowly pulled out. Sterile technique and a small syringe are necessary. Use of a guide wire, manual flushing, or injection of urokinase 5000 U (5000 U/mL) can result in embolization. These measures seldom cause any significant problem, probably because of the small volume of the embolus. The only completely safe approach, however, is aspiration. The risk of replacement of the line has to be weighed against the risk of using any of the other techniques besides aspiration. Other factors must be considered such as how long the line has been in place, whether the central line is crucial or could be dispensed with altogether, and whether there is fever or local evidence of infection.

B. **Misdirected catheter.** This usually requires removal and replacement. Sometimes with fluoroscopic assistance, a guide wire can be used to manipulate the catheter to the superior vena cava, but most often a new puncture is needed. If the catheter is in the right atrium or right ventricle and does not have to be removed for other reasons, the catheter can be partially withdrawn, using sterile technique, so that it is in the inferior or superior vena cava.

C. **Kinked catheter.** A new line that is kinked at the site of insertion can sometimes be salvaged by repositioning the line with new skin sutures. More proximal kinks can sometimes be fixed by replacing the catheter over a guide wire. If the kink is within a sheath or directly after the catheter emerges from the sheath, the sheath can sometimes be withdrawn, leaving the catheter in the same place, provided there is enough catheter left onto which the sheath can be withdrawn. The best way to deal with this problem is to prevent it. This is done by avoiding the right subclavian approach in patients who have shallow chests in the lateral dimension, in whom lines have to angulate acutely from the subclavian to the superior vena cava.

D. **Infected catheter.** An infected or possibly infected central line *must be removed.* This virtually always requires replacement elsewhere if central venous access is still desired. Intravenous line-associated sepsis is caused in large part by skin contamination. The practice of removing the line over a guide wire and traversing the same insertion site with the replacement line is not recommended. A new site is probably a better idea. It is important to draw two sets of blood cultures from the suspect line as well as two sets from the peripheral veins before the line is removed and to culture the tip of the catheter after it is removed.

E. **Thrombosis of the vein of insertion.** This also requires line removal and replacement at a site distant from the thrombosed vein. Heparin 5000 U bolus followed by 1000 U/h continuous infusion is recommended unless contraindicated for other reasons.

The PTT should be checked 6 hours after the infusion is begun and the heparin dose should be adjusted so that the PTT is one and one-half to two times the control. If sepsis is also suspected, antibiotics are necessary as is a surgical consultation for possible removal of the infected vein. Vancomycin 500 mg every 6 hours or 1000 mg every 12 hours is the preferred antibiotic if normal renal function is present. Vancomycin covers *Staphylococcus epidermidis* as well as *Staphylococcus aureus*. Be sure to decrease the dose if renal insufficiency is present.

REFERENCE

Gil RT, Kruse JA, Thill-Baharozian MC, et al. Triple- vs. single-lumen central venous catheters. *Arch Intern Med* 1989;149:1139–1143.

■ CHEST PAIN

I. Problem. A 48-year-old man with a history of tobacco abuse is admitted for elective bronchoscopy. On the evening of his admission, he develops substernal chest pain that persists approximately 15 minutes.

II. Immediate Questions. Because potentially serious conditions may cause chest pain, patients with this complaint should be evaluated on an urgent basis. By far, the most important tool in identifying the cause of chest pain is a meticulous history.

A. Does the patient have a prior history of coronary artery disease, and if so, does the current pain resemble previous episodes of angina pectoris? If the patient has a documented history of coronary artery disease, particularly if the current episode resembles previously known anginal attacks, assume the pain represents myocardial ischemia and treat accordingly.

B. What is the location, quality, and severity of the pain? Location (substernal, epigastric), radiation (jaw, arms, flank, abdomen), quality (burning, crushing, tearing, stabbing, sharp), and severity of pain are features that may suggest a particular diagnosis. Because several intrathoracic and extrathoracic structures are innervated by the same spinal cord segments, the location and quality of different causes of chest pain may overlap.

C. Are there any factors that are known to precipitate or relieve the pain? Sharp pain that is worsened by coughing or deep inspiration suggests pleuritis, pericarditis, or pneumothorax. Although classical angina is brought on by exertion, acute myocardial infarction (MI) may produce chest pain at rest. Movement of the arms or trunk that reproduces pain would indicate a musculoskeletal origin; however, pericarditis can also cause chest pain that is worsened by movement of the trunk. The pain of esophagitis is frequently exacerbated by recumbency. The relief of chest pain with sublingual nitroglycerin implies myocardial ischemia, although chest pain resulting from esophageal disease may also be relieved with nitrate therapy.

D. Has there been any recent trauma, fall, or thoracic procedure? Fractured ribs, chest wall contusions, or other musculoskeletal conditions such as recent excessive physical activity can result in chest pain.

III. Differential Diagnosis. The differential diagnosis of chest pain includes a variety of conditions ranging from musculoskeletal chest wall pain to life-threatening conditions such as acute MI and dissecting aneurysm. The clinician's initial goal is to exclude potentially catastrophic conditions, and if such conditions are identified, institute immediate therapy.

A. Cardiac causes of chest pain

1. Acute myocardial infarction

a. Pain is characterized as a severe, crushing, retrosternal pain that may radiate into the arms and neck. This pain is generally described as the worst ever experienced and generally persists 30 minutes or longer. It is seldom relieved by 1 or 2 nitroglycerin tablets and frequently requires morphine sulfate for relief. The pain of MI may begin at rest or even during sleep and is only infrequently preceded by strenuous physical activity.

b. Associated symptoms include nausea, diaphoresis, dyspnea, and palpitations.

c. Because more than 50% of the deaths caused by acute MI occur within the initial 2 hours, the physician must maintain a high index of suspicion for MI when evaluating any patient with acute chest pain.

2. Angina pectoris

a. The pain of angina is similar to that of MI although it generally lasts less than 30 minutes and is not nearly as severe. Relief can generally be obtained with sublingual nitroglycerin. The pain is generally exacerbated by exertion, but can also occur with emotional stress and at rest.

b. Any recent change in a stable pattern of angina, such as occurrence with rest or increased frequency or severity, should imply an unstable pattern that mandates close monitoring and aggressive medical therapy.

c. Although coronary artery disease is the most common cause of angina pectoris, other potential causes include coronary artery spasm, aortic stenosis, and angina precipitated by thyrotoxicosis, anemia, and low diastolic pressures.

3. Acute pericarditis

a. Pain is usually described as sharp, but may be dull, and is frequently pleuritic. The pain may be worsened by recumbency and relieved by sitting and leaning forward. Rotation of the trunk may precipitate pain.

b. Possible causes include the following:

(1) **Infection.** Most commonly viral, but may also be bacterial, fungal, or tuberculous.

(2) **Myocardial infarction.** Pericarditis may occur in the first 2–3 days after infarction or may not occur until 1–4 weeks after MI (Dressler's syndrome).

(3) **Uremia**

(4) **Malignancy.** Most often breast cancer, bronchogenic carcinoma, or lymphoma.

(5) **Connective tissue diseases.** These include rheumatoid arthritis, scleroderma, systemic lupus erythematosus, or acute rheumatic fever.

B. Vascular causes of chest pain

1. Acute aortic dissection

a. This is usually described as an excruciatingly severe pain that is tearing in nature and may radiate to the back (especially if the descending aorta is involved).

b. The condition most frequently occurs in patients with a prior history of hypertension or connective tissue disorders such as Marfan's syndrome. On presentation, however, the blood pressure may be normal or even low.

c. Aortic dissection is a potentially life-threatening condition that must be recognized and treated early.

2. Primary pulmonary hypertension. The pain in this condition is frequently similar to that of angina. It is usually mild, may be associated with syncope or dyspnea, and may occur with exertion.

C. Pulmonary causes of chest pain

1. Pulmonary embolism (PE) with infarction

a. Infarction results in inflammation of the overlying pleura and thus causes pleuritic chest pain. Embolism without infarction may cause a more vague, nondescript, substernal chest pain.

b. A number of conditions may predispose to deep venous thrombosis or PE and include the following: pregnancy, postoperative state, prolonged immobilization, malignancy (especially mucinous adenocarcinoma), obesity, exogenous estrogen use, paraplegia, cerebral vascular accident with resultant hemiplegia, and congestive heart failure.

c. Pulmonary embolism is a potentially fatal condition that is too often underdiagnosed. It should be suspected in any hospitalized patient who develops acute shortness of breath or chest pain.

2. Pneumothorax

a. This is characterized by the acute onset of pleuritic chest pain associated with dyspnea.

b. Tension pneumothorax is a potentially life-threatening condition that is characterized by hypotension, tracheal deviation, venous distension, and severe respiratory distress.

c. There are three broad categories of causes of pneumothorax:

(1) **Spontaneous causes.** This most often occurs in 20- to 30-year-old males and in older patients with bullous emphysema.

(2) **Iatrogenic causes.** Pneumothorax may be a complication of subclavian vein catheterization or thoracentesis. Barotrauma from mechanical ventilation, especially in patients requiring high inspiratory pressures, may also result in pneumothorax.

(3) **Traumatic causes.** Any patient with a penetrating chest injury, as well as patients suffering rib fractures, may sustain a pneumothorax.

3. **Pleurodynia.** This is frequently associated with Coxsackie virus.

4. **Pneumonia/pleuritis.** The pain is typically pleuritic and associated with fever, productive cough, and rigors.

D. Gastrointestinal causes of chest pain

1. **Gastroesophageal reflux.** This condition is usually described as a burning pain that is made worse with recumbency and relieved by antacids.

2. **Esophageal spasm.** This condition is easily confused with angina pectoris. It may cause substernal chest pain or tightness that is relieved by nitrates. Intermittent dysphagia, if it occurs, suggests esophageal disease; however, it may be difficult by history alone to distinguish esophageal spasm from angina. Remember that both conditions may occur together.

3. **Gastritis.** Alcoholism, steroid dependency, stress that is associated with a severe burn or intensive care unit admission, and use of nonsteroidal anti-inflammatory drugs may all induce inflammation of the gastric mucosa resulting in epigastric and lower chest pain.

4. **Peptic ulcer disease.** This is typically described as an epigastric discomfort that may be burning or gnawing. Pain may be either relieved or exacerbated by eating. It is frequently relieved by administration of antacids.

5. **Biliary colic.** This condition is characterized by postprandial pain that occurs 1–2 hours after eating and may last several hours. In contrast to the term *colic,* the pain is actually constant and may last several hours. The pain is usually located in the right upper quadrant and radiates to the scapula; however, the pain may also be perceived largely in the epigastrium and lower chest and therefore may be confused with angina.

6. **Pancreatitis.** There is usually a prior history of gallstones or

alcohol ingestion. Pain is usually midepigastric with radiation to the back. Similar to pericarditis, it may be exacerbated by recumbency and relieved by sitting upright and leaning forward. There are often associated nausea and vomiting.

E. Musculoskeletal chest pain. Pain is usually reproduced by palpation over the costochondral or sternochondral junctions. Pain is fairly well localized.

1. **Costochondritis.** Point tenderness is elicited over the costochondral junction.
2. **Muscle strain/spasm.** Most typically, there is a preceding history of exercise or overexertion.
3. **Rib fractures after trauma**

IV. Database

A. Physical examination key points

1. **Vital signs**
   a. Hypotension is an ominous sign that may result from any one of several potentially catastrophic causes including massive MI, cardiac tamponade from pericarditis, tension pneumothorax, acute massive PE, or rupture of a dissecting aneurysm.
   b. Hypertension may result from any painful condition but must be particularly looked for in the setting of acute MI or aortic dissection where emergent therapy to reduce the pressure is mandated.
   c. Fever may result from pulmonary infarction, MI, pneumonia, or pericarditis.
   d. Tachycardia may result from sinus tachycardia associated with pain, but could also indicate ventricular tachycardia that has developed because of myocardial ischemia. If untreated, ventricular tachycardia may progress into ventricular fibrillation. (See Tachycardia, p 241.)
   e. Bradycardia is a frequent occurrence with inferior MI and may result from either sinus node dysfunction or atrioventricular heart block (second or third degree). (See Bradycardia, p 35.)
2. **HEENT.** Evidence of thrush, especially in an immunosuppressed patient could indicate *Candida* esophagitis.
3. **Neck.** Significant venous distension may occur with either an acute tension pneumothorax or cardiac tamponade. Pain with hyperextension of the neck may indicate a cervical nerve or disk problem as a cause of referred shoulder and chest pain.
4. **Chest.** Localized chest wall tenderness may result from a contusion, costochondritis, or rib fracture.
5. **Lungs**
   a. Absent breath sounds, hyperresonance to percussion, and tracheal deviation all indicate a tension pneumothorax.
   b. Crackles and signs of pneumonic consolidation such as

increased tactile fremitus or egophony may occur with pneumonia or a pulmonary infarction.

- **c.** A pleural friction rub may result from pneumonia, pulmonary infarction, or any process resulting in pleuritis.
- **d.** Bibasilar crackles and/or wheezes may occur with decompensated congestive heart failure resulting from myocardial ischemia or infarction.
- **e.** Lung exam may be entirely normal in a patient with acute PE.

6. Heart

- **a.** The point of maximal impulse (PMI) may not be palpable in a patient with a pericardial effusion. The heart sounds, likewise, may be distant. In a patient with acute pericarditis, a friction rub may be present, but this is an evanescent finding and therefore the patient must be reexamined periodically.
- **b.** Most often, the cardiac exam is normal in a patient with acute MI or angina pectoris. If there is significant associated left ventricular dysfunction, an S_3 gallop may be heard. An S_4 gallop may also be present. A harsh systolic ejection murmur over the aortic outflow area may indicate aortic stenosis, which can cause angina pectoris even in the presence of normal coronary arteries. If dissection is suspected, listen for the diastolic, decrescendo murmur of aortic regurgitation which may develop if the dissection spreads to involve the aortic ring.

7. Abdomen. For a discussion of the various abdominal conditions that can also produce epigastric and lower chest pain, see Abdominal Pain, p 1.

8. Neurologic exam. A careful and detailed exam is important in any patient in whom aortic dissection is suspected. The dissection may occlude cerebral or spinal arteries and thereby cause a variety of neurologic deficits.

9. Extremities

- **a.** In a patient with suspected PE, examine for evidence of deep venous thrombosis; however, the physical exam is notoriously inaccurate in this condition and may be entirely normal despite the presence of significant venous thrombosis.
- **b.** In patients with suspected dissection, it is important to examine the pulses bilaterally in both upper and lower extremities to ascertain the presence of any pulse asymmetry.

B. Laboratory data

1. Hemogram. Leukocytosis may result from any form of inflammation such as pulmonary infarction or MI. If there is an increase in banded neutrophils, suspect a bacterial infection such as acute pneumonia.

2. **Arterial blood gases.** This should be obtained if a pulmonary process is suspected such as embolism, pneumothorax, and pneumonia. It should also be ordered for any patient with decompensated cardiac function resulting in pulmonary edema.
3. **Cardiac isoenzymes.** Serial measurements of creatine phosphokinase (CPK) every 8–12 hours over the first 24–48 hours may help to confirm or exclude an MI. It is important to note that serum levels of enzyme may not become elevated until several hours after the beginning of infarction. Therefore, a single measurement of CPK cannot be used to exclude the diagnosis of MI.

C. Radiologic and other studies

1. **Electrocardiogram.** An ECG should be obtained in any patient with a new complaint of chest pain. If available for comparison, an old ECG is helpful. New T wave changes, ST segment depression or elevation, or the presence of new Q waves may be helpful in identifying the cause of the chest pain as myocardial ischemia. Note again that patients presenting with myocardial ischemia and infarction may initially have an entirely normal ECG and that the diagnosis of MI cannot be excluded on the basis of a normal ECG.
2. **Chest x-ray.** Request a CXR in any patient in whom the etiology of the chest pain is unclear. It may be helpful in diagnosing pneumothorax, pneumonia, pleural effusion, and pericardial effusion. A widened mediastinum suggests the possibility of dissection of the thoracic aorta.
3. **Echocardiogram.** This can be performed on a nonemergent basis if pericarditis is suspected and if the patient does not appear to be in tamponade.
4. **Contrast CT scan.** This should be obtained in any patient in whom aortic dissection is suspected.
5. **Ventilation/perfusion ($\dot{V}/\dot{Q}$) lung scan.** A lung scan may be helpful if pulmonary emboli are suspected. Impedance plethysmography and Doppler ultrasound of the lower extremities may also be obtained if there is a strong suspicion for acute deep venous thrombosis.

V. Plan. In assessing any patient with acute chest pain, the physician's overriding goal is to exclude the presence of the previously mentioned life-threatening conditions. In the acute setting, it is better to maintain a high index of suspicion for these conditions and to overtreat rather than undertreat.

A. Emergency management (for all patients with chest pain)

1. Treat with oxygen. Administer oxygen therapy with 2–4 L/min by nasal cannula. If the patient has a history of chronic obstructive airway disease, it is preferable to administer 24% O_2 by Venturi face mask initially.
2. Establish an intravenous line for administration of medications should the patient deteriorate.

3. If chest pain is still present and the systolic blood pressure is above 90, administer 0.4 mg nitroglycerin sublingually.
4. Obtain a 12-lead ECG.
5. If your initial assessment suggests any evidence of a pneumothorax, pneumonia, or heart failure, obtain a stat portable CXR and ABG.

B. Myocardial ischemia. If your initial assessment suggests the possibility of acute MI, the following are brief guidelines offered for the initial treatment. A full discussion of acute MI is beyond the scope of this section.

1. **Nitrates**
   a. Nitroglycerin in a dose of 0.4–0.6 mg may be administered sublingually every 5 minutes provided that the systolic blood pressure remains above 90. It is preferable to administer the nitroglycerin while the patient is recumbent. This may provide relief for angina pectoris and possibly unstable angina pectoris.
   b. The pain of acute MI is seldom relieved by the administration of nitroglycerin sublingually and requires treatment with either morphine or nitroglycerin IV. If the nitroglycerin is effective but pain recurs, begin a nitroglycerin infusion initially at 10 μg/min and titrate to relief of pain. The systolic blood pressure must be maintained above 90 during the administration of nitroglycerin. Hemodynamic monitoring with a pulmonary artery catheter (see Chapter 3, Pulmonary Artery Catheterization, p 336) is advised.
2. **Morphine sulfate**
   a. If pain is not relieved by nitroglycerin sublingually, 3–5 mg of morphine IV every 5–10 minutes can be administered for relief. Close monitoring of the patient's blood pressure and respirations is necessary because hypotension and respiratory suppression may occur. These effects may be reversed with naloxone (Narcan) 0.4 mg IV.
   b. A few patients experience bradycardia after administration of morphine. This typically responds to 0.5–1.0 mg of atropine IV.
3. **Lidocaine**
   a. The use of prophylactic lidocaine in the management of acute MI is presently controversial.
   b. Patients are at greater risk of ventricular tachycardia and ventricular fibrillation within the first 24 hours of infarction. Ventricular tachycardia and fibrillation may develop suddenly without any preceding warning arrhythmias such as frequent premature ventricular complexes or ventricular couplets; however, the administration of lidocaine is not without potential serious side effects, including mental status changes, seizures, and asystole.

   - **c.** In a setting where the patient will be very closely monitored and where a defibrillator is readily available, it may be preferable not to administer prophylactic lidocaine.
   - **d.** In other settings where the patient may not be quite as closely monitored, lidocaine prophylaxis may be used. A loading dose of 1 mg/kg IV over 2–3 minutes should be followed by a constant infusion of 2 mg/min. The infusion should be stopped after 24 hours.
   - **e.** The continuous infusion should be reduced to 1 mg/min for elderly patients (age > 70) and patients with liver disease or heart failure.

4. Arrangements for transfer to a coronary care unit or intensive care unit should be made. This is especially important in the first 24 hours of myocardial infarction, when arrhythmia monitoring and ready access to a defibrillator are essential.

5. Discussion of thrombolytic therapy is beyond the scope of this section but should be considered in any patient in whom acute MI is suspected, especially if the onset has been within the preceding 4 hours.

C. Aortic dissection. The initial treatment goal is to reduce pain and, if the patient is hypertensive, to reduce blood pressure. Surgical correction is indicated for all ascending thoracic aneurysms.

1. Make arrangements for immediate transfer to an intensive care unit where hemodynamic monitoring can be instituted.

2. Obtain immediate vascular surgical consult.

3. A continuous infusion of nitroprusside (Nipride) 0.5–1.0 μg/kg/min should be initiated and titrated upward to control systolic blood pressure in the range of approximately 100–120 mm Hg systolic.

4. Administration of nitroprusside with the resultant short-term decrease in systolic blood pressure may result in a rebound increase in contractility and shearing force which might worsen the dissection. Propranolol (Inderal) 0.5 mg IV should therefore be administered prior to beginning nitroprusside. The initial bolus of propranolol should be followed by 1 mg IV every 5 minutes until the pulse pressure has been reduced to 60 mm Hg. Once this dose of propranolol has been established, it can be administered every 4–6 hours IV.

5. To relieve pain, morphine sulfate 3–5 mg may be administered IV every 10 minutes. Again, close monitoring of the blood pressure and respirations is necessary.

D. Pulmonary embolism

1. Ensure adequate oxygenation.

2. After checking a baseline prothrombin time and partial thromboplastin time, administer a bolus of heparin 10,000 U IV and follow it with a continuous IV infusion of 1000 U/h. Repeat the

PTT in approximately 4–6 hours and adjust the heparin to maintain a PTT approximately 1.5–2 times the control value.

3. If systemic anticoagulation is contraindicated, surgical consultation will be necessary to place a venocaval filter.

E. Acute pneumothorax

1. An acute tension pneumothorax should be treated by immediate placement of a 16-gauge needle into the second intercostal space in the midclavicular line. This potentially life-saving measure can be instituted while awaiting placement of a chest tube.
2. A spontaneous pneumothorax occurring in an otherwise healthy person and involving 20% or less of the lung can usually be followed simply by observation and oxygen. All other pneumothoraces should be treated by chest tube insertion.

F. Pericarditis

1. If tamponade is suspected, an emergent echocardiogram should be performed. If tamponade is confirmed, consultation with cardiology for pericardiocentesis should be requested.
2. Indomethacin (Indocin) 50 mg TID is generally effective for pain relief in most cases of pericarditis.

G. Gastritis/esophagitis

1. Antacids such as Mylanta-II 30 mL every 4–6 hours may provide immediate relief.
2. H2 antagonists such as cimetidine (Tagamet) and ranitidine (Zantac) may also relieve symptoms.
3. Elevating the head of the bed on 6-in. blocks may help to reduce the reflux that occurs with recumbency.

H. Costrochondritis. Treat with nonsteroidal anti-inflammatory drugs such as ibuprofen (Motrin) 400–600 mg every 6 hours.

REFERENCE

Fortuin NJ, Walford GD. Thoracic pain and anginal pectoris. In: Harvey AM, Johns RJ, McKusick VA, et al, eds. *The Principles and Practice of Medicine.* 22nd ed. Norwalk, Conn: Appleton & Lange; 1988:88–98.

■ COAGULOPATHY

I. Problem. After placement of a Tenckhoff catheter, a patient has bleeding from the incision as well as oozing from an intravenous site.

II. Immediate Questions

A. What is the patient's blood pressure? Determine immediately if the bleeding is extensive enough to cause hypovolemia and shock. Assess volume status by blood pressure, urine output, and central pressures if available. If the patient has a tachycardia (pulse over 100) or hypotension (blood pressure of 90 or less), then immediate establishment of intravenous access and fluid resuscitation is required. If central lines need to be placed, determine extent of the coagulopathy before inserting needles into major noncompressible vessels.

B. **How much external bleeding is there?** Look at wounds or needle puncture sites to see if there is active bleeding. Ask to have any old dressings saved so that you can see the amount and the nature of the bleeding.

C. **Do factors exist that increase the likelihood of generalized bleeding?** In the example given, the patient might be suspected of having disseminated intravascular coagulation. In general, when confronted with a bleeding patient, inquire about liver disease, nutritional status, relatives with bleeding disorders, any bleeding with prior surgical procedures (dental extractions, cholecystectomy), and use of medications such as aspirin, nonsteroidal anti-inflammatory drugs (NSAIDs), or anticoagulants.

III. **Differential Diagnosis**

A. **Inadequate surgical hemostasis.** Most common cause of localized bleeding in the postoperative patient. In most cases, the bleeding is minimal.

B. **Platelet disorders**

1. **Thrombocytopenia** (See Thrombocytopenia, p 246.)

A. **Decreased production.** Often secondary to chemotherapy or bone marrow replacement by fibrosis or neoplasia. Tuberculosis and histoplasmosis are two granulomatous diseases that can invade the bone marrow. Vitamin B_{12} or folic acid deficiency may result in decreased production as can iron deficiency.

b. **Sequestration.** Caused by splenic enlargement resulting from portal hypertension, neoplasia, infection or storage diseases.

c. **Destruction.** Idiopathic thrombocytopenic purpura (ITP), thrombotic thrombocytopenic purpura (TTP), collagen vascular diseases, and drug reactions to penicillins, sulfa drugs, thiazides, and heparin can cause platelet destruction.

d. **Dilution.** May occur in patients who have been transfused with large volumes of blood over a short interval.

2. **Qualitative platelet disorders**

a. **von Willebrand's disease.** Generally an autosomal dominant disease with decreased platelet adhesion. Many different variants.

b. **Acquired disorder.** Results from interference with cyclooxygenase metabolism by aspirin and NSAIDs. Aspirin will affect platelet function for the life of the platelet (7–10 days after aspirin is discontinued); NSAIDs affect platelet function only in the presence of the drug.

c. **Glanzmann's thrombasthenia.** Inherited abnormality in which platelets do not aggregate.

d. **Bernard-Soulier syndrome.** Inherited abnormality characterized by giant platelets with abnormal platelet adhesion.

e. **Uremia.** Abnormal platelet aggregation arising by an unknown mechanism.

C. Coagulation defects

1. Congenital

a. **Hemophilia A.** Factor VIII deficiency, X-linked recessive. Incidence of 1/10,000 male births.

b. **Hemophilia B.** Factor IX deficiency, X-linked recessive. Incidence of 1/100,000 male births.

c. **Congenital deficiencies of other coagulation factors.** Much less common than factor VIII and IX deficiency.

2. Acquired

a. **Disseminated intravascular coagulation (DIC).** Associated with sepsis, trauma, burns, and malignancy. A complication of pregnancy and delivery, liver disease, and heat stroke.

b. **Vitamin K deficiency.** Required for synthesis of factors II, VII, IX, and X. Most frequent setting is malnourished patient receiving antibiotics.

c. **Severe liver disease.** Cirrhosis, hepatitis, hemochromatosis, biliary cirrhosis, or cancer. Coagulopathy caused by decreased production of coagulation factors, production of abnormal coagulation factors, and/or a failure to clear activated coagulation factors.

IV. Database. The most important factor in diagnosing a coagulopathy is understanding and utilizing appropriate laboratory tests. It is imperative to draw blood for needed tests prior to instituting therapy or transfusions.

A. Physical examination key points

1. **Vital signs.** Orthostatic hypotension signifies a major loss of blood, and by definition is a decrease of 10 mm Hg in the systolic blood pressure and/or an increase in the heart rate of 20 beats per minute on movement from a supine to a standing position after one minute. Also look for tachycardia or hypotension.
2. **Skin.** Petechia, purpura, easy bruising, and oozing from intravenous sites suggest a systemic rather than a local cause.
3. **Incision.** Examine any incision for hematoma or active bleeding.
4. **Abdomen.** Splenomegaly, hepatomegaly, or ascites suggest cirrhosis.
5. **Extremities.** Hemarthrosis may be seen with hemophilia or other causes of coagulopathy.
6. **Neurologic exam.** Needed as a baseline and to assess for central nervous system bleeding.

B. Laboratory data

1. **Hemogram.** Follow serial hematocrits in ongoing bleeding.
2. **Platelet count.** An adequate platelet count does not imply adequate function of platelets. Generally, platelet counts of 50,000–100,000 are adequate to maintain hemostasis if function is normal.
3. **Prothrombin time and partial thromboplastin time.** The PTT assess all coagulation proteins except factors VII and XIII. The PT is elevated if there is a deficiency of factor I, II, V, VII, or X. Factor VII has the shortest half-life and a deficiency in factor VII is the usual cause in generalized problems such as liver disease. In lupus erythematous, there can be circulating anticoagulant, which usually prolongs the PTT and, less frequently, prolongs the PT. This generally does not cause a bleeding diathesis but may predispose to thrombosis.
4. **Thrombin time.** Assays functional fibrinogen level and can assay for heparin effect and presence of fibrinogen degradation products.
5. **Fibrinogen and fibrin split products.** In DIC, fibrinogen may be decreased and fibrin split products are increased. The absolute fibrinogen level may be normal but a downward trend is helpful.
6. **Bleeding time.** Evaluates platelet function. Uremia, liver disease, and aspirin therapy within the last week may adversely affect function. Bleeding time is also prolonged by rare disorders of collagen that may impair integrity of the vessel wall. Thrombocytopenia by itself will also increase the bleeding time.
7. **Peripheral blood smears.** May reveal fragments and helmet cells in DIC and TTP. May suggest other causes of thrombocytopenia such as vitamin B_{12} or folate deficiency. Presence of nucleated red blood cells might suggest the presence of marrow infiltrative disorders such as prostate cancer as a cause of DIC.
8. **Blood replacement.** Type and crossmatch if needed.
9. **Future studies.** Save one or two tubes of blood prior to transfusion therapy to assay for any coagulation factors or other studies that may be decided on later.

C. Radiologic and other studies

1. **Chest x-ray.** If there is indication of intrathoracic bleeding.
2. **Bone marrow aspiration and biopsy.** Might be performed to assess platelet production in the presence of unexplained thrombocytopenia or if leukemia or another infiltrative marrow disorder is suggested.

V. Plan. Assess the rate of bleeding and differentiate between mechanical bleeding and a true coagulopathy. Almost all external bleeding that is mechanical can be controlled by applying direct pressure and elevation. Treatment of coagulopathy requires the appropriate laboratory tests to make the diagnosis and then institution of the correct treatment. In any case, in the acute setting assess the amount of blood loss and the volume status and treat with intravenous fluids if hypovolemia is present. For further information regarding transfusion of blood products, refer to Chapter 5—Blood Component Therapy, p 349.

A. Thrombocytopenia

1. Use random donor platelet transfusion, usually 5–10 U at a time, for a platelet count below 20,000 or with a lesser degree of thrombocytopenia if there is ongoing bleeding. Platelet transfusions are generally not indicated in immune thrombocytopenias unless there is active bleeding. Patients receiving multiple platelet transfusions may develop HLA antibodies and have better increments with HLA-matched single donor platelets. Immunocompromised patients should receive irradiated platelets to avoid a graft-versus-host reaction (bone marrow transplant patients, possibly patients with acute leukemia or aggressive lymphoma undergoing aggressive therapy).
2. For a drug reaction, discontinue the drug and transfuse platelets if necessary.
3. In the presence of ITP, no treatment is usually needed until the platelet count is below 10,000 unless there is bleeding. Chronic ITP is treated with prednisone, cyclophosphamide (Cytoxan), azathioprine (Imuran), or danazol (Danocrine). The best long-term results are obtained with splenectomy. Platelet transfusions prior to splenectomy in these patients are very short-lived.
4. Document functional defect with bleeding time and treat underlying condition such as uremia. Discontinue drugs adversely affecting function.

B. von Willebrand's disease (VWD)

1. Cryoprecipitate or fresh-frozen plasma are plasma products of choice. (See Chapter 5, Blood Component Therapy, p 352.)
2. Deamino-8-D-arginine vasopressin (DDAVP), a vasopressin analog, increases von Willebrand factor levels by releasing stores from endothelium. Can be effective for certain types of VWD for mild bleeding, but is contraindicated in type II_B since it may exacerbate thrombocytopenia.

C. Hemophilia A. Specific recommendations for factor replacement depend on site of bleeding and severity of factor deficiency and are beyond the scope of this book. The reader is referred to a standard hematology text for this information. The half-life of factor VIII is about 8–12 hours. As many factor VIII concentrates are now available, the treatment of choice should be with a heat-treated preparation, preferably one heat-treated in solution that should minimize risk of transmission of hepatitis and HIV virus.

D. Hemophilia B. As with hemophilia A, the reader is referred to a standard hematology text for specific recommendations for factor replacement. Factor IX concentrate has a half-life of approximately 24 hours. Several factor IX preparations are available. There is concern about some preparations containing activated coagulation factors which may induce thrombosis or DIC. New preparations probably avoid this risk. Newly diagnosed patients should receive only heat-treated products to avoid transmission of hepatitis or HIV virus.

E. Disseminated intravascular coagulation. Treat the underlying cause. Support the bleeding patient with fresh-frozen plasma, platelet transfusions, and blood transfusions.

F. Vitamin K deficiency/liver disease. If immediate treatment is needed, transfuse with 2–4 units of fresh-frozen plasma and follow the PT/PTT. As factor VII, which has a half-life of 6 hours, is metabolized quickly, repeat infusions may be needed 6–12 hours later. In all cases, begin treatment with vitamin K 10 mg SC every day for 3 consecutive days. Vitamin K may be given intravenously, but because of rare anaphylactic reactions, it must be given slowly over several minutes. If the coagulopathy is secondary to vitamin K deficiency, a response to vitamin K should be evident after 24 hours. If there is no response to vitamin K, the coagulopathy is not due to vitamin K deficiency.

REFERENCE

Colman RW, et al. *Hemostasis and Thrombosis.* 2nd ed. Philadelphia: Lippincott; 1987.

■ COMA, ACUTE MENTAL STATUS CHANGES

I. Problem. You are called to evaluate a 63-year-old woman in the emergency room because of disorientation and lethargy.

II. Immediate Questions

A. What are the vital signs? Shock of any etiology can cause poor cerebral perfusion and altered mental status. A changing respiratory pattern may indicate increased intracranial pressure, with an initial slowing followed by a rapid respiratory rate. Fever could result from an infectious process which frequently in the elderly can cause an acute confusional state.

B. What is the time course of the mental status changes? If the disorientation is long-standing, then the patient may have Alzheimer's disease or some other cause of dementia.

C. What medications is the patient taking? Medications, especially in the elderly, can cause mental status changes. The following are but a few of the medications that can cause mental status changes: narcotics (morphine, codeine, meperidine), phencyclidine (PCP), cocaine, barbiturates, amphetamines, atropine, scopolamine, and commonly prescribed medications such as H2 blockers (cimetidine, ranitidine), digitalis, sedatives (benzodiazepines), tricyclic antidepressants, and steroids. If the patient is hospitalized, look at the medication records to see how much pain medication and sedatives the patient has actually received, not just how much was ordered.

D. **Was there a traumatic event?** Especially in a patient receiving anticoagulant therapy, recent head trauma may result in a subdural or epidural hematoma, often resulting in increasing lethargy and coma.

E. **Is there evidence of central nervous system pathology such as headache, hemiparesis, ataxia, or vomiting?** A cause of increased intracranial pressure such as tumor, subdural hematoma, or cerebral hemorrhage may cause delirium, lethargy, or coma as well as the previously mentioned symptoms.

F. **Does the patient drink?** Intoxication with ethanol or other substances as well as alcohol withdrawal or delirium tremens (see p 79) can cause disorientation.

G. **Is the patient a diabetic?** Either hypoglycemia (see p 156) or hyperglycemia (see p 136) may cause altered mental status.

H. **Does the patient have any known systemic illnesses?** Severe liver disease, renal failure, hypothyroidism, and respiratory failure can cause mental status changes and lethargy.

I. **Is there a history of psychiatric illness?** Patients with depression may present with confusion and disorientation.

J. **In the perioperative patient, did the patient receive any anticholinergic medications or was there any prolonged hypotension during surgery?** Delirium postoperatively is common and there are many potential causes including hypotension, anoxia, myocardial ischemia/infarction, and medications including anticholinergics, sedatives, and narcotics.

K. **Does the patient have a prior history of pulmonary problems?** Hypoxemia can cause acute confusion but patients are initially agitated rather than lethargic.

III. Differential Diagnosis

A. Trauma

1. **Subdural hematoma.** The most common intracranial mass lesion resulting from head injury.
2. **Epidural hematoma.** Usually associated with a skull fracture and a lacerated meningeal vessel.
3. **Concussion.** A clinical diagnosis of cerebral dysfunction that clears within 24 hours.
4. **Contusion.** Usually associated with neurological deficits that persist longer than 24 hours after injury. Small hemorrhages are present in the cerebral parenchyma on CT scan.

B. Metabolic causes

1. Exogenous. Intoxication with ethanol or alcohol withdrawal (either minor withdrawal or delirium tremens, see p 79), drugs (see Section II.C) including drug withdrawal, anesthetic agents with delayed clearance postoperatively, carbon monoxide poisoning, and poisoning from plants such as *Psilocybe* or *Paneolus* mushrooms that often cause hallucinations and inability to concentrate.

2. Endogenous

a. Endocrine

(1) Pancreas. Hypoglycemia (most often secondary to treatment of diabetes) or marked hyperglycemia resulting in a hyperosmolar state.

(2) Pituitary. Hypopituitarism leading to adrenal insufficiency and hypothyroidism.

(3) Thyroid. Hyperthyroidism and hypothyroidism. Both may have associated mental status changes. Hyperthyroidism is associated with agitation and nervousness, whereas hypothyroidism is associated with lethargy. Must have a high index of suspicion in elderly because mental status changes may be the only sign.

(4) Parathyroid. Either hyperparathyroidism resulting in hypercalcemia or hypoparathyroidism resulting in hypocalcemia can cause mental status changes.

b. Fluids/electrolytes

(1) Sodium. Hyponatremia (see p 167) and hypernatremia (see p 145) may cause confusion. With hyponatremia, the severity of the mental status changes is related to the level and the rate of decrease of sodium.

(2) Potassium. Hypokalemia (see p 159) or hyperkalemia (see p 142). Potassium abnormalities infrequently cause mental status changes. Hypokalemia may precipitate hepatic encephalopathy in cirrhotics.

(3) Calcium. Hypocalcemia (see p 153) or hypercalcemia (see p 132.)

(4) Magnesium. Hypomagnesemia (see p 163). Often there is associated hypokalemia and hypocalcemia. In addition to being delirious, the patient may be anxious or psychotic.

(5) Acidosis or alkalosis. Mental status changes often result from the underlying cause of acidosis/alkalosis. Acute, and to a lesser extent, chronic hypercapnia can cause confusion, hallucinations, and coma.

(6) Hypoxia

(7) Osmolarity disturbances. Hyperosmolar coma. Common causes are hypernatremia and marked hyperglycemia as well as foreign substances such as mannitol.

(8) **Thiamine deficiency (Wernicke's encephalopathy).** Often seen in alcoholics but also observed in other conditions such as hyperemesis gravidarum. Mental status changes range from mild confusion to coma. Patients presenting in coma with Wernicke's encephalopathy are often not diagnosed until autopsy. Ataxia and ophthalmoplegia (usually bilateral nystagmus) are also frequently present.

C. **Organ failure**

(1) **Renal failure.** Usually with markedly elevated blood urea nitrogen.

(2) **Hepatic encephalopathy.** Seen in fulminant hepatitis and cirrhosis. Often precipitated by worsening hepatic function, gastrointestinal bleeding, dehydration, azotemia, hypokalemic alkalosis, constipation, and medications such as sedatives.

(3) **Respiratory failure.** Hypoxia and/or hypercapnia.

C. **Infection**

1. **Central nervous system infections (meningitis, encephalitis)**
2. **Sepsis**

D. **Tumors**

1. **Primary or metastatic to CNS**
2. **Hypercalcemia from metastatic disease**
3. **Paraneoplastic syndromes.** Hypercalcemia from parathyroid-like substance (squamous cell carcinoma) or hyponatremia from syndrome of inappropriate antidiuretic hormone (SIADH) release.

E. **Psychiatric causes**

1. **Psychogenic coma.** The neurologic and laboratory profile is completely normal.
2. **Depression.** May cause dementia, especially in the elderly. Also called pseudodementia.
3. **Intensive care unit psychosis**

F. **Miscellaneous**

1. **Seizures.** Including postictal confusion.
2. **Cerebrovascular disease**
   a. **Infarction or hemorrhage.** Will often have focal neurologic findings.
   b. **Arteriovenous malformation**
   c. **Hypertensive encephalopathy.** Blood pressure is markedly elevated and fundoscopic exam is notable for exudates, hemorrhages, and often papilledema.
3. **Syncope** (See Syncope, p 236.)

4. **Decreased cardiac output (shock)** (See Hypotension, p 174.)
5. **Other CNS diseases**
   a. **Alzheimer's dementia**
   b. **Normal pressure hydrocephalus.** Triad of ataxia, incontinence, and dementia.
   c. **Korsakoff's psychosis (thiamine deficiency).** Result of untreated, unrecognized Wernicke's encephalopathy. Anterograde amnesia and confabulation. Irreversible.
6. **Hypothermia** (See p 180.) Most commonly from exposure.
7. **Hyperthermia** (See Fever, p 98.) Most commonly from heat stroke.

IV. Database

A. Physical examination key points

1. **Vital signs.** Hypotension can cause decreased cerebral perfusion. Bradyarrhythmias or tachyarrhythmias may cause hypotension. Tachycardia may be associated with other causes of mental status changes such as sepsis, pulmonary embolus, and myocardial infarction. Severe hypertension may indicate hypertensive encephalopathy. Bradycardia in association with hypertension may indicate central nervous system pathology (Cushing's reflex). Bradypnea may indicate ethanol intoxication or barbiturate overdose. Tachypnea may indicate significant hypoxia or sepsis. A fever suggests infection or possibly loss of thermoregulation associated with thyroid storm; a markedly elevated temperature from heat stroke or malignant hyperthermia can cause mental status changes. The elderly may not have a fever in response to an infection/sepsis. Hypothermia may suggest hypothyroidism (myxedema coma), sepsis, or exposure.
2. **HEENT**
   a. **Head.** Look for evidence of trauma that may point to a subdural or epidural bleed or a cerebral contusion.
   b. **Eyes.** Pinpoint pupils may indicate narcotic use. Unilateral, fixed, and dilated pupils suggest herniation. Bilateral, fixed, and dilated pupils suggest anoxia and brain death. Pupils may be dilated or sluggish to direct and indirect light in hypothermia or hyperthermia. Nystagmus is seen with Wernicke's encephalopathy. Conjunctival or fundal petechiae suggest fat embolism or endocarditis. Papilledema suggests a mass, an intracranial bleed, or hypertensive encephalopathy.
   c. **Ears.** Blood behind the tympanic membranes suggests head trauma with a basilar skull fracture. An otitis media could be a source for meningitis.
   d. **Nasopharynx.** A fruity odor suggests diabetic ketoacidosis.

e. **Neck.** Nuchal rigidity is evidence for meningitis or subarachnoid bleed. Bruits suggest a stroke; however, many patients have incidental bruits. Thyroid enlargement points to hypothyroidism or hyperthyroidism. A bruit over an enlarged thyroid gland is pathognomonic of Grave's disease.

3. **Chest.** Thorough exam to rule out significant pulmonary disease resulting in hypoxia or hypercapnia.
4. **Heart.** An irregularly irregular apical pulse (atrial fibrillation) points to embolization from a mural thrombus. A new murmur with fever and/or leukocytosis suggests endocarditis. Also, a right-to-left shunt may cause hypoxia.
5. **Abdomen.** Splenomegaly, ascites, and other evidence of chronic liver disease suggest hepatic encephalopathy.
6. **Skin.** Jaundice, spider angiomata, and palmar erythema point to hepatic encephalopathy.
7. **Neurologic exam**
   a. A thorough neurologic exam including mental status examination is essential in any patient with coma or mental status changes, acute or chronic. Focal findings suggest an intracranial process. Hyperreflexia may be seen with upper motor neuron lesions or hyperthyroidism. Clonus is absent with hyperthyroidism and present in upper motor neuron lesions. Absent or sluggish reflexes are seen in hypothyroidism and hypothermia.
   b. In evaluating the comatose patient, the Glasgow Coma Scale is helpful. It assesses spontaneous movement and response to pain. See the Appendix, Table A–3, p 502. Testing the oculocephalic reflex is also helpful. Hold the eyes open and turn the patient's head quickly to one side. The eyes should move toward the midline as if staring at a fixed point (intact doll's eyes). Movement of the eyes in the direction the head is turned (absent doll's eyes) suggests a brainstem lesion.

B. **Laboratory data**

1. **Complete blood count with differential, platelet count.** To evaluate for infection and anemia.
2. **Complete blood chemistry.** Includes electrolytes, glucose, blood urea nitrogen, creatinine, total bilirubin, alkaline phosphatase, and transaminases (ALT and AST [SGOT and SGPT]), calcium, magnesium, and osmolality. Will rule out many of the organ-failure or metabolic causes. A serum glucose can be rapidly checked with a "fingerstick" glucometer available on most nursing units.
3. **Arterial blood gases.** Along with serum bicarbonate, will uncover a metabolic or respiratory acid-base disturbance, which may point to the underlying cause. Also necessary to rule out hypoxemia.

4. **Serum ammonia.** Elevation indicative of hepatic failure; however, not all patients with hepatic encephalopathy have an elevated ammonia.
5. **Thyroid-stimulating hormone (TSH) and thyroxine (T4) levels.** To rule out suspected hypothyroidism or hyperthyroidism. Must have high index of suspicion.
6. **Urine and serum toxicology screening.** If there is an unexplained metabolic gap acidosis, salicylate, ethanol, methanol, and ethylene glycol ingestion/overdose must be ruled out.
7. **Blood and urine cultures.** If sepsis is suspected.

C. Radiologic and other studies

1. **Chest x-ray.** Especially if an infectious or pulmonary source is possible.
2. **CT scan of the head.** If there are any indications of a CNS etiology, especially in the presence of headache, vomiting, focal signs, or papilledema.
3. **Lumbar puncture** (See Chapter 3, p 330.) Should be performed in any patient with unexplained fever and mental status changes.
4. **Electrocardiogram.** Look for myocardial infarction or atrial fibrillation. Myocardial infarction, especially in the elderly, may present with acute mental status changes.
5. **Electroencephalogram.** Diffuse theta and delta changes may be present with most metabolic causes. Often not diagnostic except for herpes encephalitis.

V. Plan. Although the therapy of changing neurological status must be directed at the underlying cause, certain steps should be taken immediately: ensure adequate airway, breathing, and circulation (the ABCs of basic life support). Intubation may be necessary to protect the airway.

A. Metabolic causes. Treat the underlying defect. Refer to specific abnormality in the index. Anyone in coma should receive 1 ampoule of 50% dextrose if the etiology is unknown. The effect on a patient in diabetic ketoacidosis is minimal, so it is always safe to give the dextrose. Any patient in coma should also receive thiamine 100 mg slow IV push.

B. Exogenous causes. Any suspicion of narcotic-induced somnolence can be safely treated with naxolone 0.4–0.8 mg IV push. A repeat dose may be necessary (up to 4–5 ampoules are commonly given in this situation).

C. Tumor. Somnolence in the presence of metastatic or primary CNS tumors is an emergency usually treated by radiotherapy; however, the intracranial pressure must be acutely decreased. This can be done with steroids, hyperventilation, and osmotic diuresis. Give dexamethasone intravenous bolus 0.1–0.2 mg/kg. The patient should be intubated to protect the airway and can be hyperventilated by increasing the rate of the respirator and following the pCO_2. You should attempt to decrease the pCO_2 to 20–25 mm Hg. Osmotic diuresis with mannitol 1–1.5 g/kg over 20 minutes is also beneficial if there is associated cerebral edema.

D. **Infection.** Treat with appropriate antibiotics. A gram stain may help direct initial antibiotic therapy prior to culture results.

E. **Cardiac syncope or low cardiac output.** Treat the underlying cardiac problem.

F. **Vascular problems.** Intracranial bleeding is usually treated like other causes of increased intracranial pressure. Contact the neurosurgical consultant immediately. Increased intracranial pressure should be emergently treated to circumvent herniation. Intubation with hyperventilation, osmotic diuresis with mannitol 1–1.5 g/kg over 20 minutes, and dexamethasone 0.1–0.2 mg/kg may acutely decrease intracranial pressure.

REFERENCES

Adams RD, Victor M. Coma and related disorders of consciousness. In: *Principles of Neurology.* 4th ed. New York: McGraw-Hill Information Services Co; 1989:273–290.

Adams RD, Victor M. Delirium and other acute confusional states. In: *Principles of Neurology.* 4th ed. New York: McGraw-Hill Information Services Co; 1989:323–333.

Plum F, Posner J. *The Diagnosis of Stupor and Coma.* Philadelphia: FA Davis; 1980.

■ CONSTIPATION

I. **Problem.** A 75-year-old bedridden woman from a nursing home admitted with dehydration and a urinary tract infection has not had a bowel movement in 7 days.

II. **Immediate Questions**

A. **What is the patient's normal bowel habits?** Normal bowel habits vary from three stools per day to three stools per week. Some individuals develop a dependence on bowel stimulants and other laxatives.

B. **What medications is the patient taking?** Constipation is a side effect of many medicines including narcotics, antidepressants, nonabsorbable antacids, diuretics, and calcium channel blockers (especially verapamil [Calan, Isoptin]).

C. **Is the abdomen distended, tender, or tense? Is the patient passing flatus? Is the patient vomiting?** Mechanical obstruction from sigmoid volvulus, intussusception, and hernia can lead to constipation. Mechanical obstruction often has other symptoms. Flatus signifies an intact, working gastrointestinal tract.

D. **Does the patient have a history of hemorrhoids or rectal bleeding?** Rectal lesions including hemorrhoids, proctitis, and fissures may induce constipation.

E. **Has the patient undergone any procedures recently?** Barium from x-ray studies can cause constipation. Many postoperative patients will have an ileus resulting in constipation.

III. Differential Diagnosis

A. Systemic disorders

1. **Drugs.** Constipation is a side effect of multiple medications including narcotics, aluminum and calcium antacids, anticholinergics, diuretics, calcium channel blockers (especially verapamil), antidepressants, and iron supplements.
2. **Endocrine disorders.** Includes hypothyroidism, diabetes, and hyperparathyroidism.
3. **Metabolic disorders.** Hypercalcemia and hypokalemia.
4. **Volume status.** Patients with dehydration, especially the elderly, can become constipated.

B. Gastrointestinal disorders

1. **Tumors.** Benign or malignant tumors lead to constipation through obstruction by mass effect.
2. **Inflammatory lesions.** With induction of pain, the patient suppresses the urge to defecate, resulting in constipation. Common inflammatory disorders include diverticulitis, proctitis, hemorrhoids, fissure-in-ano, and inflammatory bowel diseases such as ulcerative colitis and Crohn's disease.
3. **Mechanical obstruction.** Constipation can be secondary to physical blockage from adhesions, incarcerated hernias, volvulus, or intussusception.

C. Neurologic conditions

1. **Spinal or pelvic trauma.** Can result in colonic dysmotility or anal sphincter dysfunction.
2. **Autonomic neuropathy.** Results in colonic dysmotility and can even cause pseudo-obstruction.
3. **Cerebral vascular accident.** Can lead to constipation via an associated decrease in activity level.

IV. Database

A. Physical examination key points

1. **Vital signs.** Fever suggests an inflammatory source such as diverticulitis or inflammatory bowel disease (IBD). Orthostasis leads one to consider dehydration.
2. **Abdomen.** Distension may result from obstruction. Evidence of prior surgery suggests adhesions. Listen for bowel sounds and quality to assess for ileus or obstruction. Absence of bowel sounds is consistent with any cause of complete obstruction. On palpation, look for tenderness or rebound. Rebound suggests peritoneal inflammation. Feel for stool-filled colon.
3. **Rectum.** Rule out external lesions (hemorrhoids or fissures) as the cause. Be sure the anal canal is not stenotic. Check the quality of sphincter tone. Absence of sphincter tone suggests a

spinal cord lesion. Rule out any rectal lesions. Presence of blood suggests an inflammatory cause or a benign or malignant tumor.

4. **Neurologic exam.** Look for evidence of prior cerebrovascular accident or spinal injury such as decreased motor function or asymmetric reflexes. A delay in the relaxation phase of the reflexes points to hypothyroidism.

B. Laboratory data

1. **Electrolytes and calcium.** Hypokalemia is a rare cause of constipation. Check calcium to rule out hypercalcemia.
2. **Complete blood count.** Elevated white blood cell count may indicate an inflammatory disorder. A low hemoglobin accompanies blood loss and can be from a variety of causes such as benign or malignant tumors, diverticulitis, or IBD.
3. **Sedimentation rate.** With active IBD, the sedimentation rate is elevated, but it can be elevated with any inflammatory process.
4. **Stool for occult blood.** Inflammatory disorders and tumors result in blood loss.
5. **Thyroid function studies.** If history and physical examination are consistent with hypothyroidism, TSH and T4 levels should be obtained.

C. Radiologic and other studies

1. **Acute abdominal series.** If acute obstruction is considered likely.
2. **Proctosigmoidoscopy.** To further assess if obstructing or inflammatory lesions are present.
3. **Barium enema.** For demonstrating partial obstruction or mass lesion. Colonoscopy is the procedure of choice if colon carcinoma or colonic polyps are suspected.
4. **CT scan of abdomen.** To further evaluate for partial obstruction.

V. Plan. Once the etiology is demonstrated, the underlying cause should be corrected. Medicines inducing constipation should be discontinued whenever possible. Electrolyte abnormalities should be corrected or obstruction relieved.

A. Prevention. Patients on narcotics should be started on stool softeners and bowel stimulants. Bedridden patients should also be on stool softeners. Use high-fiber diets; encourage activity and adequate fluid intake.

B. Laxatives and enemas. There are several modalities from which to choose depending on preference and etiology (Table 1–5). Use bulk laxatives (psyllium) and high-fiber diets for control and prevention of constipation. Surfactants or wetting agents, osmotic laxatives, and colonic stimulants for rapid action can also be used to relieve constipation. Suppositories or enemas such as gentle

TABLE 1–5. Laxatives

Type	Name	Dosage
Bulk—daily use	Effersyllium	1 teaspoon (6–7 g) in fluid 1 or 2 times daily
	Metamucil	1 teaspoon (6–7 g) in fluid 1 or 2 times daily
Softeners/wetting agents—daily use	Docusate sodium (Colace)	50–200 mg 1 or 2 times daily Available: Capsules 50–100 mg Solution 10 mg/mL Syrup 25 mg/mL
	Docusate calcium (Surfac)	240 mg 1 or 2 times daily
	Lactulose (Cronulac)	15–30 mL 1 or 2 times daily
	Mineral oil	15–45 mL; one-time dose
Stimulants—prn	Biscadyl (Dulcolax)	Oral 5–15 mg, 5-mg tablets Rectal 10 mg, 10-mg suppository
	Senna (Senakot)	1 tablet 1 or 2 times daily
	Glycerine suppository	3 g; 1 rectally
Osmotic—prn	Milk of Magnesia	15–30 mL 1 or 2 times daily
	Magnesium citrate	200 mL; one-time dose
Enema—prn	Fleet enema	120 mL rectally
	Oil retention enema	

tap water enema, oil retention enema, and glycerin suppositories are useful for rapid action.

C. Disimpaction. Digital disimpaction is occasionally required when hard stool will not pass through the rectum. This is more common in the elderly. After disimpaction, the patient should receive laxatives or preferably enemas to relieve the constipation. Use stool softeners or bulk laxatives to prevent recurrence.

D. Other. If obstructing or inflammatory lesions are demonstrated, they should be treated with surgery, anti-inflammatory medicines, or antibiotics.

REFERENCES

Portenoy RK. Constipation in the cancer patient: Causes and management. In: Payne R, Foley KM, eds. *Medical Clinics of North America*. Vol. 71, No. 2: *Cancer Pain*. Philadelphia: WB Saunders; 1987:303–311.

Read NW, Timms JM. Defecation and the pathophysiology of constipation. In: Mendeloff AI, ed. *Clinics in Gastroenterology*. Vol. 15, No. 4: *Pathophysiology of Nonneoplastic Colonic Disorders*. London: WB Saunders; 1986:937–965.

Rousseau P. Treatment of constipation in the elderly. *Postgraduate Medicine* 1988;83(4):339–349.

■ COUGH

I. Problem. A nurse notifies you that one of your patients is unable to sleep because of a persistent cough.

II. Immediate Questions

A. Is the cough acute or chronic? Acute onset of cough most often results from infections such as the common cold, but can result from urgent conditions such as acute bronchospasm (see Wheezing, p 257), pulmonary embolus, aspiration (see Aspiration, p 32) or decompensated congestive heart failure. A chronic cough is unlikely to represent a condition that could pose immediate danger to the patient.

B. Is the cough productive of sputum? If so, what does the sputum look like? A productive cough implies an inflammatory condition such as infection. Blood in the sputum leads to consideration of several other causes. (See Hemoptysis, p 128.)

C. Is the patient tachypneic or dyspneic? Either of these could suggest a significant underlying respiratory disease such as pulmonary embolus or pneumonia.

III. Differential Diagnosis. Cough reflex receptors are present in the ear, pharynx, sinuses, nose, larynx, trachea, bronchi, and pleural surfaces. Thus, disorders stimulating receptors in these locations can result in cough.

A. Ear. Impacted cerumen, foreign body, or hair in the ear can produce cough.

B. Oropharynx/nasopharynx. Postnasal drip from allergic and nonallergic rhinitis or sinusitis is a common cause of cough.

C. Larynx. Acute viral laryngitis can produce cough.

D. Tracheobronchial tree. Any process irritating the mucosal receptors or preventing clearance of secretions can result in cough.

1. **Bronchospasm.** Asthma is a frequent cause of nonproductive cough, especially nocturnal cough. Wheezing may be absent.
2. **Bronchitis.** Both acute and chronic bronchitis can cause irritation of mucosal receptors and result in cough.
3. **Pneumonia.** Viral, bacterial, tuberculous, and fungal causes should all be considered, especially in any immunocompromised patient. These patients include those who have acquired immunodeficiency syndrome, those who are receiving immunosuppressive treatment, or those who have an underlying lymphoproliferative or hematologic malignancy.
4. **Gastroesophageal reflux.** Aspiration of oropharangeal and gastric contents can produce cough. Symptoms are typically worse at night or while eating.
5. **Inhaled irritants.** The most common cause of a chronic cough is inhaled tobacco smoke.
6. **Bronchogenic carcinoma.** Produces mechanical irritation of

mucosal receptors. The majority of patients with bronchogenic carcinoma develop chronic cough as a symptom at some point.

E. **Others.** There is a long list of other causes of cough. A few of these are listed here.
   1. **Congestive heart failure.** A nocturnal cough may be the only manifestation of early congestive heart failure.
   2. **Interstitial lung disease.** This includes interstitial fibrosis and granulomatous disease such as tuberculosis and sarcoidosis.
   3. **Thoracic aneurysm.** This can cause cough by producing bronchial or tracheal compression.

IV. Database

A. Physical exam key points

1. **Vital signs.** Fever occurs with infection and pulmonary infarction. Tachypnea and accessory respiratory muscle use suggest significant underlying pulmonary disease.
2. **HEENT**
   a. Examine the ears for impacted cerumen, foreign body, or hair in the external auditory canal.
   b. Examine the posterior pharynx for evidence of sinusitis or rhinitis, such as a postnasal drip or cobblestoning resulting from lymphoid hyperplasia.
   c. Check for evidence of sinus tenderness or opacification.
3. **Lungs**
   a. **Stridor.** This is a manifestation of upper airway obstruction resulting from largngeal edema or epiglottitis.
   b. **Rhonchi.** Occurs with bronchitis and inhalation injuries.
   c. **Signs of consolidation.** Peripheral bronchial breath sounds, egophony, and increased tactile fremitus occur with pneumonia.
   d. **Crackles.** Occurs in congestive heart failure, pneumonia, and interstitial lung disease.
   e. **Wheezing.** Occurs in asthma. If localized, may signify a foreign body or obstructing neoplasm.
4. **Heart.** Jugular venous distension, displaced point of maximal impulse, and third heart sound (S_3) gallop indicate congestive heart failure.
5. **Lymph nodes.** Lymphadenopathy suggests metastatic carcinoma, a lymphoproliferative disorder, or a granulomatous disease such as sarcoidosis.
6. **Extremities.** Clubbing occurs in patients with bronchiectasis, bronchogenic carcinoma, or severe chronic obstructive airway disease.

B. Laboratory data

1. **Hemogram.** Leukocytosis and left shift occur with infectious diseases. Thrombocytosis may result from underlying malignancy.

2. **Arterial blood gases.** This should be obtained only if the patient appears dyspneic or cyanotic.

C. Radiologic and other studies

1. **Chest x-ray.** Evidence of congestive heart failure, neoplasm, pneumonia, interstitial lung disease, hilar adenopathy and thoracic aortic aneurysm may appear on CXR.
2. **Ventilation/perfusion ($\dot{V}/\dot{Q}$) scan.** Should be obtained if there is a high suspicion for pulmonary embolism.
3. **Sputum.** Examine for color, viscosity, odor, and amount. Perform a gram stain, acid fast stain, and fungal stain. If asthma is suspected, perform a Wright stain looking for eosinophils. If neoplasm is a possibility, request sputum cytology.
4. **Purified protein derivative (PPD) skin test.** Should be performed if tuberculosis is a possibility.
5. **Pulmonary function tests.** A restrictive pattern occurs in interstitial lung disease. A restrictive pattern is a decrease in all lung volumes: forced expiratory volume at 1 second (FEV_1), functional vital capacity (FVC), total lung capacity (TLC), and other lung volumes. The FEV_1/FVC ratio is maintained near normal (~70%). A reversible obstructive defect (a decrease in the FEV_1 and FEV_1/FVC ratio) would suggest underlying emphysema or asthma. Bronchial provocation with methacholine may be necessary to diagnose occult asthma if baseline pulmonary function tests are normal.
6. **Bronchoscopy.** This is of value only if there is an abnormality noted on CXR.

V. Plan. The treatment of cough is dependent on identifying the etiology and then directing treatment toward that cause.

A. Infectious conditions (See Chapter 7 for drug dosages.)

1. **Community-acquired pneumonia.** Penicillin is recommended for pneumococcal infections; however, erythromycin should be used in those situations in which mycoplasma or Legionnaires' pneumonia is a diagnostic possibility.
2. **Acute bronchitis.** Most often, acute bronchitis is of a viral etiology; however, in those instances in which mycoplasma or bacteria is suspected, erythromycin or ampicillin can be given.
3. **Chronic bronchitis.** Most often occurs in smokers. Cough resolves with cessation of smoking.

B. Rhinitis/sinusitis. In these instances, cough is best managed by treatment with an antihistamine and decongestant. Antibiotics are indicated if bacterial sinusitis is suspected.

C. Asthma. Inhaled bronchodilators such as metaproterenol (Alupent) and albuterol (Ventolin) represent the best treatment for those whose cough is due to asthma. Oral bronchodilators may be necessary for patients in whom inhalational therapy provokes cough.

D. Gastroesophageal reflux. These patients should have the head of their beds elevated and should not eat before retiring for bed. Antacids and histamine H2 antagonists such as cimetidine (Tagamet) and ranitidine (Zantac) may also be required.

E. General measures. In patients with a nonproductive cough in whom infection is not a concern, cough suppression can provide much needed symptomatic relief.

1. **Cough suppression**
   - **a.** Codeine phosphate in a dosage of 30 mg is the most effective cough suppressant.
   - **b.** Dextromethorphan, a codeine derivative, acts centrally and is the best nonnarcotic for cough suppression.
2. **Expectorants.** Have been shown to be of no value and should not be used.

REFERENCES

Irwin RS, et al. Persistent cough in the adult: Spectrum and frequency of causes and successful outcome of specific therapy. *Am Rev Resp Dis* 1981;123:413.

Poe, RH, et al. Chronic persistent cough: Experience in diagnosis and outcome using an anatomic diagnostic protocol. *Chest* 1989;95:723–728.

■ DELIRIUM TREMENS (DTs): MAJOR ALCOHOL WITHDRAWAL

I. Problem. A 55-year-old intoxicated man is admitted with abdominal pain and an elevated amylase. Narcotic analgesia is initiated. On the third hospital day, he is found talking to the walls and shaking violently.

II. Immediate Questions

A. What are the patient's vital signs? Hypertension, tachycardia, and fever may represent signs of autonomic overactivity, common in DTs. A fever may also point to an infectious etiology as the cause of the delirium.

B. What is the patient's mental status? Altered levels of consciousness and impaired cognitive function define delirium. Hallucinations and confusion are important observations. These coupled with autonomic hyperactivity are typical of DTs. Delirium tremens can also present as unresponsiveness. Visual hallucinations, "pink elephants," are more commonly associated with toxic psychosis (eg, ethanol), and auditory hallucinations are more commonly associated with psychiatric illness.

C. What is the patient's airway status? Any patient with an altered level of consciousness is at increased risk of aspiration.

D. What medications is the patient taking? This is extremely important because medications may cause disorientation. Medications that can cause disorientation include narcotics (morphine, codeine, meperidine), phencyclidine (PCP), cocaine, barbiturates, amphetamines, atropine, scopolamine, and commonly prescribed medications such as H2 blockers (cimetidine, ranitidine) or aspirin and especially in the elderly, digitalis, sedatives (benzodiazepines), tricyclic antidepressants, and steroids. Individuals who abuse one substance are more likely to abuse other substances. A thorough drug history including illicit drugs is essential. Ask specifically regarding the use of narcotics, sedatives, barbiturates, and atropine.

E. **Is there a history of alcohol abuse?** This is central to an accurate diagnosis.

F. **Is there a history of DTs in the past?** Many times there is a past history of DTs. The absence of such a history does not exclude DTs as the cause of the delirium.

III. **Differential Diagnosis.** DTs is a manifestation of diffuse cerebral dysfunction. Focal neurologic deficits point to a structural abnormality (stroke, brain tumor, and so on). The differential diagnosis of delirium is more extensive than that given here and includes any source of diffuse cerebral dysfunction. (See Coma, Acute Mental Status Changes, p 65.) The patient presenting with DTs may have a wide range of other concomitant problems. The patient described in this case may be delirious because of any of the following diagnoses.

A. **Withdrawal syndromes**

1. **Minor alcohol withdrawal.** A less severe form of alcohol withdrawal. Occurs between 8 and 48 hours after the last drink. Disorientation is usually mild. Tachycardia, diaphoresis, and tremor are often present. Seizures and hallucinations may occur.
2. **Barbiturate withdrawal.** Indistinguishable from DTs clinically.
3. **Opioid withdrawal.** Occurs up to 48 hours after cessation of agent (most rapid with heroin). Symptoms include restlessness, rhinorrhea, lacrimation, nausea, diarrhea, and hypertension.

B. **Metabolic abnormalities.** There are multiple metabolic abnormalities that can cause altered levels of consciousness and impaired cognitive function similar to DTs.

1. **Fever** (See Fever, p 98.)
2. **Hepatic encephalopathy**
3. **Hypercalcemia** (See Hypercalcemia, p 132.)
4. **Hyperkalemia** (See Hyperkalemia, p 142.)
5. **Hyperosmolar states.** Can result in delirium. Most common causes are hypernatremia and hyperglycemia but can also include hyperproteinemia and foreign substances such as mannitol.
6. **Hypocalcemia** (See Hypocalcemia, p 153.)
7. **Hyponatremia** (See Hyponatremia, p 167.)
8. **Hypothermia** (See Hypothermia, p 180.)
9. **Hypoxia.** Congestive heart failure can produce hypoxia and delirium in an indolent fashion.

10. **Uremia**
11. **Wernicke's encephalopathy.** Results from nutritional deficiency of the vitamin thiamine. Characterized by a triad of changes: (1) mental status (confusion to coma); (2) ataxia; and (3) ophthalmoplegia (most commonly bilateral nystagmus).

C. Endocrine abnormalities

1. **Hypoglycemia** (See Hypoglycemia, p 156.) Either from an insulin-secreting tumor or from intentional or accidental insulin overdose.
2. **Hyperglycemia** (See Hyperglycemia, p 136.) Extreme hyperglycemia, especially in the elderly, can result in delirium.
3. **Hyperthyroidism.** The signs/symptoms of hyperthyroidism may mimic alcohol withdrawal syndrome. There may be mental status changes, diaphoresis, tachycardia, tremor, and agitation. There is often a history of weight loss, hot weather intolerance, and hyperdefecation. The thyroid gland is often enlarged. The T4 will be elevated and the TSH level suppressed. The signs and symptoms of hyperthyroidism are usually more subacute or chronic; however, thyroid storm can develop acutely if there is a precipitating event such as an operation or infection. Thyroid storm is characterized by thermoderegulation (hyperthermia), mental status changes, and an identifiable precipitating event.

D. Hypertensive encephalopathy. Encephalopathy induced by poorly controlled hypertension. Headache is often present. Exudates and hemorrhages are present on fundoscopic examination. Papilledema may be present.

E. Central nervous system infections. In anyone with disorientation, consider infectious causes including meningitis, brain abscess, and encephalitis. With bacterial causes, fever and leukocytosis with a left shift are often present as are other signs (meningism or papilledema). If there are focal findings or papilledema, initially a CT scan should be performed. Meningitis is diagnosed by lumbar puncture.

F. Intensive care unit psychosis. Secondary to unfamiliar setting. Often seen in elderly patients. May be secondary to or aggravated by medications such as lidocaine and digoxin.

G. Sepsis. Sepsis can cause mental status changes. A fever and elevated white blood cell count with an increase in the percentage of early neutrophils (bands) are common. A source for sepsis is often evident, such as pyuria or an infiltrate on chest x-ray.

H. Sundowning. Nighttime agitation and confusion are common problems, especially in the elderly. The agitation and confusion resolve in the morning.

I. Low cardiac output states. Either from ischemia or cardiomyopathy. Can cause confusion secondary to decreased cerebral perfusion and may result in agitation. A history of chest pain or myocardial infarction may be present. Previous symptoms of congestive heart failure (orthopnea, paroxysmal nocturnal dyspnea, dyspnea on exertion) may be present. On physical examination, hypotension or relative hypotension is present as are increased jugular vein distension and rales.

IV. Database

A. Physical examination key points

1. **Vital signs.** Tachycardia, hypertension, and fever are common manifestations of DTs. Severe hypertension and delirium suggest hypertensive encephalopathy. Fever may also be a manifestation of a localized infection or sepsis. Hypothermia could be associated with sepsis or could be the cause of the delirium. Carpal spasm with inflation of the blood pressure cuff between the diastolic and systolic blood pressure for 3 minutes (Trousseau's sign) is seen in hypocalcemia.
2. **Eyes.** Nystagmus suggests Wernicke's encephalopathy. Lid lag or proptosis suggests hyperthyroidism. Papilledema may be seen in meningitis or hypertensive encephalopathy or with a space-occupying lesion.
3. **Neck.** Thyromegaly suggests hyperthyroidism as a cause of the delirium. Jugular venous distension points toward congestive heart failure as the cause.
4. **Chest.** Signs of congestive heart failure and other causes of pulmonary edema and hypoxia should be sought.
5. **Abdomen.** Check for bladder distension, a common cause of agitation in the elderly.
6. **Skin.** Profuse sweating is typical of DTs. Telangiectasia and gynecomastia are associated with chronic ethanol use and chronic liver disease.
7. **Neurologic exam.** Mental status changes define delirium. Hallucinations, confusion, and disorientation are typical. Reflexes will be exaggerated but symmetrical. Hyperreflexia is also seen in hyperthyroidism. Twitching at the corner of the mouth with tapping over the facial nerve (Chvostek's sign) is seen in hypocalcemia. Any focal findings on motor, sensory, deep tendon, or cranial nerve examination point to a structural abnormality, either spinal or intracranial.

B. Laboratory data.

There are multiple electrolyte abnormalities that can cause delirium or that can be associated with heavy ethanol use.

1. **Sodium.** Hyponatremia could be the etiology of the delirium.
2. **Glucose.** To eliminate hypoglycemia or hyperglycemia as a cause of delirium. Both can be associated with heavy ethanol ingestion.
3. **Calcium.** May reveal hypocalcemia or hypercalcemia as causes of the delirium.

4. **Potassium.** Hyperkalemia may result in delirium. Hypokalemia often complicates heavy ethanol ingestion.
5. **Blood urea nitrogen and creatinine.** May point to uremia/renal failure as etiology of the delirium.
6. **Liver function tests.** Transaminases (AST [SGOT] and ALT [SGPT]), total bilirubin, and alkaline phosphatase to rule out hepatic failure as a cause of the delirium. Liver dysfunction is common in patients who chronically use alcohol.
7. **Arterial blood gases.** To eliminate hypoxemia as a cause.
8. **Complete blood count with differential.** An elevated white blood cell count with an increase in banded neutrophils suggests an infectious etiology. An elevated mean corpuscular volume may be from associated folate or vitamin B_{12} deficiency. Anemia from a variety of causes is commonly seen in heavy ethanol use.
9. **Thyroid function tests.** Thyroid-stimulating hormone is suppressed and thyroxine is usually elevated with hyperthyroidism.
10. **Phosphorus.** Hypophosphatemia is associated with heavy ethanol use as a result of either poor nutritional intake, diarrhea, vomiting, or refeeding after prolonged starvation.
11. **Magnesium.** Hypomagnesemia is often seen with heavy ethanol use. Hypomagnesemia may result from poor intake, diarrhea, renal losses, and excessive sweating.

C. Radiologic and other studies

1. **Chest x-ray.** May reveal cardiomegaly, pulmonary edema, or pneumonia.
2. **Electrocardiogram.** To rule out myocardial ischemia as an etiology of delirium. Also tachyarrhythmias are associated with alcohol withdrawal (major or minor).
3. **CT scan of head.** Indicated if there is a focal finding on examination or seizures associated with DTs.
4. **Lumbar puncture.** Indicated in any patient with mental status changes and fever. May be difficult to rule out meningitis in a patient with DTs without a lumbar puncture.
5. **Electroencephalogram.** May help diagnose encephalitis. Usually increased activity and nonfocal with DTs. Rarely is an electroencephalogram needed.

V. Plan

A. Prevention. Patients at risk for DTs (those with a history of ethanol withdrawal, minor or major, or heavy ethanol ingestion) should be treated while hospitalized with around-the-clock benzodiazepines, most commonly oxazepam (Serax) 15–30 mg PO every 4–6 hours or chlordiazepoxide (Librium) 25–50 mg PO every 6–8 hours.

B. Delirium tremens. Sedation and correction of associated metabolic disturbances are the primary goals in treatment. The patient should be calm but still be arousable.

1. Benzodiazepines given intravenously initially: diazepam (Valium) 5–10 mg IV every 4–6 hours, followed by oral treatment with diazepam, lorazepam (Ativan), chloridiazepoxide (Librium), or oxazepam (Serax) in the nonvomiting patient. Oxazepam is preferred with suspected cirrhosis because it is renally excreted.
2. If benzodiazepines do not achieve the level of sedation desired, a short-acting barbiturate such as pentobarbital (Nembutal) 200 mg IM or IV, then 100 mg every hour prn, can be administered.
3. Ethanol itself can be used. Because of its short half-life, it must be given as a drip and the usual dose is 20–60 mg/kg/h. Ethanol levels of 2–10 mg/dL are adequate to prevent DTs. Most authors discourage the use of ethanol to treat DTs because of its direct toxicity on organs, its short half-life, and its usage promoting the "acceptability of alcohol."
4. Restraints to prevent injury may be needed, often in the prone position.
5. Intravenous fluid replacement for volume and correction of electrolyte abnormalities are usually needed.
   a. **Hypokalemia.** Replacement with potassium supplements either orally or intravenously. A total replacement dose of 100 mEq of potassium is required to raise a potassium of 3.0 mEq/L to 4.0 mEq/L. Intravenous replacement is generally 10–20 mEq per hour. Oral replacement is 20–60 mEq per dose and can be repeated in 2–4 hours.
   b. **Hypophosphatemia.** Intravenous replacement is reserved for severe, life-threatening hypophosphatemia (levels less than 1 mg/dL). Intravenous replacement is with 5–10 mmol over 4–6 hours. Oral replacement can be with "Neutra phos" capsules (250 mg per capsule) or skim milk (1 quart contains 1 g of phosphorus or about 30 mmol).
   c. **Hypomagnesemia.** Replacement is generally either intravenously or intramuscularly. The oral route often causes diarrhea. Magnesium sulfate can be given 1 g IM in each hip or 1 g IV per hour for 4 hours. The magnesium level should be checked 1 to 2 hours after the fourth gram finishes infusing. More may need to be given. Magnesium is mostly an intracellular cation. With extremely low levels of magnesium, often 10–15 g will be required.
   d. **Thiamine deficiency.** Thiamine 100 mg IM should be given prior to the administration of any intravenous fluids containing glucose. Large boluses of glucose can precipitate Wernicke's encephalopathy in a patient with marginal thiamine stores.
6. Antipyretics (Tylenol, aspirin) and a cooling blanket may be required because of the fever often seen in patients with DTs.

REFERENCES

Kraus ML, Gottlieb LD, Horwitz RI, et al. Randomized clinical trial of atenolol in patient with alcohol withdrawal. *N Engl J Med* 1985;313:905–909.

Lerner WD, Fallon HJ (eds). The alcohol withdrawal syndrome. *N Engl J Med* 1985;313:951–952.

Turner RC, Lichstein PR, Peden JG, et al. Alcohol withdrawal symptoms: A review of pathophysiology, clinical presentations, and treatment. *J Gen Intern Med* 1989;4:432–444.

West LJ, Maxwell DS, Noble EP, et al. Alcoholism. *Ann Intern Med* 1984;100:405–416.

■ DIARRHEA

I. **Problem.** A 50-year-old woman is admitted with a history of diarrhea for 36 hours.

II. **Immediate Questions**

A. **What are the patient's vital signs?** Hypotension suggests volume depletion or possible septic shock. Fever implies an infectious etiology. Diarrhea with associated hypotension and/or fever should be evaluated immediately.

B. **Is the diarrhea grossly bloody?** This usually is seen with ischemic bowel or infarction, invasive infections, neoplasms, or inflammatory bowel disease. Bloody diarrhea requires more active and immediate intervention.

C. **Is this an acute or chronic problem? Acute diarrhea** is usually a self-limited disease and can often be treated symptomatically. The most common cause of acute diarrhea in the outpatient setting is infection, and in the inpatient setting, drugs. **Chronic diarrhea** is diarrhea that has been present 4–6 weeks or longer. Common causes include lactose intolerance, irritable bowel syndrome, inflammatory bowel disease (IBD), postsurgical procedures, malabsorptive syndromes, drugs, and various infections. Some causes of chronic diarrhea can present with an acute phase.

D. **Are there risk factors that suggest a specific cause?** Risk factors include drug-induced diarrhea, travel, homosexuality, abdominal surgery, vascular disease, and various endocrine disorders such as diabetes and Addison's disease.

E. **Is there associated abdominal pain?** Absence of pain makes inflammatory causes such as ischemic bowel disease or ulcerative colitis less likely.

F. **What is the volume of the stool?** Large volumes suggest small bowel or right colon; small volumes suggest left colon.

III. **Differential Diagnosis**

A. **Infection**

1. **Viruses.** Viral syndromes usually resolve in a few days and

can be treated symptomatically. Rotavirus and Norwalk virus are the most common viruses causing diarrhea.

2. **Bacteria.** *Shigella dysenteriae, Salmonella typhimurium, Campylobacter jejuni, Yersinia species, Staphylococcus aureus, Vibrio cholerae, Vibrio parahaemolyticus, Escherichia coli, Bacillus cereus, Clostridium perfringens,* and *Clostridium difficile* all cause diarrhea by producing enterotoxins or enteroinvasion. The spectrum of illness may range from asymptomatic to a life-threatening illness with diarrhea and abdominal pain. *S. aureus, B. cereus,* and *C. perfringens* are often associated with food poisoning. *C. jejuni* often causes a bloody diarrhea. *V. cholerae* can cause severe, life-threatening diarrhea and is commonly associated with consumption of raw shellfish.
3. **Parasites.** *Giardia lamblia, Entamoeba histolytica,* and *Cryptosporidium. G. lamblia* is often contracted by drinking contaminated water. *E. histolytica* is seen in travelers to Third World countries and in institutionalized patients. *Cryptosporidium* can cause a self-limited diarrhea in individuals who work with animals, especially livestock. *G. lamblia, E. histolytica,* and *Cryptosporidium* are common etiologic agents causing diarrhea in homosexual men. *Cryptosporidium* results in a severe, unremitting diarrhea in patients infected with human immunodeficiency virus.

B. Inflammatory diseases

1. **Ischemic bowel** secondary to thrombosis, embolism, or vasculitis such as polyarteritis nodosa and systemic lupus erythematous can result in bloody or guaiac-positive diarrhea. Atrial fibrillation is a common source of embolism.
2. **Inflammatory bowel disease.** Ulcerative colitis (UC) begins in the rectum, spreads proximally in a continuous manner. Presenting complaints begin abruptly and usually include rectal bleeding and diarrhea. Patients with Crohn's disease may also present with diarrhea; however, the onset of symptoms is more insidious than with UC, and the diarrhea is less often bloody.

C. Tumor

1. **Malignant carcinoid syndrome.** Flushing is also common.
2. **Colon carcinoma.** Bright red blood per rectum as well as occult blood loss or anemia is common.
3. **Medullary thyroid carcinoma**
4. **Lymphoma involving the bowel**
5. **Villous adenomas**
6. **Gastrinomas**

D. Endocrinopathies

1. **Hyperthyroidism.** Hyperdefecation (loose, frequent stools) rather than diarrhea. Diarrhea may be present with thyroid storm.

2. **Diabetes.** Associated with long-standing diabetes.
3. **Hypoparathyroidism**
4. **Addison's disease.** Associated nausea, vomiting abdominal pain, weight loss, and lethargy along with diarrhea.

E. **Drugs**

1. **Laxatives.** Chronic laxative abuse causes chronic diarrhea.
2. **Antacids.** Magnesium-containing antacids can cause osmotic diarrhea.
3. **Lactulose.** Used to treat hepatic encephalopathy. Should be titrated to two to three loose stools per day but can result in severe, life-threatening hypernatremia secondary to an osmotic diarrhea if not dosed properly.
4. **Quinidine.** Diarrhea is a common reason why quinidine is discontinued.
5. **Colchicine.** In treatment of acute gout, diarrhea can occur with increasing doses.
6. **Antibiotics.** Antibiotics can produce diarrhea by altering gut flora, leading to malabsorption or inducing *C. difficile* overgrowth and toxin production which can result in pseudomembranous colitis. Pseudomembranous colitis is most often secondary to antibiotics, especially broad-spectrum antibiotics such as clindamycin and the cephalosporins.

F. **Abdominal surgery.** Can cause chronic diarrhea.

1. **Gastric surgery.** Either vagotomy, resection, or bypass procedures.
2. **Cholecystectomy**
3. **Bowel resection**

G. **Malabsorption.** A common cause of chronic diarrhea that may result in deficiencies of fat-soluble vitamins A, D, E, and K; weight loss; and hypoalbuminemia.

1. **Chronic pancreatitis**
2. **Bowel resection**
3. **Bacterial overgrowth**
4. **Celiac or tropical sprue**
5. **Whipple's disease**
6. **Eosinophilic gastroenteritis**

H. **Lactose intolerance.** A common cause of chronic diarrhea resulting from lactose enzyme deficiency. Often associated flatulence.

I. **Irritable bowel syndrome.** Intermittent diarrhea may alternate with constipation. Symptoms are aggravated by stress. Abdominal pain may be present. Physical examination and routine laboratory tests are normal.

J. **Fecal impaction.** Can present with diarrhea. Often occurs in older age group.

K. **Human immunodeficiency virus (HIV) infection.** Diarrhea is common in patients positive for HIV or with acquired immunodeficiency syndrome (AIDS). Parasitic infections mentioned in Section III.A.3 are common in homosexual men with or without HIV infection. *Isospora belli* and *Microsporidia* are two other parasites that can cause diarrhea in HIV patients. Other nonparasitic etiologies associated with HIV infection include *Salmonella typhimurium,* which often results in bactremia, *Campylobacter jejuni, Mycobacterium avium-intracellulare,* and cytomegalovirus. Often the diarrhea is idiopathic and associated with fever and weight loss and may precede other manifestations of AIDS by months.

IV. Database

A. Physical examination key points

1. **General.** Cachexia suggests a chronic process such as carcinoma, AIDS, IBD, or malabsorption.
2. **Vital signs.** Hypotension or postural changes suggest significant sepsis or volume depletion. Tachycardia implies volume depletion or infection, or could be secondary to pain. Tachypnea may indicate fever, anxiety, pain, or sepsis or may represent compensation for a metabolic acidosis from a variety of causes including sepsis and bowel infarction.
3. **HEENT.** Aphthous ulcers are associated with IBD. An enlarged thyroid suggests hyperthyroidism or medullary carcinoma.
4. **Abdomen.** Look for surgical scars. Distension may be from carbohydrate malabsorption. Absent bowel sounds suggest bowel infarction or associated peritoneal infection. Metastatic cancer can result in hepatomegaly.
5. **Rectum.** Rule out rectal carcinoma. Look for fissures suggesting UC. Fecal impaction can present with diarrhea.
6. **Musculoskeletal exam.** Arthritis is associated with IBD, Whipple's disease, and *Yersinia enterocolitica* infection.
7. **Skin.** Hyperpigmentation can be seen with Addison's disease or celiac sprue. Erythema nodosum and pyoderma gangrenosus point to IBD. Dermatitis herpetiformis suggests celiac sprue, a rare cause of diarrhea.

B. Laboratory data

1. **Electrolytes.** With severe diarrhea various electrolyte abnormalities can occur including hypokalemia, metabolic acidosis, hypernatremia, and hyponatremia.
2. **Complete blood count with differential.** An elevated hematocrit suggests volume depletion. An anemia (See Anemia, p 25) may be associated with IBD, carcinoma, or HIV infection. A microcytic anemia suggests chronic gastrointestinal blood loss or malabsorption of iron. Macrocytic anemia may be secondary to vitamin B_{12} deficiency after gastric surgery or folate and vitamin B_{12} malabsorption.
3. **Sedimentation rate.** Expect to be increased in IBD, metastatic carcinoma, and systemic infections.
4. **Prothrombin time and partial thromboplastin time.** An el-

evated PT and PTT could be secondary to vitamin K deficiency from malabsorption or associated liver disease.

5. **Albumin.** Expect a low albumin in diarrhea secondary to malabsorption, IBD, and metastatic carcinoma.
6. **Calcium.** To rule out hypoparathyroidism as a cause. Hypocalcemia associated with vitamin D deficiency secondary to steatorrhea also may be seen.
7. **Endocrine tests.** Helpful as clinically indicated. Include thyroid tests (thyroxine, thyroid-stimulating hormone), parathyroid hormone, cortrosyn stimulation test, and gastrin.
8. **24- to 72-hour collection of stool for fecal fat.** Essential for workup of malabsorption.
9. **Stool for occult blood.** Follow with serial exams to increase sensitivity. Occult blood suggests UC, neoplasm, ischemic bowel, or various infections such as *C. jejuni.*
10. **Stool for leukocytes.** Presence of fecal leukocytes suggests a bacterial cause or IBD. In the absence of fecal leukocytes, viruses, enterotoxic food poisoning, or parasites can be suspected as can drugs, causes of malabsorption or endocrinopathies, cancer, irritable bowel, lactose intolerance, and abdominal surgery.
11. **Stool cultures.** Indicated for clinical dysentery (fever, abdominal cramps, fecal leukocytes) suggestive of inflammatory causes, prolonged diarrhea (longer than 7–14 days), symptoms suggestive of acute proctitis, or a prolonged illness.
    a. Contact lab regarding special procedures to identify *Yersinia, Vibrio,* or invasive *E. coli* if clinically indicated.
    b. If cultures remain negative, must consider invasive *E. coli.*
12. **Stool for ova and parasites** (O&P)
    a. Parasitic infections often require a "fresh" specimen within several hours of collection.
    b. Amebic dysentery diagnosed with presence of trophozoites. Cysts suggest the carrier state in the absence of trophozoites. Serology may help in the diagnosis.
    c. Identification of *Giardia* cysts is diagnostic of active infection. A small bowel aspirate may be required to recover *Giardia.*
13. ***Clostridia difficile* toxin.** If antibiotics given in the last 2 to 4 weeks. The presence of *C. difficile* without the toxin should not cause diarrhea.

C. Radiologic and other studies

1. **Proctosigmoidoscopy.** Indicated if pseudomembranous colitis is a possible etiology, if patient remains ill with negative stool cultures, or if diarrhea is bloody. An unprepped study is useful in determining the presence of mucosal inflammation suggesting inflammatory bowel disease, obtaining cultures and biopsies,

and examining for masses or stool impaction. Enemas or suppositories may obscure the presence of disease.

2. **Colonoscopy.** May be indicated if bleeding is seen proximal to the colon visualized on sigmoidoscopy.
3. **Barium enema.** May reveal carcinoma or IBD.
4. **Upper gastrointestinal series with small bowel follow-through.** May suggest Crohn's disease, celiac sprue, Whipple's disease, or lymphoma.
5. **D-Xylose test.** Abnormal in diseases involving the small bowel mucosa such as Crohn's disease, celiac sprue, Whipple's disease, and lymphoma.

V. Plan. Symptomatic treatment with fluids and electrolytes and antidiarrheal agents is usually all that is required. The initial use of antibiotic therapy should be avoided and implemented only in specific situations guided by stool culture results. Many causes of diarrhea resolve with treatment or removal of the underlying cause, eg, discontinuation of a drug like quinidine. For further recommendations regarding treatment other than those listed, please refer to any general medicine text.

A. Fluid replacement. This is the most important early intervention in diarrhea.

1. **Oral.** Helpful if given as hyposmolar solution and with glucose to facilitate uptake of sodium and water.
2. **Intravenous.** Necessary if patient is markedly volume depleted or has accompanying nausea and vomiting. May need potassium replacement as well.

B. Diet. Place patient on a lactose-free diet to prevent the development of diarrhea secondary to lactose deficiency which may be transient as a result of acute gastroenteritis. Diarrhea could also be secondary to lactose intolerance. Consider clear liquid diet for 24–48 hours, and then advance diet slowly.

C. Anitdiarrheal agents. Often helpful but should not be used if invasive diarrhea is clinically suspected. Antimotility drugs are contraindicated in patients with pseudomembranous colitis or IBD because of the risk for precipitating toxic megacolon. Commonly used agents include kaolin and pectin (Kaopectate) 60 mL every 4 hours prn, bismuth subsalicylate (Pepto-Bismol) 30–60 mL every 4 hours, diphenoxylate with atropine (Lomotil) 2 tablets or 10 mL every 4 hours, and loperamide (Imodium) 4 mg initially then 2 mg every 4 hours prn.

D. Antibiotics. Usually does not shorten the duration of illness and may select out resistant strains of organisms and often lead to pseudomembranous colitis.

1. **Salmonella.** Does not usually require antibiotics unless the patient remains ill or is predisposed to osteomyelitis from sickle cell disease or endocarditis. Treatment is chloramphenicol, ampicillin, or trimethoprim-sulfamethoxazole (Bactrim or Septra).
2. **Shigellosis.** Antibiotics recommended to decrease duration of

illness and fecal shedding. Antibiotic sensitivity is crucial because resistance is common. Treatment is with trimethoprim-sulfamethoxazole BID for 7 days or ampicillin 500 mg QID for 7 days.

3. **Pseudomembranous colitis.** Recommended treatment with vancomycin 125 mg PO every 6 hours or metronidazole (Flagyl) 500 mg PO every 6 hours for 7–10 days. Metronidazole is less expensive and is as effective. Addition of cholestyramine (Questran) QID may help control diarrhea if given with antibiotics.
4. ***Campylobacter infection.*** Often self-limiting illness. With severe or persistent diarrhea, erythromycin or ciprofloxacin for 5–7 days is effective.

REFERENCES

Ahnen DJ. Disorders of nutrient assimilation. In: Kelly WN (editor-in-chief). *Textbook of Internal Medicine.* Philadelphia: JB Lippincott; 1989;522–534.

Dobbins J. Approach to the patient with diarrhea. In: Kelly WN (editor-in-chief). *Textbook of Internal Medicine.* Philadelphia: JB Lippincott; 1989;669–680.

Reilly BM. *Practical Strategies in Outpatient Medicine.* Philadelphia: WB Saunders; 1984;100–163.

■ DYSPNEA

I. **Problem.** A patient admitted to the coronary care unit to rule out a myocardial infarction complains of difficulty breathing.

II. **Immediate Questions**

A. **Was the onset of dyspnea acute or gradual?** The differential diagnosis for acute dyspnea differs from that for subacute or chronic dyspnea. Causes of acute dyspnea include bronchospasm, pulmonary embolism (PE), pneumothorax, and acute pulmonary edema.

B. **Are there other associated symptoms such as chest pain?** The patient may focus on the shortness of breath and fail to disclose chest pain or discomfort unless specifically asked. Some patients may also perceive acute myocardial ischemia as dyspnea rather than angina (anginal equivalent).

C. **Is the patient cyanotic?** Hypoxemia is a potentially lethal condition. If cyanosis is noted, immediate therapy is indicated.

III. **Differential Diagnosis.** Dyspnea is awareness of an increased difficulty in breathing. It may occur through increased respiratory muscle work, stimulation of neuroreceptors throughout the respiratory tract, or stimulation of peripheral chemoreceptors. Causes of dyspnea can be broadly categorized into cardiac and pulmonary.

A. **Pulmonary**

1. **Pulmonary embolism.** This diagnosis must be considered in any patient presenting with acute dyspnea. Also, recurrent pul-

monary emboli can cause intermittent dyspnea at rest. This diagnosis should be especially considered in any patient with risk factors such as prolonged immobilization, recent surgery, obesity, malignancy, or high-dose estrogen therapy.

2. **Pneumothorax.** This can occur after trauma or spontaneously in patients with bullous emphysema, or in males with a tall, thin body habitus. Patients on ventilators receiving positive end-expiratory pressure ventilation are at increased risk of pneumothorax.
3. **Asthma/chronic obstructive airway disease.** These patients usually have a prior history of dyspnea; however, anaphylaxis can also produce acute asthma. (See Anaphylactic Reaction, p 22.) In addition to bronchospasm, these patients often demonstrate other evidence of anaphylaxis such as stridor and urticaria.
4. **Aspiration** (See Aspiration, p 32.)
5. **Pneumonia.** Characterized by fever, productive cough, radiographic infiltrates, and leukocytosis.
6. **Interstitial lung disease.** This usually produces progressive dyspnea and is caused by a large number of diseases.
7. **Pleural effusion.** This also is more likely to cause a chronic or subchronic dyspnea rather than acute dyspnea.

B. Cardiac

1. **Acute myocardial infarction.** As mentioned earlier, patients experiencing acute myocardial ischemia can present complaining of dyspnea rather than chest pain. In addition, patients with acute myocardial infarction (MI) can develop acute PE.
2. **Congestive heart failure.** Accumulation of fluid in the interstitial spaces of the lung stimulates neuroreceptors, which produce a sensation of dyspnea. These patients frequently experience orthopnea and paroxysmal nocturnal dyspnea. Orthopnea also occurs in patients with chronic obstructive airway disease.
3. **Pericardial tamponade.** Dyspnea is frequently a significant complaint in patients with this problem.

C. Psychogenic breathlessness

1. Dyspnea associated with hyperventilation can be difficult to separate from organic causes. Typically, these patients are anxious and develop acral paresthesias and lightheadedness. Their dyspnea is often worse at rest and improved with exercise. In patients with this history, one should strongly suspect a psychogenic origin. Nevertheless, this diagnosis should not be made until organic causes have been excluded.

IV. Database

A. Physical examination key points

1. **Vital signs.** Fever may signify infection but also occurs with pulmonary and myocardial infarction. Tachypnea occurs in most cases of dyspnea; however, dyspnea can occur in pa-

tients with a normal respiratory rate. Hypotension may result from a tension pneumothorax, anaphylaxis, pericardial tamponade, or acute MI. Pulsus paradoxus may occur in patients with acute exacerbations of asthma, chronic obstructive pulmonary disease, or pericardial tamponade.

2. **Lungs.** Observe for accessory muscle use. Listen for wheezes, stridor, crackles, and absent breath sounds. Paradoxic abdominal movement during respiration suggests diaphragmatic and respiratory muscle fatigue.
3. **Heart.** Elevated jugular venous pressure, a displaced point of maximal impulse, or an S_3 gallop suggest decompensated heart failure.
4. **Extremities.** Examine for swelling or other evidence of deep venous thrombosis which would predispose to pulmonary embolus. Also evaluate for peripheral cyanosis.
5. **Neurologic exam.** Confusion and impaired mentation may signify severe hypoxemia.

B. **Laboratory data**

1. **Hemogram.** Leukocytosis occurs with pneumonia. Anemia can cause dyspnea on exertion.
2. **Arterial blood gases.** Should be obtained in any patient with significant dyspnea or if hypoxemia is suspected.
3. **Sputum gram stain and culture.** Obtain in patients with suspected pneumonia.

C. **Radiologic and other studies**

1. **Chest x-ray.** If a patient is in obvious distress, obtain a stat portable upright chest x-ray. If the patient is unable to sit for an adequate film, obtain lateral decubitus films to rule out the possibility of a basilar pneumothorax.
2. **Electrocardiogram.** Should always be obtained in any patient with acute dyspnea to rule out the possibility of pericarditis or myocardial ischemia.
3. **Pulmonary function tests.** These are not applicable to the acute situation but can assist in the evaluation of patients with obstructive or restrictive lung disease. (See Cough, Section IV.C.5, Pulmonary Function Tests, p 78.)
4. **Ventilation perfusion ($\dot{V}/\dot{Q}$) scan.** To evaluate for PE.
5. **Pulmonary angiogram.** In patients with a non–high-probability lung scan in whom there still exists a suspicion for PE, this test is necessary to establish a diagnosis.
6. **Echocardiogram.** Should be obtained emergently if there is a strong clinical suspicion for cardiac tamponade. Otherwise, echocardiography can be useful for assessing left ventricular function and whether or not cardiac disease is responsible for the dyspnea.

V. Plan

A. **Emergent therapy**

1. **Oxygen supplementation.** The initial goal of treatment in pa-

tients with acute dyspnea should be to ensure adequate oxygenation; thus, the majority of patients should be treated with 100% oxygen therapy. In those patients with a history of chronic obstructive airway disease in whom one is concerned about the possibility of suppression of their hypoxemic ventilatory drive, therapy should be initiated with 24% oxygen by Venturi mask. In either case, an ABG should be obtained to direct subsequent adjustments of the oxygen.

2. Stat portable chest x-ray, ECG, and ABG. Indicated in any patient who complains of acute dyspnea.

B. Asthma

1. Request a stat nebulizer treatment with metaproterenol (Alupent) 0.3 mL in 2–3 mL normal saline.
2. In patients with anaphylaxis or in young patients with acute asthma, epinephrine 0.25–0.4 mL of a 1:1000 concentration can be given subcutaneously.

C. Anaphylaxis (See Anaphylactic Reaction, Section V, p 24.)

D. Myocardial ischemia. If initial assessment suggests myocardial ischemia, administer sublingual nitroglycerin provided the systolic blood pressure is above 100. (See Chest Pain, Section V, p 57.)

E. Acute congestive heart failure. Furosemide (Lasix) 40–80 mg IV may be given provided the patient is not hypotensive. Morphine sulfate 2–5 mg IV may also be helpful initially if acute pulmonary edema is present.

F. Pneumonia. Treat with pulmonary toilet and antibiotics as directed by results of the sputum gram stain.

G. Pleural effusion. Removal of pleural fluid by thoracentesis can oftentimes produce a significant improvement in a patient's dyspnea. (See Chapter 3, Thoracentesis, p 343.)

H. Aspiration (See Aspiration, Section V, p 34.)

REFERENCE

Ingram RH, Braunwald E. Dyspnea and pulmonary edema. In: Braunwald E, Isselbacher KJ, Petersdorf RG, et al, eds. *Harrison's Principles of Internal Medicine.* 11th ed. New York: McGraw-Hill; 1987:141–143.

■ DYSURIA

I. Problem. A 28-year-old diabetic woman complains of pain with urination.

II. Immediate Questions

A. How long has this symptom been present? A gradual onset of several days' duration suggests a chlamydial infection. Prostatitis and subclinical pyelonephritis may also present with several days of symptoms.

B. Does the patient have a prior history of urinary tract infection

(UTI) or urologic abnormality? Women and patients with urinary tract abnormalities are prone to recurrent UTIs.

C. **Are there any other associated symptoms?** Fever, chills, nausea and vomiting, and back pain are often signs of upper UTIs such as pyelonephritis. Frequency, urgency, and dysuria are lower UTI signs and occur in cystitis, prostatitis, and urethritis. A vaginal discharge would suggest vaginitis as a cause of dysuria. In men, ask about a history of recent penile discharge.

D. **Has the patient recently had a Foley catheter removed?** A catheter may result in an infection or urethral irritation.

III. **Differential Diagnosis.** The principal causes of dysuria differ for men and women.

A. **Female.** Women presenting with acute dysuria may have one of seven conditions, each of which may require different management.

1. **Acute pyelonephritis.** Suggested by fever, flank pain, rigors, nausea, and vomiting.
2. **Subclinical pyelonephritis.** As many as 30% to 80% of patients presenting only with signs of lower UTI (dysuria, frequency, urgency) in fact have an upper UTI as well. This condition should be especially suspected in patients with urinary tract abnormalities, diabetes, or history of relapsing infection, or when symptoms have been present for 7–10 days.
3. **Lower UTI.** These patients have either cystitis or urethritis, with bacteria confined to either the bladder or the urethra.
4. **Chlamydial urethritis.** This is characterized by a prolonged onset over several days. The patient often reports a partner who has similar symptoms. An associated mucopurulent endocervical secretion may be noted on pelvic exam.
5. **Other urethral infections.** Urethritis may also be caused by *Neisseria gonorrhoeae* and *Trichomonas.*
6. **Vaginitis.** In contrast to the sensation of an internal, dull pain experienced with the dysuria of cystitis, vaginitis causes external burning as the urinary stream flows past inflamed labia.
7. **No recognized pathogen.** These patients have no pyuria and no evidence of infection. The most common cause is atrophic vaginitis. Consider bladder or urethral carcinoma.

B. **Male**

1. **Cystitis/pyelonephritis**
2. **Urethritis**
   a. **Nongonococcal.** Discharge occurs 8 to 21 days after exposure and is typically thin and clear.
   b. **Gonococcal.** In contrast, in this condition the discharge is heavy and purulent. Symptoms occur 2 to 6 days after exposure.
   c. **Nongonococcal/gonococcal.** Recall that both conditions frequently coexist.

3. **Prostatitis.** Symptoms include vague groin or back pain. The diagnosis is confirmed by palpation of a tender, boggy prostrate.
4. **Cancer (bladder, prostate, urethral)**
5. **Urethral stricture**

IV. Database

A. Physical examination key points

1. **Vital signs.** Check for fever, tachycardia, or hypotension which suggest urosepsis.
2. **Abdomen.** Examine for evidence of suprapubic tenderness or costovertebral angle tenderness.
3. **Genitalia.** In women who present with acute dysuria and also report a vaginal discharge, pelvic examination is mandatory to rule out vaginitis or cervicitis. In men with a history of urethral discharge, penile stripping may be necessary to produce a discharge. Examine for evidence of epididymitis or orchitis.
4. **Prostate.** In acute prostatitis, the gland is swollen, tender, and boggy. In patients with chronic prostatitis, examination of the prostate may be unremarkable.

B. Laboratory data

1. **Urinalysis.** Pyuria, defined as >5 white blood cells per high-power field, suggests a treatable infectious cause of dysuria. Bacteriuria confirms a bacterial cause. Also examine for white blood cell casts, which occur with pyelonephritis. Hematuria frequently occurs with cystitis/pyelonephritis but is seldom seen with urethritis. Gram stain of the urine sediment is useful in confirming or excluding the presence of gram-positive cocci, which suggests enterococcus. This organism requires different treatment as compared to other urinary tract pathogens.
2. **Urine culture.** Although useful in determining a bacterial cause of dysuria, in women a urine culture is usually indicated only if acute pyelonephritis or subclinical pyelonephritis is suspected or if the patient is presenting with a relapse from a UTI. In men, a urine culture should always be obtained to confirm and direct subsequent treatment.
3. **Blood cultures.** Should be ordered in all patients who appear septic and are admitted for presumed acute pyelonephritis.
4. **Leukocytosis and left shift.** Observed with acute pyelonephritis and sometimes with acute prostatitis but is seldom seen in urethritis, chronic prostatitis, or cystitis.
5. **Urethral discharges.** In both men and women, the discharge should be gram stained and cultured on Thayer–Martin medium. The presence of intracellular gram-negative diplococci on gram stain is sufficient presumptive evidence of gonorrhea in men and warrants therapy. In women with endocervical discharge, cultures for gonorrhea should be obtained.
6. **Vaginal discharge.** Wet mount to look for *Trichomonas vagi-*

nalis, which have flagella and, when viewed on wet mount, move rapidly and erratically. Clue cells or squamous cells "salt and peppered" with bacteria indicate infection with *Gardnerella vaginalis.* Hyphae indicating infection with *Candida albicans* should be looked for on a slide of the vaginal discharge treated with 2 to 3 drops of 10% potassium hydroxide.

C. **Radiologic and other studies.** Full urologic evaluation is indicated in all men presenting with a UTI. Women who have had more than three UTIs in 1 year should also probably undergo full urologic evaluation; however, these studies are seldom performed acutely unless there is a strong clinical suspicion of urinary tract obstruction, or a renal stone is believed to be present. An ultrasound or intravenous pyelography should be obtained in patients admitted for acute pyelonephritis if they remain febrile after 3 days of treatment with an appropriate antibiotic.

V. Plan

A. Acute pyelonephritis

1. In patients who appear septic or are unable to tolerate oral medications, administer gentamicin 1.5–2.0 mg/kg IV loading dose and then about 1.5 mg/kg every 8–24 hours depending on renal function. (See Aminoglycoside Dosing in Tables 7–13 and 14, p 499.) A third-generation cephalosporin such as ceftriaxone 1 g IV every 12 hours is an alternative. The latter may be preferred in patients who are elderly, have associated renal insufficiency, or have indwelling Foley catheters favoring the growth of antibiotic-resistant organisms. After the patient is afebrile and clinically improved, and results of urine culture and sensitivity testing are known, a switch to PO medications such as Bactrim can be made. Duration of therapy should be at least 14 days.
2. In patients who do not appear septic and are able to tolerate oral medications, a 14-day course of trimethoprim (320 mg daily), sulfamethoxazole (1600 mg daily) or Bactrim DS 1 tablet BID should be administered.
3. Patients should have urine cultures checked 2 to 3 weeks after completion of therapy.

B. **Subclinical pyelonephritis.** These patients should be treated with a 14-day course of Bactrim PO as described above.

C. **Uncomplicated lower UTI.** In patients presenting with acute dysuria who are noted to have pyuria and bacteriuria on urinalysis, but do not have the clinical picture of acute pyelonephritis, uncomplicated lower UTI can be presumed and treated. A urine culture is not mandatory in these patients. Studies indicate that Bactrim is the most efficacious treatment. At present, the duration of therapy is controversial, with evidence suggesting that Bactrim DS 2 tablets as a single dose is sufficient for uncomplicated lower UTI. Such short-course regimens avoid the toxicity of a 7- to 10-day course of antibiotics. An acceptable middle-of-the-road approach might be to administer Bactrim DS 1 tablet BID for 3 days. The patient should be instructed to return for follow-up if symptoms persist or recur after therapy. Follow-up culture is not necessary.

D. **Vaginitis.** Therapy is directed to the specific cause of the vaginitis. For patients with candidal vaginitis, miconazole (Monistat) cream topically for 7 days is effective. Metronidazole (Flagyl) 500 mg BID for 7 days is effective for bacterial vaginosis. For trichomonal vaginitis, metronidazole 2 g PO in a single dose is recommended. Topical Premarin cream is effective for atrophic vaginitis which should be applied nightly for 1 week and two or three times weekly thereafter.

E. **Chlamydial urethritis.** This should be suspected in patients who have dysuria and pyuria but no bacteriuria and who have a partner with symptoms. Doxycycline 100 mg BID for 7 days is effective. An alternative therapy is tetracycline 500 mg QID for 7 days. These patients should have their partner evaluated and treated as well.

F. **Gonococcal urethritis.** With the emergence of penicillin resistance, ceftriaxone 125 mg IM is now recommended. Because of the frequent coexistence of chlamydial urethritis, a course of doxycycline as suggested in Section V.E is recommended.

G. **Acute prostatitis.** For patients who do not appear septic, Bactrim DS 1 tablet BID for 21 days may be used. Patients who are septic should be admitted and a regimen of either Ampicillin and gentamicin or a third-generation cephalosporin instituted.

REFERENCES

Johnson JR, Stamm WE. Urinary tract infections in women: Diagnosis and treatment. *Ann Intern Med* 1989;111:906–917.

Komaroff AL. Acute dysuria in women. *N Engl J Med* 1984;310:368–375.

Komaroff AL. Urinalysis and urine culture in women with dysuria. *Ann Intern Med* 1986;104:212–218.

■ FEVER

I. **Problem.** You are called to see a 57-year-old man who has been hospitalized for 3 days and now has a fever of 39.5°C (103.1°F).

II. **Immediate Questions**

A. **How long has the patient been febrile and how high is the temperature?** It is important to know if this elevation in temperature signals the abrupt onset of fever or represents the gradual worsening of a prior fever. Fever above 40.0°C (104.0°F) requires immediate action.

B. **What is the fever pattern?** Is the fever intermittent (it falls to normal at some time during the day), sustained (it remains elevated), or relapsing (febrile periods are followed by one to several days of normal temperatures)? Drug fever is often sustained but can be intermittent. Examples of relapsing fever include malaria and the Pel-Ebstein fever of Hodgkin's disease.

C. **Does the patient have any other pertinent medical illnesses or is he or she immunocompromised?** Such information is vital before you can properly assess the patient.

D. **Are any intravenous lines in place?** Indwelling Foley catheters, intravenous access sites, nasogastric tubes (which can predispose to sinusitis), and central venous catheter sites are frequent sources of nosocomial fever.

E. **Are there any associated symptoms?** The symptoms to ask about are many and include chills, rigors, rash, myalgias, arthralgias, cough, chest pain, headache, dysuria, abdominal pain, pain at an intravenous site, night sweats, and change in mental status. Such questions may point you toward a specific cause of the fever.

F. **What medications is the patient taking?** Ask first if the patient is taking any antipyretics or any current antibiotics. Also consider a drug-induced fever and review *all* medications.

G. **Have any recent procedures been done such as bronchoscopy or has the patient received blood recently?** A fever to 38.3°C (101°F) is common after bronchoscopy. A fever is also common after transfusions.

III. **Differential Diagnosis.** The list is extraordinarily long so the major categories are presented here:

A. **Infections**
   1. **Pyogenic**
   2. **Viral**
   3. **Mycobacterial**
   4. **Fungal**
   5. **Parasitic**

B. **Neoplasms.** Solid tumors, lymphoma, Hodgkin's disease, leukemia. Fever with leukemia is often due to infection but may be caused by the primary disease, especially in chronic myelogonous leukemia.

C. **Connective tissue disease**
   1. **Acute rheumatic fever**
   2. **Rheumatoid arthritis**
   3. **Adult Still's disease**
   4. **Systemic lupus erythematosus**
   5. **Vasculitis.** Including hypersensitivity vasculitis, polymyalgia rheumatica, temporal arteritis, and polyarteritis nodosa.

D. **Thermoregulatory disorders.** Heat stroke, malignant hyperthermia, thyroid storm, and neuroleptic malignant syndrome. Thyroid storm may be a postoperative complication in a hyperthyroid patient. Features of neuroleptic malignant syndrome include hyperthermia, hypertonicity of skeletal muscle, mental status changes, and autonomic nervous system instability in patients on neuroleptics.

E. **Drug fever.** Potential culprits include antibiotics, methyldopa (Aldomet), quinidine, hydralazine (Apresoline), procainamide, phenytoin (Dilantin), chlorpromazine (Thorazine), carbamazepine (Tegretol), anti-inflammatory agents such as ibuprofen (Motrin), antineoplastic agents, and allopurinol (Zyloprim).

F. **Miscellaneous disorders.** Including pulmonary embolus with infarction, myocardial infarction, hyperthyroidism (thyroid storm), atrial myxoma, inflammatory bowel disease, and Addisonian crisis.

G. **Fever of unknown origin.** Manifested by fever greater than 38.3°C (101.0°F) on several occasions for a duration of at least 3 weeks, with no definite etiology.

H. **Unknown source.** Eighteen percent in one series of inpatients.

I. **Factitious fever**

IV. Database

A. Physical examination key points

1. **Vital signs.** Take temperature both orally and rectally. (Neutropenia is a contraindication to a rectal temperature.) A rectal temperature should be taken to make sure the oral temperature is not falsely elevated secondary to recent consumption of a hot liquid or smoking. A rectal temperature is usually 1° greater than an oral temperature. Check pulse and blood pressure to make sure the patient is hemodynamically stable.
2. **Skin.** Check the intravenous site. Look for a rash. If there is a rash, involvement of the palms and soles may suggest Rocky Mountain spotted fever, secondary syphilis, and Stevens-Johnson syndrome which can result from a hypersensitivity drug reaction. Look for flame hemorrhages under the fingernails suggesting endocarditis.
3. **HEENT.** Look for evidence of sinusitis (can be caused by an indwelling nasogastric tube), otitis, pharyngitis, conjunctivitis, and cotton-wool spots on fundoscopic examination could indicate systemic candidiasis, endocarditis, or cytomegalovirus.
4. **Neck.** Check for neck stiffness or meningism. Check for Kernig's and Brudzinski's signs, which may occur with meningitis.
5. **Lymph nodes.** Including cervical, supraclavicular, epitrochlear, axillary, and inguinal.
6. **Lungs.** Listen for crackles or signs of consolidation indicating pneumonia.
7. **Heart.** A murmur, especially a regurgitant murmur, suggests endocarditis.
8. **Abdomen.** Listen for bowel sounds, palpate and percuss for signs of tenderness, and check for Murphy's sign (tenderness in the right upper quadrant on inspiration while palpating in

the right upper quadrant), which is seen in cholecystitis. Examine for costovertebral angle tenderness indicating pyelonephritis.

9. **Genitourinary system.** Necessary to exclude pelvic inflammatory disease or tubo-ovarian abscess in a female and epididymitis or orchitis in a male. Also check prostate for tenderness.
10. **Extremities.** Check intravenous site. Look for joint effusions or tenderness.

B. Laboratory data

1. **Complete blood count with differential.** An elevated WBC count and left shift suggest infectious etiology. Eosinophilia suggests drug reaction or parasitic infection. A low WBC count may suggest overwhelming sepsis, a collagen vascular disease such as lupus, a viral infection, or a process that has replaced the normal bone marrow such as a lymphoma or carcinoma.
2. **Blood cultures.** Usually two sets; four sets if endocarditis is suspected.
3. **Culture tips of central lines.** If a patient with a central venous catheter becomes febrile and diagnostic workup fails to reveal a source of infection, the venous catheter must be assumed to be the culprit and must be removed.
4. **Sputum gram stain.** Request gram stain if there is a productive cough.
5. **Urinalysis and culture.** Rule out cystitis, prostatitis, or pyelonephritis. Eosinophils in the urine suggest a drug reaction.
6. **Miscellaneous tests.** In certain circumstances and only if clinically indicated: liver function tests, erythrocyte sedimentation rate, hepatitis serologies, PPD and anergy, culture for tuberculosis and fungus, examination of peripheral blood smear, complement fixation, *Legionella* titers, viral titers, fungal serologies, VDRL, antistreptolysin-O (ASO) titer, antinuclear antibody (ANA), lumbar puncture.

C. Radiologic and other studies

1. **Chest x-ray.** Should be obtained with a fever of unknown source.
2. **Sinus films.** If sinus tenderness or discharge is present or if a nasogastric tube has been in place.
3. **Acute abdominal series.** Should be considered and obtained if clinically indicated.
4. **Ultrasound.** To assess the gallbladder and biliary tree. Can also be used to detect abdominal, renal, and pelvic masses.
5. **HIDA scan.** If acute cholecystitis is suspected.
6. **Bone scan.** If osteomyelitis is suspected.
7. **CT scans.** To detect subphrenic, abdominal, pelvic, and intracranial lesions.

8. **Gallium scan.** To detect an abscess.
9. **Echocardiogram.** Especially if blood cultures are positive. Sensitivity is not high enough that a normal echocardiogram rules out endocarditis.

V. Plan. The plan is dependent on the clinical setting. Many of the previously mentioned tests should be obtained only in certain circumstances and only if a previous workup has been unrevealing. The *initial* workup of a febrile patient late at night will not be as exhaustive as a more leisurely performed FUO evaluation.

A. Initial assessment

1. Rule out hemodynamic instability.
2. Carefully review medications, especially looking for any recent changes.
3. Obtain appropriate cultures.
4. Reduce temperature. Give antipyretics such as acetaminophen 650 mg PO or rectally. If the fever is above 40.0°C (104.0°F), consider a cooling blanket. If the patient has underlying cardiac disease, the temperature should be brought down quickly to avoid cardiac decompensation.
5. Consider antibiotics. If the patient is hemodynamically stable and there is no apparent source of infection, it is often prudent to withhold antibiotics. As noted in the differential, the causes of fever are many and oftentimes nonbacterial. Empiric antibiotics will many times confuse the issue.

B. Fever with hypotension. Septic shock is a medical emergency. Begin fluid resuscitation through a large-bore IV, place the patient in Trendelenburg, begin appropriate antibiotics, and transfer to an ICU. If the patient's blood pressure fails to respond to fluids, begin a dopamine infusion at 2–5 μg/kg/min. The use of IV steroids is controversial but probably not warranted unless you suspect Addisonian crisis.

C. Intravenous catheter infection. Remove the offending IV, apply local heat, use anti-inflammatory agents if it is a peripheral site, and consider antibiotics. If you feel a warm, tender, swollen vein and/or the patient has a history of IV drug abuse, suspect septic thrombophlebitis and immediately obtain a surgery consult and begin antibiotics. If a central line is in place, change all sites, culture the catheter tips, and begin antibiotics.

D. Pneumonia. Initial treatment of pneumonia should be based on the gram stain and clinical picture. Community-acquired pneumonia in a normal host can be treated with penicillin G 600,000–1,000,000 U IV every 4 hours or erythromycin 500 mg to 1 g every 6 hours (to cover for *Mycoplasma* and *Legionella*). If the gram stain reveals gram-positive diplococci, indicating *Streptococcus pneumoniae,* penicillin is preferred unless the patient has a penicillin allergy. Other agents can be used to treat *Streptococcus* including first-generation cephalosporins such as cefadyl (Cephapirin) and cefazolin (Ancef, Kefzol). Hospital-acquired pneumonia or pneumonia in an immunocompromised host requires broader coverage. The gram stain can also be helpful. If there are gram-positive cocci in clusters, the chosen antibiotic regimen should include either naficillin 1.0–2.0 IV every 4 hours or vancomycin 500 mg IV every 6 hours or 1000 mg IV every 12 hours in a patient with normal renal function. Be sure to adjust the dose of vancomycin with renal insufficiency. For gram-negative organisms, an aminoglycoside such as tobramycin or gentamicin should be administered. In patients with renal insufficiency, an alternative to aminoglycosides such as aztrenonam (Azactam) should be considered or a third-generation cephalosporin such as cefotaxime (Claforan), ceftazidime (Fortaz), or ceftriaxone (Rocephin) should be included.

E. **Febrile, neutopenic patient.** Culture completely and empirically begin antibiotics such as tobramycin and ticarcillin, **even if a source of infection is not apparent.** Add Flagyl if anaerobes are suspected and a first-generation cephalosporin such as cephalothin if staphylococcal infection is likely.

F. **Meningitis.** A medical emergency. A lumbar puncture should be done as quickly as possible, especially if there is no history of bleeding disorder and no focal deficits or papilledema, and you have no reason to suspect an intracranial abscess. Begin antibiotics as you are doing the lumbar puncture. If for any reason there is a delay in doing the lumbar puncture (such as obtaining a CT scan of the head because of papilledema), the antibiotics should be administered immediately and **not** delayed until after the lumbar puncture. A third-generation cephalosporin such as cefotaxime or ceftazidime should be given for meningitis of unknown etilogy; otherwise, antibiotic therapy should be guided by the gram stain.

G. **Cholecystitis.** Obtain an ultrasound and/or HIDA scan, begin antibiotics, and consult surgery.

H. **Drug fever.** Discontinue all drugs possibly causing a drug fever and substitute an appropriate alternative.

I. **Thyroid storm.** Treat with hydration, apply cooling blanket, and give saturated solution of potassium iodide (SSKI), beta blockers, propylthiouracil, and glucocorticoids.

J. **Addisonian crisis.** Treat immediately with IV steroids (hydrocortisone 100 mg IV push, then 100 mg IV every 8 hours continuous infusion).

K. **Neuroleptic malignant syndrome.** Treatment consists of discontinuation of the neuroleptics, general supportive measures, and consideration of dantrolene (Dantrium) 50 mg PO every 12 hours.

L. **No or unknown diagnosis.** Remember to consider pulmonary infarction and myocardial infarction.

REFERENCES

Guze BH, Baxter LR. Neuroleptic malignant syndrome. *N Engl J Med* 1985; 313:163–166.

Mackowiak PA, LeMaistre CF. Drug fever: A critical appraisal of conventional concepts. *Ann Intern Med* 1987;106;728–733.

May DC, Morris SH, Stewart RM, et al. Neuroleptic malignant syndrome: Response to dantrolene sodium. *Ann Intern Med* 1983;98:183–184.

McGowan JE, Rose RC, Jacobs NF, et al. Fever in hospitalized patients. *Am J Med* 1987;82:580–586.

Petersdorf RG, Root RK. Chills and fever. In: Braunwald E, Isselbacher KJ, Petersdorf RG, et al, eds. *Harrison's Principles of Internal Medicine.* 11th ed. New York: McGraw-Hill Book Co; 1987:50–57.

Petersdorf RG, Root RK. Disturbances of heat regulation. In: Braunwald E, Isselbacher KJ, Petersdorf RG, et al, eds. *Harrison's Principles of Internal Medicine.* 11th ed. New York: McGraw-Hill Book Co; 1987:43–50.

Swartz MN, Simon HB. Pathophysiology of fever and fever of undetermined origin. In: Rubenstein E, editor-in-chief; Federman DD, ed. *Scientific American.* Sect. 7: *Infectious Diseases.* vol 2, pt XXIV. New York: Scientific American Inc; 1989:1–12.

■ FOLEY CATHETER PROBLEMS

(See also Chapter 3, Bladder Catheterization, p 311.)

I. **Problem.** The Foley catheter is not draining in a patient admitted 2 days previously for congestive heart failure.

II. **Immediate Questions**

A. **What has the urine output been?** If the urine output has slowly tapered off, then the problem may be oliguria rather than a nonfunctioning Foley. A catheter that has never put out urine may not be in the bladder.

B. **Is the urine grossly bloody, or are there any clots in the tubing or collection bag?** Clots or tissue fragments can obstruct the flow of urine in a Foley catheter.

C. **Is the patient complaining of pain?** Bladder distension often causes severe lower abdominal pain; bladder spasms are painful and may cause urine to leak out around the catheter rather than through the catheter.

D. **Was any difficulty encountered in catheter insertion?** Problematic urethral catheterization should raise the possibility that the catheter is not in the bladder.

III. **Differential Diagnosis**

A. **Low urine output.** This may be due to volume depletion, hemorrhage, acute renal failure, septic shock, or several other causes. (See Oliguria/Anuria, p 213.)

B. **Obstructed Foley catheter**

1. **Kinking of catheter or tubing**
2. **Clots, tissue fragments.** Most common after transurethral resection of the prostate or bladder. Grossly bloody urine suggests that a clot is obstructing the catheter. "Tea"-colored or

"rusty" urine suggests that an organized clot may be present even though the urine is no longer grossly bloody. Bleeding often accompanies "accidental" catheter removal with the balloon still inflated and any coagulopathy.

3. **Sediment/stones.** Chronically indwelling catheters (usually longer than 1 month) can become encrusted and obstructed. Calculi can lodge in the catheter.

C. **Improperly positioned Foley catheter.** These problems are much more common in males. In traumatic urethral disruption associated with a pelvic fracture, the catheter can pass into the periurethral tissues. Strictures or prostatic hypertrophy may cause the end of the catheter to be placed in the urethra and not the bladder.

D. **Bladder spasms.** The patient may complain of severe suprapubic pain, pain radiating to the end of the penis, or urine leaking from around the catheter. Spasms are common after bladder or prostate surgery. Spasms may be the only catheter-related complaint or may be so severe as to obstruct the flow of urine.

IV. Database

A. Physical examination key points

1. **Vital signs.** Check for tachycardia and/or hypotension characteristic of hypovolemia.
2. **Abdomen.** Determine if the bladder is distended (suprapubic dullness to percussion with or without tenderness). May be indicative of an obstructed Foley catheter.
3. **Genitalia.** Bleeding at the meatus suggests urethral trauma or partial removal of the catheter with the balloon inflated.
4. **Rectum.** A "floating prostate" suggests urethral disruption.

B. **Laboratory data.** Most problems are usually mechanical in nature so that laboratory data are somewhat limited in this setting.

1. **Blood urea nitrogen, serum creatinine.** Elevations may be seen with cases of renal insufficiency.
2. **Prothrombin time, partial thromboplastin time, platelet count.** Especially if there is severe bleeding present.

C. **Radiologic and other studies.** In the acute setting of a Foley catheter problem, radiologic studies are usually not needed. Ultrasound may demonstrate hydronephrosis in cases of obstructive uropathy.

V. Plan

A. **Verify function.** A rule of thumb is that a catheter that will not irrigate is in the urethra and not in the bladder. Start by irrigating the catheter with aseptic technique using a catheter-tipped 60-mL syringe and sterile normal saline. This may dislodge any clots obstructing the catheter. If sterile saline cannot be satisfactorily instilled and aspirated, the catheter should be replaced.

B. **Oliguria.** If the catheter irrigates freely, work up the patient for oliguria/anuria. (See Oliguria/Anuria, p 213.)

C. **Spasms.** Bladder spasms can be treated with oxybutynin (Ditropan) or propanthline (Pro-Banthine). Be SURE to discontinue these medications before removing the catheter to allow normal bladder function.

REFERENCE

Andriole UT. Care of the indwelling catheter. In: Kayes D, ed. *Urinary Tract Infection and Its Management.* St. Louis, Mo: CV Mosby; 1973:256–260.

■ HEADACHE

I. **Problem.** A 72-year-old man is admitted to the hospital for elective cardiac catheterization. You are called by the nurses to evaluate the patient because he is complaining of a severe headache.

II. **Immediate Questions**

   A. **Has the patient experienced similar headaches before?** If the headache is similar to previous tension or migraine headaches, then the situation is unlikely to be urgent; however, if the headache is new or has changed from a previous pattern, a number of potentially serious conditions should be considered including acute glaucoma, sinusitis, subarachnoid hemorrhage, meningitis, and early hypertensive encephalopathy.

   B. **What are the patient's vital signs?** Although essential hypertension of itself infrequently causes headache, it may exacerbate a preexisting vascular or tension headache. Diastolic blood pressures above 140 can cause severe headache. A fever should alert one to the possibility of subarachnoid hemorrhage, meningitis, and acute sinusitis.

III. **Differential Diagnosis.** The history is the most important tool for evaluating headache. The great majority of headaches are secondary to either chronic tension or migraine headaches. A headache may also be the only symptom of a patient with a more serious condition such as an intracranial mass, temporal arteritis, meningitis, and subarachnoid hemorrhage. These are all potentially dangerous conditions that the physician must not miss on the initial assessment.

   A. **Tension headache**

      1. **Acute tension headache.** This is frequently described as a squeezing, "bandlike" tightness that is felt bilaterally and may occur in the occipital, frontal, or bitemporal regions. Occasionally, patients with tension headaches may describe a throbbing-type pain. This form of headache may last minutes to days. It is frequently precipitated by fatigue, emotional crisis, and stressful workloads.

      2. **Chronic tension headache.** This headache is similar to the acute tension headache in quality but its duration may be months or even years. Depression, personality problems, and a history of narcotic use frequently occur in these patients.

B. Migraine headache. Although the exact pathophysiology has not been fully ascertained, it is thought to be secondary to cerebral vasoconstriction followed by vasodilation. The initial vasoconstriction may be associated with a variety of neurologic deficits including visual disturbances (scotoma, zig-zag lines, bright lights), dysarthria, hemiparesis, and hemianesthesia. Of these, the visual phenomena are most common. These neurologic features generally last 5 to 30 minutes and are then followed by headache. The headache is usually pounding or throbbing but may be dull and boring. It is usually unilateral but may also occur bilaterally in any location. Anorexia, nausea, and vomiting are frequent. The attack may last several hours to 2 or 3 days and occasionally longer. Migraines are much more common in women. Three characteristic patterns of migraine are recognized:

1. **Common migraine.** This vascular headache is **not** preceded by neurologic deficits or visual disturbances. It is the most frequent type.
2. **Classic migraine.** Headache is preceded by visual deficits such as scotoma and field deficits.
3. **Complicated migraine.** In this form of migraine, the headache is accompanied by neurologic symptoms including hemiplegia and ophthalmoplegia.

C. Cluster headaches

1. These headaches are excruciating, usually unilateral, and frequently associated with ipsilateral nasal congestion, lacrimation, and conjunctival injection. Nausea and vomiting are unusual. Cluster headaches are not preceded by any neurologic symptoms.
2. Each headache typically lasts less than 2 hours; however, multiple attacks can occur within a 24-hour period.
3. Unlike migraine, cluster headaches most often affect men between the ages of 20 and 40.

D. Temporal arteritis

1. Temporal arteritis should be considered in any patient older than 50 years presenting with a recent history of headache.
2. Other symptoms such as malaise, weight loss, fever, and myalgias are frequently present. Jaw claudication may also occur.
3. It is especially important to ask the patient if he or she has experienced any new visual problems such as double or blurred vision. Temporal arteritis can cause sudden blindness as a result of inflammation of the ophthalmic artery.

E. Trigeminal neuralgia. This condition is more common in the elderly. The pain is described as brief but severe jabs of pain. Pain is usually unilateral and localized to one or more divisions of the trigeminal nerve. Precipitants include talking, chewing, or physical pressure exerted on a specific trigger area. Etiology is unknown.

F. Pseudotumor cerebri. This is an uncommon cause of headache usually seen in obese women. Etiology is believed to be impaired drainage of cerebral spinal fluid.

G. **Sinusitis**

1. Headache is usually dull, aching, and frontally located. Pain is frequently worse in the morning when the patient awakens but improves as the sinuses drain during the day.
2. If the patient displays an altered mental status or complains of a stiff neck, a complicated sinus infection should be suspected (brain abscess, meningitis, septic cavernous sinus thrombophlebitis).

H. **Eye disease.** Glaucoma, keratitis, and uveitis may all cause headaches. Pain is usually dull and located in the periorbital or retro-orbital regions.

I. **Dental disease**

1. Innervation of the teeth is by the second and third divisions of the trigeminal nerve; therefore, disease involving these structures may cause referred pain to the face or head. Secondary muscle spasm may result.
2. Temporomandibular joint disease may produce excessive muscle contraction and headache.

J. **Mass lesions.** Both neoplasm and brain abscess can produce headache as a result of either increased intracranial pressure or distension of local structures.

1. Any new neurologic deficit such as visual or motor loss or change in mental status should alert one to the possibility of a mass lesion.
2. The new onset of headache in a patient over the age of 50 suggests the possibility of a mass lesion.
3. Nonspecific features of headache resulting from a mass lesion include progressive worsening despite administration of analgesics, early-morning awakening because of headache, headache that is exacerbated by coughing or sneezing, and the presence of anorexia, nausea, and vomiting. It is important to note that these features also occur frequently with other types of headache, including chronic tension headache, migraine headache, cluster headache, and sinus headache.

K. **Subarachnoid hemorrhage.** The rupture of a cerebral aneurysm is associated with the acute onset of a violent headache. The patient may also quickly develop neurologic deficits or lose consciousness. Blood in the subarachnoid space may induce fever and nuchal rigidity, resembling acute meningitis. Sentinel leaks (warning leaks) from a cerebral aneurysm are more subtle and frequently precede subsequent rupture. These headaches may be difficult to distinguish from tension headaches and may cause nonspecific symptoms such as myalgias or a stiff neck which may be erroneously attributed to an acute viral illness.

L. Acute febrile illness

1. Fever may cause a vascular-type throbbing headache that remits as the illness resolves.
2. Any febrile patient in whom headache is a major complaint should also be suspected of having meningitis, especially if nuchal rigidity or other signs of meningeal irritation are present.

IV. Database

A. Physical examination key points

1. **Vital signs** (See Section II.B.)
2. **HEENT**
   - **a.** Patients with both migraine and chronic tension headaches frequently complain of scalp tenderness, which may also suggest temporal arteritis.
   - **b.** Palpate the temporal arteries. A diminished pulse or tender temporal arteries suggest arteritis; however, temporal arteries may feel normal to palpation in 30% to 40% of patients with temporal arteritis.
   - **c.** Examine the eyes for injected conjunctivae and excessive lacrimation which occur with cluster headaches. Examine the fundi for any signs of papilledema or optic nerve atrophy resulting from an intracerebral mass. Retinal hemorrhage may be observed after subarachnoid hemorrhage.
   - **d.** Palpate and/or percuss the maxillary and frontal sinuses for tenderness.
   - **e.** Examine the ears for any signs of otitis media.
   - **f.** Examine the dentition for painful teeth and the temporomandibular joint for any crepitus or pain.
3. **Neck.** Examine for any nuchal rigidity, which would suggest meningeal irritation from either subarachnoid hemorrhage or meningitis.
4. **Neurologic exam.** A detailed exam is mandated in any patient with a complaint of headache to identify localizing signs that would suggest a CNS mass lesion, meningitis, or intracerebral hemorrhage.

B. Laboratory data

1. **Complete blood count.** An elevated leukocyte count could suggest infection such as sinusitis or meningitis.
2. **Erythrocyte sedimentation rate (ESR).** Almost always greater than 50 mm/h in patients with temporal arteritis; however, on occasion the ESR may be normal. If clinical suspicion is high, a temporal artery biopsy should never be deferred simply because of a normal ESR.

C. Radiologic and other studies

1. **Sinus films.** Should be obtained if sinusitis is suspected.
2. **Head CT scan.** Should be obtained in any patient with a chronic headache pattern that has recently changed in frequency or

severity, in any patient over the age of 50 with a new onset of headache, or if the neurologic exam reveals any focal findings.

3. **Lumbar puncture.** If meningitis is suspected, lumbar puncture should be performed and not delayed for a CT scan when papilledema is absent and the neurologic examination is nonfocal.

V. Plan. The initial goal in the management of headache is to exclude the rare but potentially serious causes of headache such as brain tumor, subarachnoid hemorrhage, brain abscess, and meningitis. Once these conditions have been excluded, treatment can be directed according to the type of headache. Only the management of tension headache, migraine headache, and cluster headache is discussed here.

A. Acute tension headache

1. Typically resolves with removal of the inciting situation such as fatigue, emotional crisis, or stressful workload.
2. Relief can also be obtained by administration of aspirin or acetaminophen.

B. Chronic tension headache

1. This condition is notoriously difficult to manage. The physician must attempt to avoid the chronic use of narcotic analgesics which frequently results in narcotic dependence.
2. A tricyclic antidepressant such as amitriptyline (Elavil) 75 mg nightly is one of the most useful agents for treating chronic tension headache. This medication should be used regardless of whether depression is overtly present.
3. Nonsteroidal anti-inflammatory drugs (NSAIDs) such as aspirin 325–650 mg PO every 6 hours, indomethacin (Indocin) 25 mg PO TID, or ibuprofen (Motrin) 400–600 mg PO every 6 hours may also be beneficial.
4. If suboccipital or cervical muscle spasm is present, muscle relaxants such as cyclobenzaprine (Flexeril) 10 mg TID may be useful.
5. Psychotherapy and biofeedback may also be used in those patients who fail to respond to the preceding measures.

C. Migraine headache. A number of different medications can now be administered in the management of acute migraine.

1. **NSAIDs.** For an early, mild attack, treatment with a NSAID such as ibuprofen 400–600 mg every 4–6 hours or naproxen (Naprosyn) 500 mg every 12 hours may be effective.
2. **Ergotamine tartrate (Cafergot) 1 mg**
   a. Two tablets orally at the beginning of the headache followed by two tablets every 30 minutes to a maximum of six tablets in 24 hours. This medication should be used at the onset of headache rather than waiting for the headache to progress. Because gastric atony may occur during acute

migraine and thus impair absorption of orally administered drugs, some physicians also give metoclopramide (Reglan) 10 mg PO and repeat every 6 hours if needed.

  b. Dihydroergotamine 1 mg IV every 30 minutes for three doses can also be administered. This regimen is especially useful in patients whose headache has been present for several hours or who cannot tolerate oral drugs because of nausea.
  c. It is important to avoid administration of ergotamine in patients with peripheral vascular disease, coronary artery disease, hypertension, and hyperthyroidism, and in pregnant patients.

3. **Isometheptene 65 mg/dichloralphenazone 100 mg/acetaminophen 325 mg (Midrin).** Two capsules are given at the beginning of the headache followed by 1 capsule every hour to maximum of 5 capsules in 24 hours.
4. **Prochlorperazine (Compazine) 25 mg IV.** Some studies have indicated that this medication is just as effective as meperidine (Demerol) in achieving acute relief of migraine headache.
5. **Prednisone.** A few patients with a severe attack who fail to respond to the preceding measures may benefit from the administration of prednisone 60 mg PO daily for 3–4 days followed by rapid tapering.
6. **Prophylactic therapy.** A number of medications can be used for prophylaxis of migraine including propranolol (Inderal), amitriptyline (Elavil), and verapamil (Calan). These medications are less useful in the management of an acute attack of migraine and are not further discussed here.

D. Cluster headaches

1. Ergotamine is often effective in the treatment of cluster headaches and is administered in the same fashion as described for migraine headache.
2. Oxygen inhalation by face mask at 7 L/min for 15 minutes has been reported to be successful in aborting a cluster headache if administered early in the attack.
3. Prednisone is useful in the management of cluster headaches and is administered at a dose of 60 mg daily for 3–4 days followed by rapid tapering.

REFERENCES

Gordon B, Barker LR, Bleecker ML. Headaches and facial pain. In: Barker LR, Burton JR, Zieve PD, eds. *Principles of Ambulatory Medicine.* 2nd ed. Baltimore: Williams & Wilkins; 1986:810–824.

Kumar KL, Cooney TG. Vascular headache. *J Gen Intern Med* 1988;3:384–395.

Speed WG, McArthur JC. Headache. In: Harvey AM, Johns RJ, McKusick VA, et al, eds. *The Principles and Practice of Medicine.* 22nd ed. Norwalk, Conn: Appleton & Lange; 1988:1046–1052.

■ HEART MURMUR

I. **Problem.** You are asked to see a middle-aged man on the ward who "looks sick." The nursing staff notes a loud murmur.

II. **Immediate Questions**

A. **Is the murmur the problem itself, or is it a manifestation of some other underlying problem?** Acute aortic or mitral regurgitation from endocarditis or acute mitral regurgitation resulting from rupture of a papillary muscle after a myocardial infarction (MI) could explain the patient's condition. Underlying medical conditions such as a severe anemia, hyperthyroidism, and pregnancy can also have associated innocent flow murmurs related to increased cardiac output.

B. **Does the patient have known valvular disease?** Progression of valvular disease could be a likely cause of deterioration in a patient with a history of known valvular disease.

C. **Does the patient have known congenital heart disease?** In a patient with a history of a murmur, a bicuspid aortic valve, an atrial septal defect (ASD), a ventricular septal defect (VSD), a patent ductus arteriosus (PDA), and pulmonic stenosis (PS) should always be considered. Often, patients with mild PS or a small ASD will be asymptomatic.

D. **Has the deterioration been chronic or acute?** Acute decompensation would suggest an arrhythmia or ischemia, whereas chronic deterioration would suggest increasing left ventricular dysfunction in a patient with preexisting valvular disease.

E. **Is there a history of intravenous drug abuse, recent dental work, invasive procedures such as a sigmoidoscopy or cystoscopy, or a history of fever or chills?** These would suggest endocarditis.

F. **Does the patient have any chest pain?** It is important to characterize the chest pain. Chest pain is often seen with angina, aortic dissection, and pericarditis. Ischemic chest pain is a heavy, pressurelike sensation, usually not sharp; radiation to the jaw is very suggestive (radiation to the midscapular area of the back is not uncommon); shortness of breath, nausea, and diaphoresis often accompany the chest discomfort. A sharp, pleuritic, left anterior or substernal pain that improves with sitting up and leaning forward is consistent with pericarditis. A pericardial friction rub may be mistakenly identified as a murmur. Pain associated with dissection usually begins abruptly, reaches maximum intensity quickly, and is often continuous.

G. **Does the patient have coronary artery disease, and if so, is this the etiology of the murmur?** A recent MI with papillary muscle dysfunction or rupture may result in acute mitral regurgitation. An acute ventricular septal defect or free wall rupture following a MI may be present. Previously unrecognized aortic stenosis can also cause classic angina and may result in a myocardial infarction. Hypertrophic obstructive cardiomyopathy, also called idiopathic hypertrophic subaortic stenosis, and aortic dissection can cause angina.

III. Differential Diagnosis

A. Murmur aggravated by an underlying problem

1. **Flow murmur.** A flow murmur is aggravated by significant anemia and/or high-outflow congestive heart failure (CHF)..
2. **Congestive heart failure with "secondary" mitral regurgitation** can occur from a variety of possible etiologies.
3. **Murmur of aortic insufficiency in the face of possible aortic dissection.** In this setting, always consider an underlying connective tissue disorder such as Marfan's disease as well as severe hypertension.
4. **Noncardiac murmur.** A thyroid bruit, subclavian artery stenosis, venous hum, and pericardial or pleural friction rub can be mistaken for a cardiac murmur.
5. **A new murmur** with bacterial endocarditis is an ominous finding.

B. Coronary artery disease

1. **Acute ischemia/injury with papillary muscle dysfunction** can cause reversible mitral regurgitation.
2. **Recent myocardial infarction**
   a. **Acute severe mitral regurgitation secondary to a ruptured chordae tendineae or head of a papillary muscle**
   b. **Acute VSD**
   c. **Acute rupture of the ventricular wall**
3. **Acute ischemia.** Leading to immediate, severe left ventricular dysfunction with pulmonary edema and new or worsening mitral regurgitation.

C. Valvular heart disease

1. **Mitral valve prolapse with ruptured chordae/papillary muscle head and congestive heart failure.** Arrhythmias (ventricular or atrial) may occur leading to decompensation.
2. **Mitral stenosis.** New-onset atrial fibrillation can lead to decompensation.
3. **Aortic stenosis.** With progression may result in angina, left ventricular dysfunction, syncope, or arryhthmias (especially ventricular) leading to sudden death.
4. **Hypertrophic obstructive cardiomyopathy.** Arrhythmias, angina, and dyspnea are common. Sudden death can occur and is often related to exertion.
5. **Prosthetic valve dysfunction**
6. **Severe stenotic or regurgitation lesion on any valve (especially mitral or aortic)** may lead to left ventricular dysfunction.

D. Congenital heart disease

1. ASD/VSD with right-to-left shunt, Eisenmenger's physiology, and decompensation

2. New dysrhythmias in a patient with previously stable congenital defects

E. Myxoma. A rare cause of a murmur. Can present with CHF, chest pain, syncope, arrhythmias, or an embolic event.

IV. Database

A. Physical examination key points

1. General. Inability to lie flat suggests pulmonary edema or possibly pericarditis.

2. Vital signs

a. Temperature. Elevated temperature might indicate infection although postinfarct patients can have a moderate fever for up to a week.

b. Heart rate and rhythm. Tachycardia (See Tachycardia, p 241) is often associated with congestive heart failure, pain, infection, pericarditis, and perhaps dysrhythmias. Irregular rhythm may suggest the presence of atrial fibrillation or frequent premature atrial or ventricular beats as well as second-degree atrioventricular block.

c. Blood pressure. Hypertension or hypotension is often associated with angina or MI. Hypotension could reflect sepsis or hemodynamic collapse. Pulsus paradoxus (a difference of 10 mm Hg in systolic blood pressure between tidal inspiration and expiration) suggests tamponade in the face of acute free wall rupture.

d. Tachypnea. Suggests CHF.

3. Neck

a. Elevated jugular venous distension suggests right-sided or biventricular failure or pericardial tamponade.

b. A decrease in the carotid upstroke is seen in significant aortic stenosis. Also, the murmur of aortic stenosis radiates to the carotids bilaterally but should not be confused with bilateral carotid bruits, a venous hum, or a thyroid bruit.

4. Heart. Careful cardiac examination is essential. First (S_1) and second (S_2) heart sounds and splitting of S_2 must be characterized. The presence of a fourth heart sound may suggest a recent MI or long-standing hypertension. A third (S_3) heart sound is consistent with ventricular dysfunction.

a. Aortic insufficiency. A diastolic blowing murmur heard best at the right second intercostal space down to the left lower sternal border with the patient leaning forward in full expiration. This may be seen in the face of aortic dissection or acute bacterial endocarditis, or may be chronic and yet give a clue to the left ventricular dysfunction that is causing the patient's deterioration. The aortic component of S_2 may be soft or absent. The murmur of acute aortic insufficiency is usually soft in intensity and in duration, is heard best at the left lower sternal border, and can easily be missed.

b. **Aortic stenosis.** The murmur is crescendo-decrescendo and harsh and is heard best at the right second intercostal space. A diminished aortic component of S_2, palpable S_4, late-peaking of the murmur, a thrill, and delayed and diminished carotid upstroke suggest critical aortic stenosis.

c. **Mitral regurgitation.** Heard best as a blowing pansystolic murmur at the apex and radiating to the axilla, and occasionally into the midback. An intermittent murmur of mitral regurgitation might suggest intermittent papillary muscle dysfunction secondary to ischemia. The murmur of acute, severe mitral regurgitation may be short in duration and soft in intensity. Other findings suggestive of severity include an S_3 gallop, tachycardia, pulmonary rales, and signs of poor peripheral perfusion.

d. **Mitral valve prolapse.** A mid systolic click followed by a late systolic murmur suggests mitral valve prolapse. A click or murmur may be present together or singly.

e. **Mitral stenosis.** Heard best with the patient lying in left lateral decubitus position with the bell positioned over the apex. Mitral stenosis is often missed, particularly in a sick patient. It is always an important consideration and a confirmatory echocardiogram is usually indicated. An otherwise stable patient with mitral stenosis will decompensate quickly when atrial fibrillation develops. Control of the heart rate to permit adequate diastolic filling is imperative.

f. **Hypertrophic cardiomyopathy.** Characteristically causes a systolic murmur that might be confused with aortic stenosis, but actually represents left ventricular outflow track obstruction secondary to hypertrophy of the interventricular septum. The murmur is a crescendo-decrescendo systolic murmur that increases in intensity with the Valsalva maneuver and standing, and decreases in intensity with squatting. The murmur is best heard at the apex and left lower sternal border. An S_4 gallop is usually present. A bisferiens contour to the carotid pulse is characteristic (double peaking of the pulse). Again, a stable person with this can decompensate rapidly in the face of new atrial fibrillation.

g. **Atrial septal defect/ventricular septal defect.** Usually heard over the entire precordium and the murmur is both systole and diastole. An ASD murmur may be difficult to hear. Widely fixed splitting of S_2 is a clue to the presence of an ASD.

5. **Extremities.** Distal pulses—look for evidence of a pulse deficit that might suggest the presence of dissection or embolic phe-

nomenon. **Quincke's sign** is seen in chronic aortic insufficiency and is the to-and-fro movement seen in the capillary bed of the fingers when light pressure is applied to the distal finger tip.

6. **Neurologic exam.** Focal neurologic deficits suggest subacute bacterial endocarditis, myxoma, and thrombus formation with embolus.
7. **Skin.** Look for any evidence of intravenous drug use that might suggest the presence of bacterial endocarditis.

B. **Laboratory data.** Clearly, this would depend on the history and exam. The order in which laboratory data are acquired depends on the clinical picture at the bedside.

1. **Complete blood count with differential.** Anemia can be the cause of high-output congestive heart failure. A significantly elevated WBC count with an increase in the percentage of banded neutrophils may indicate the presence of an infectious process. An elevated WBC count may accompany an acute MI.
2. **Blood culture.** Should be obtained if there is any question of endocarditis. Three sets of two cultures should be obtained over several hours if the patient is stable. If the patient is unstable, at least one set of blood cultures should be obtained before any antibiotic therapy is initiated.
3. **Arterial blood gases.** Acidosis (see Acidosis, p 9) and hypoxia suggest the presence of significant left ventricular compromise and pulmonary congestion in the sick patient with a new murmur.
4. **Thyroid function tests, electrolytes including magnesium, renal function tests.** May provide clues as to the reason for decompensation in any particular patient.

C. **Radiologic and other studies**

1. **Electrocardiogram.** The most useful test to screen for ischemia, myocardial infarction, or dysrhythmia, particularly atrial fibrillation. Recall that the abrupt onset of atrial fibrillation in a person with compensated CHF, stable hypertrophic cardiomyopathy, or stable valvular disease may cause rapid decompensation.
2. **Chest x-ray.** The cardiac silhouette may give a clue to valvular disease. Increased vascularization, pleural effusion, Kerley A and B lines, and confluent alveolar densities are radiographic evidence of pulmonary edema. Other signs to look for are cardiac chamber enlargement and mediastinal widening.
3. **Echocardiogram.** In evaluating an acutely ill patient with a murmur that is not readily identified, the echocardiogram may be the single best source of information. It can accurately determine the presence and quantify the degree of valvular stenosis and regurgitation. The etiology of the valvular problem can also be suggested. Atrial and ventricular septal defects can be diagnosed.

4. **Swan-Ganz catheterization.** From a diagnostic standpoint, one can obtain right atrial and pulmonary artery blood samples to diagnose a stepup in oxygen saturation, confirming the diagnosis of acute VSD. Acute or severe mitral regurgitation can be suggested by the presence of a significant V wave in the pulmonary capillary wedge pressure tracing.

V. Plan. Treatment is generally aimed at the condition that is either causing the murmur (myocardial infarction, papillary muscle dysfunction, VSD, aortic insufficiency in the face of aortic root dissection) or aggravating the condition for which the murmur is an examination finding (hyperthyroidism, atrial fibrillation with mitral stenosis, hypertrophic obstructive cardiomyopathy, endocarditis, thrombus on a mechanical valve or anemia). While initiating therapy, consultation should be considered. When a patient is symptomatic from a cardiac murmur, a formal cardiology consult is appropriate.

A. Relieve angina. This can result in prompt improvement in the setting of recurrent pulmonary edema secondary to ischemia. (See Chest Pain, p 51.)

B. Maintain hemodynamic support

1. Dopamine can be used if an arterial vasoconstricting agent is needed. (See Hypotension, p 174.)
2. Dobutamine should be used if a positive inotropic drug is required.

C. Intensive care monitoring. Certain pathologic conditions may require arterial pressure monitoring (see Chapter 3, Arterial Line Placement, p 305) and/or continuous monitoring of right heart pressures and pulmonary wedge pressure (see Chapter 3, Pulmonary Artery Catheterization, p 336).

D. Treatment of acute myocardial infarction

1. **Pain relief with nitroglycerin, intravenous beta blockers, and morphine sulfate** (See Chest Pain, Section V, p 57, or Chapter 7, Commonly Used Medications, p 371, for doses.)
2. **Thrombolysis.** If indicated and if the patient is an appropriate candidate.

E. Treatment of suspected endocarditis. Initiate antibiotic therapy after obtaining four sets of blood cultures.

F. Arrange for invasive evaluation if warranted. The evaluation of an unknown heart murmur in a critically ill patient can be extremely complex. The basic goal is to determine the possible etiologies as quickly as possible. Emergent evaluation with an echocardiogram, aortic root contrast injection, or consultation may be indicated if the patient's condition is unstable.

■ HEMATEMESIS, MELENA

I. Problem. You are called to see a 39-year-old black male with lymphoma who is "vomiting blood."

II. Immediate Questions

- **A. What are the patient's vital signs?** This establishes hemodynamic stability. If the patient has tachycardia (pulse over 100) or hypotension (BP of 90 or less), immediate establishment of IV access and fluid resuscitation is required.
- **B. Does the patient have intravenous line access?** If not, ask the nurse to place an IV with D5 normal saline at a KVO rate with a 16- or 18-gauge needle.
- **C. Is there a history of peptic ulcer disease or esophageal varices?** A previous history of these disorders may indicate the etiology; however, in only 50% of patients with known esophageal varices can upper gastrointestinal bleeding be attributed to variceal bleeding.
- **D. Is the patient on any medications?** Review the drug history, taking note particularly of nonsteroidal anti-inflammatory drugs, steroids, and anticoagulants. Anticoagulants may unmask significant pathology.
- **E. Does the patient have a history of alcohol abuse?** This suggests gastritis or varices as the source of bleeding. Ethanol alone is not an etiologic factor for peptic ulcer disease. Cirrhotics have an increased incidence of duodenal ulcers.
- **G. Is there a previous hematocrit?** It will be important to establish a baseline with which to monitor the patient.
- **H. What is the volume of hematemesis?** Ask the nurse to save the emesis. This is important to establish the volume of hematemesis as well as to validate the presence of blood. A large amount indicates more urgency.
- **I. Has there been any melena or bright red blood per rectum?** Acute upper GI tract blood loss of about one unit results in melena and loss of two units may cause hematochezia.

III. Differential Diagnosis

- **A. Peptic ulcer disease.** Accounts for 40% to 50% of upper GI tract hemorrhages.
- **B. Esophageal varices.** Accounts for 10% to 15% of upper GI tract bleeding. Esophageal varices are associated with the highest morbidity and mortality of all causes of upper GI bleeding, with a 30% to 40% mortality rate. (See Hematochezia, p 121.)
- **C. Mallory-Weiss tear.** Causes approximately 15% of upper GI tract bleeding and is associated with recent alcohol intake in more than 70% of cases.
- **D. Acute hemorrhagic gastritis.** Accounts for 5% of community-acquired upper GI tract hemorrhage. It is much more common in patients who are in the ICU and is associated with stress (20% of septic ICU patients develop this complication). Often associated with alcohol or NSAID intake.
- **E. Carcinoma.** Accounts for approximately 1% to 2% of upper GI tract bleeding.

F. **Arterial enteric fistula.** Not a common cause of upper GI tract hemorrhage, but can be quite dramatic in presentation. Should be suspected in patients who have had aortic bypass graft surgery.

IV. Database

A. Physical examination key points

1. **Vital signs.** Recheck vital signs including orthostatic blood pressure and heart rate. Orthostatic changes are a decrease in systolic blood pressure of 10 mm Hg and/or an increase in heart rate of 20 per minute 1 minute after movement from the supine to the standing position.
2. **Skin.** Spider telangiectasia, palmar erythema, and jaundice indicates underlying cirrhosis and possible varices. Poor skin turgor and absent axillary sweat may indicate volume depletion.
3. **Chest.** Gynecomastia suggests cirrhosis.
4. **Eyes.** Scleral icterus suggests chronic liver disease.
5. **Abdomen.** Examine for tenderness or masses. Look for evidence of chronic liver disease such as ascites and hepatomegaly.
6. **Genitourinary system.** Perform a rectal examination looking for melena. Testicular atrophy may be secondary to cirrhosis/chronic liver disease and may point to varices as an etiology of the bleeding.

B. Laboratory data

1. **Stat complete blood count.** This can be done by phlebotomy before your arrival if available.
2. **Type and cross-match.**
3. **A large-bore Ewald or Edlich tube with gastric lavage.** It is essential for accurate diagnosis. The possibility of varices is **not** a contraindication to this procedure.
4. **Hematocrit.** Serial hematocrits are helpful, but do not always reflect the amount of blood loss as equilibration with extravascular fluid may take several hours.
5. **Blood urea nitrogen and creatinine.** A significant increase in the BUN or an elevated BUN-to-creatinine ratio may indicate blood in the GI tract.
6. **Clotting studies.** Knowledge of a coagulation disorder is essential in the treatment of the patient.
7. **Platelet count.** If a lesion is present thrombocytopenia could cause a significant bleed as well as make it difficult to stop the bleeding.

C. Radiologic and other studies.

The source of bleeding must be identified so specific therapy can be instituted.

1. **Upper GI endoscopy.** This is the cornerstone of diagnosis of upper GI tract bleeding. Removal of blood and clots from the stomach and duodenum is essential for accurate diagnosis.
   - **a.** The timing of upper GI endoscopy is not well established.

Most gastroenterologists believe that upper GI endoscopy should be performed within 24 hours of the patient's presentation. Emergent endoscopy is indicated if it will change the treatment plan.

b. The most common situation is a patient with known alcoholic liver disease and upper GI tract bleeding. These patients are at risk for peptic ulcer disease in addition to rebleeding from esophageal varices. As the therapy for these two entities is quite different, emergent upper GI endoscopy is generally indicated.

2. **Colonoscopy.** Should be done if the upper GI endoscopy is entirely negative and the patient has melena. To rule out a right-sided colon lesion which can be associated with melena.
3. **Technetium-labeled bleeding scan.** Should be done if the upper GI endoscopy and colonoscopy are negative.

V. Plan

A. Monitoring. The first step in the management is to determine whether the patient should be monitored in an ICU. The following are indications for monitoring in an intensive care unit overnight.

1. Anyone with frank hematemesis that is clearly documented
2. Anyone with coffee-ground emesis **and** either melena or bright red blood per rectum
3. Anyone with hemodynamic instability, either hypotension or orthostatic hypotension
4. Anyone with a greater than 5-point drop in hematocrit
5. Anyone with a significant unexplained increase in the BUN where GI bleeding is suspected

B. Volume resuscitation. If massive bleeding is evident, place two large-bore (14- or 16-gauge) lines. Begin IV fluids containing normal saline at a rate to maintain hemodynamic stability. Transfuse packed red cells when available with massive bleeding.

C. Surgical consult. Essential in the management of upper GI tract hemorrhage. Should be obtained within the first few hours of the patient's arrival.

D. Specific treatment. The management of various sources of upper GI tract hemorrhage is dependent on the diagnosis.

1. **Peptic ulcer disease.** Acid reduction therapy with any H_2 antagonist prior to esophagogastroduodenoscopy (EGD) and both antacids and H_2 receptor antagonists after EGD. Cimetidine (Tagamet) 300 mg IV every 6 hours or rantidine (Zantac) 50 mg IV every 6–8 hours is the standard. Both can be given as continuous drips.
2. **Acute hemorrhagic gastritis.** Acid reduction therapy. (See Section V.D.1.)
3. **Mallory-Weiss tear.** Antireflux precautions and acid therapy reduction. (See Section V.D.1.)
4. **Esophageal varices.** Vasopressin beginning at a dose of 0.1–

0.2 U/min up to 0.5–0.6 U/min along with nitropaste 1 in. every 6 hours. If bleeding continues, then a Blakemore tube needs to be placed.

5. In patients in the ICU, nasogastric tubes are necessary for monitoring bleeding and gastric pH. Maintenance of a pH of 4–4.5 is desirable.

REFERENCE

Peterson WL. Gastrointestinal bleeding. In: Sleisinger MH, Fortran JS, eds. *Gastrointestinal Disease.* 4th ed. Philadelphia: WB Saunders; 1989:397–427.

■ HEMATOCHEZIA

I. **Problem.** You are called to see a 58-year-old white man who has been under your care for the last 3 days for exacerbation of chronic obstructive pulmonary disease. The nurse calls you and tells you that the patient has just passed a bloody bowel movement.

II. **Immediate Questions**

A. **What are the patient's vital signs?** Establish hemodynamic stability. If the patient has tachycardia (pulse greater than 100) or hypotension (blood pressure 90 or less), you need to go to the patient's bedside immediately.

B. **Does the patient have intravenous line access?** If not, ask the nurse to place an intravenous (IV) with D5 normal saline at a KVO rate with a 16- or 18-gauge needle.

C. **Is there a history of gastrointestinal tract bleeding?** If so, determine the nature of the previous bleeding. Ask about a history of diseases associated with GI tract bleeding such as diverticular disease, polyps or carcinoma, inflammatory bowel disease, hemorrhoids, and other anal diseases.

D. **What medications is the patient taking?** Specifically, steroids, nonsteroidal anti-inflammatory drugs, and anticoagulants.

E. **Does the patient have a history of alcohol abuse?** This suggests an upper GI source of bleeding such as varices or gastritis.

F. **What is the most recent hematocrit?** Find out from the chart the most recent hematocrit. This will establish the baseline value with which to compare the complete blood count you will be obtaining.

G. **What is the volume of bright red blood per rectum?** Ask the nurse to save the specimen or specimens for your review. This is important for establishing the presence and volume of blood loss. A large volume of blood suggests immediate action.

H. **Has there been hematemesis?** Acute upper GI blood loss may result in hematochezia.

III. **Differential Diagnosis**

A. **Hemorrhoids.** Usually not a source of hemodynamically significant bleeding but can be significant in patients with portal hypertension. Causes 98% of all lower GI tract bleeding, most of which is not significant or brought to the attention of a physician.

B. **Diverticular disease.** Most common etiology for significant lower GI bleeding, causing up to 70% of cases.

C. **Angiodysplasia.** Much more common in the elderly, causing approximately 10% of significant lower GI bleeding.

D. **Upper GI bleed** (See Hematemesis, Melena, p 117.) Remember that upper GI bleeding can present as bright red blood per rectum 5% of the time. Indicates at least an acute two-unit bleed and is virtually always associated with hemodynamic instability.

E. **Neoplasia including carcinoma and polyps.** Causes 3% of **significant** lower GI tract bleeding.

F. **Inflammatory bowel disease.** Infrequent cause of significant lower GI tract bleeding. But when bleeding is the initial symptom, think of ulcerative colitis.

G. **Ischemic colitis.** Unusual cause of lower GI tract bleeding. Think of this when the patient has abdominal bruits or peripheral vascular disease with a history of abdominal operations for vascular disease.

IV. Database

A. Physical examination key points

1. **Vital signs.** Including orthostatic blood pressure.
2. **Skin.** Telangiectasias or melanotic lesions on palms or soles suggest Osler-Weber-Rendu disease and Peutz-Jeghers syndrome, respectively.
3. **HEENT.** Vascular malformations on lips or buccal mucosa suggest angiodysplasia or Osler-Weber-Rendu disease.
4. **Heart.** Aortic stenosis is associated with angiodysplasia.
5. **Abdomen.** Bruits may point to ischemic colitis. Hyperactive bowel sounds may indicate blood in the upper GI tract. Check for masses or tenderness.
6. **Rectum.** Check for hemorrhoids and also to document blood in the rectal vault.

B. Laboratory data

1. **Nasogastric tube placement.** Obtain a quick aspirate looking for coffee-ground material (testing for occult blood confirms the presence of bleeding and is not performed if coffee-ground material is not aspirated).
2. **Stat complete blood count and type and cross match.** This can be done before you arrive if phlebotomy is available.
3. **Serial hematocrits.** Helpful but do not always reflect the amount of blood loss as equilibration with extravascular fluid may take several hours. Changes in the indices may also be helpful in differentiating acute from chronic bleeding.

5. **Platelet count.** Thrombocytopenia could interfere with stabilization of the patient.

C. Radiologic and other studies

1. **Proctoscopy.** Very easy test that can document the presence of blood or melena and frequently leads to diagnosis.
2. **Anoscopy.** Look for bleeding hemorrhoids.
3. **Upper GI endoscopy.** Must rule out an upper GI source prior to surgery. Ten percent of upper GI bleeds will have a negative nasogastric aspirate.
4. **Technetium-labeled bleeding scan.** Can detect very slow bleeding (0.5 mL/min). Localization is only fair and needs to be documented with endoscopy or angiography.
5. **Angiography.** Localization is very good but patients must be bleeding fairly briskly (2 mL/min) to detect site. Can also give intra-arterial pitressin therapeutically.

V. Plan

A. Monitoring. The first step in the management is to determine whether the patient should be monitored in an ICU. The following are indications that the patient be transferred to an ICU for overnight observation.

1. Anyone who has more than 100 mL of bright red blood per rectum
2. Anyone with a positive nasogastric aspirate for coffee-ground material and bright red blood per rectum
3. Anyone with an unexplained increase in BUN
4. Anyone with a greater than 5-point drop in hematocrit on CBC
5. Anyone with hypotension on initial examination or orthostatic hypotension

B. Volume resuscitation. If massive bleeding is evident, place two large-bore (14- or 16-gauge) peripheral or central lines. Begin IV fluids containing normal saline at a rate to maintain hemodynamic stability. Transfuse packed red cells when available with massive bleeding.

C. Surgical consult. Contact early in the management, especially if brisk bleeding is encountered.

D. Establish source of bleeding. The source of bleeding must be identified so specific therapy can be instituted.

1. If bleeding is brisk and the nasogastric aspirate negative, start with proctoscopy and anoscopy. If negative, proceed to upper GI endoscopy. If bleeding slows, proceed to colonoscopy; if not, proceed to technetium-labeled bleeding scan with follow-up angiography (can proceed directly to angiography if very brisk). If bleeding site is found on angiography, vasopressin can be given. If this fails to stop bleeding or if bleeding site cannot be found and bleeding continues, then patient will require exploratory laparotomy.
2. If the bleeding has stopped and the nasogastric aspirate is negative, proceed first with proctoscopy and anoscopy. If negative, observe the patient for 48 hours with no procedures.

If the patient rebleeds, do an endoscopy followed by colonoscopy or angiography. If the colonoscopy is negative, do an upper GI endoscopy and then angiography. Remember, at any point, if the patient becomes unstable and difficult to stabilize with IV fluids and blood, surgery is indicated.

3. Remember that the tempo of the evaluation is dictated by the tempo of the patient's bleeding and overall stability.

REFERENCE

Peterson WL. Gastrointestinal bleeding. In: Sleisinger MH, Fortran JS, eds. *Gastrointestinal Disease.* 4th ed. Philadelphia: WB Saunders; 1989:397–427.

■ HEMATURIA

I. Problem. A 51-year-old male patient has red blood cells noted on urinalysis 3 days after undergoing a total hip replacement.

II. Immediate Questions

A. Is there a history of gross hematuria? Microscopic hematuria may have been present for a long time without the patient's being aware of it, suggesting a chronic or acute process. Gross hematuria will not have gone unnoticed by the patient and likely represents an acute process.

B. Does the patient have a Foley catheter in place? Irritation of the bladder mucosa by a Foley catheter is a common cause of hematuria, as are trauma during placement and manipulation of the catheter by the patient. Other causes should be investigated if the hematuria does not completely clear after removal of the catheter.

C. Has the patient had recent abdominal surgery? This always raises the question of an inadvertently nicked ureter or kidney, and would usually be apparent by the night of surgery.

D. Does the patient have abdominal pain or fever? Abdominal pain may suggest an inflammatory or infectious cause. Colicky pain radiating from the flank to the groin suggests a renal stone. Infection is often accompanied by fever.

E. Has there been a significant change in urine output? A sudden decrease in urine output may indicate acute oliguric renal failure, obstruction, or renal vein thrombosis. (See Oliguria/Anuria, p 213.)

F. Does the patient have symptoms suggestive of urinary tract infection? Dysuria, frequency, and urgency are common symptoms associated with urinary tract infections.

G. Is the patient on anticoagulants? Anticoagulation may cause hematuria by unmasking significant urinary tract pathology.

H. **Has the patient been treated with antineoplastic agents such as cyclophosphamide (Cytoxan)?** These patients are at risk for developing hemorrhagic cystitis or secondary genitourinary tract tumors.

III. Differential Diagnosis

A. Blood

1. **Coagulopathy** (See Coagulopathy, p 60.) Inheritable defects such as hemophilia, severe liver dysfunction, and pharmacologic anticoagulation are potential etiologies.
2. **Hemoglobinopathy.** Sickle cell disease with crisis is frequently associated with gross hematuria.

B. Kidneys

1. **Glomerular disease**
   a. **Primary.** Poststreptococcal glomerulonephritis, IgA nephropathy, Goodpasture's syndrome, idiopathic rapidly progressive glomerulonephritis. Characterized by red cell casts.
   b. **Secondary.** Vasculitis associated with systemic lupus erythematosus, scleroderma, Wegener's granulomatosis, polyarteritis, hypersensitivity vasculitis, subacute bacterial endocarditis.
   c. **Hereditary.** Alport's syndrome associated with sensorineural hearing loss and ocular abnormalities.
2. **Interstitial disease**
   a. **Consequence of systemic diseases.** Diabetic nephrosclerosis, accelerated hypertension, systemic lupus erythematosus.
   b. **Consequence of pharmacologic therapy.** Analgesic nephropathy, heavy metals, heroin nephropathy.
3. **Infections**
   a. **Pyelonephritis**
   b. **Tuberculosis.** Characterized by sterile pyuria.
4. **Malformations**
   a. **Cystic.** Familial polycystic kidney disease, ruptured solitary cysts, medullary sponge kidney.
   b. **Vascular.** Suggested by findings of hemangiomas or telangiectasias elsewhere.
5. **Neoplasms.** Particularly renal cell carcinoma and more rarely transitional cell carcinoma.
6. **Ischemia**
   a. **Embolism.** Aortic atherosclerosis, cardiac arrhythmias, manipulation of the aorta (aortography, coronary angiography).
   b. **Thrombosis.** Nephrotic syndrome, neoplastic disease, coagulation disorders (antithrombin III, protein C, or protein S deficiencies).

7. **Trauma**

C. **Postrenal**

1. **Mechanical**
   a. **Kidney stones.** Nephrolithiasis and urolithiasis.
   b. **Obstruction.** Prostatic hypertrophy, mass effect, posterior urethral valves, retroperitoneal fibrosis, ureteropelvic junction abnormalities.
2. **Inflammatory.** Infection or regional inflammation.
   a. **Periureteritis.** Diverticulitis, pelvic inflammatory disease.
   b. **Cystitis.** Infectious or inflammatory such as cyclophosphamide-induced hematuria, which is a medical emergency.
   c. **Prostatitis**
   d. **Urethritis**
3. **Neoplasm.** Transitional cell carcinoma, adenocarcinoma of the prostate, squamous cell carcinoma of the penis.
4. **Exercise.** Especially marathon runners.

D. **False hematuria**

1. **Vaginal/rectal bleeding**
2. **Factitious.** Especially in patients demonstrating drug-seeking behavior and requesting narcotics for renal stones.

IV. **Database**

A. **Physical examination key points**

1. **Abdomen.** Examine for palpable masses indicative of tumors, polycystic kidneys, or diverticular abscess. Tenderness will accompany infection, infarction, sickle cell crisis, inflammatory processes, and obstruction.
2. **Urethral meatus.** Look for gross blood, especially in trauma patients, and evidence of recent instrumentation or superficial lesions.
3. **Rectum.** Critical in the trauma patient when a "free-floating" prostate may be found, signifying urethral disruption. More commonly, prostatitis or prostatic carcinoma is uncovered. Attention should also be given to possible hemorrhoids.
4. **Pelvis.** Look for another source of bleeding such as vaginitis, cervicitis, and menorrhagia.
5. **Skin.** Ecchymoses, petechiae, and rash are suggestive of vasculitis or a coagulation disorder.

B. **Laboratory data**

1. **Urinalysis.** Red cell casts are seen only with glomerulonephritis. White blood cells and/or bacteria suggest an infectious cause; WBC casts suggest pyelonephritis. Crystals may be seen in association with stones. Red discoloration without cells should suggest myoglobinuria and a urine myoglobin should be checked.
2. **Coagulation studies.** Prothrombin time, partial thromboplastin time, platelets.

3. **Hemogram.** An elevated WBC count will suggest an infectious or inflammatory process. A microcytic anemia may suggest chronic blood loss; however, hematuria is an unusual cause of microcytic anemia.
4. **Urine culture.** Rule out bacterial infection. Cultures for acid-fast bacilli should be done if there is pyuria and bacteria cultures are sterile off antibiotics. An acid-fast stain may be helpful; however, some common saprophytes are acid-fast staining.
5. **Blood urea nitrogen and creatinine.** To be used as baseline evaluation of renal function or to assess any change in renal function.
6. **Sickle cell screen.** Useful if the status of the patient was previously unknown and this is being entertained as a cause of the patient's hematuria.
7. **Urinary cytology.** May diagnose transitional cell carcinoma.

C. **Radiologic and other studies**

1. **Abdominal plain x-ray (kidney/ureter/bladder [KUB]).** Eighty percent of the urinary calculi are radiodense. Also, the KUB may show an inflammatory process (ileus or loss of psoas shadow).
2. **Excretory urography (intravenous pyelography).** A part of the evaluation in all patients without an active infection who can receive intravenous contrast without undue risk.
3. **Retrograde urethrogram/cystogram.** Second-line study to be used in cases where tumor, vesicoureteral reflux, posterior urethral valves, or traumatic disruption is suspected.
4. **Further studies.** Should be directed by clinical suspicion and the results of initial studies. May include a CT scan of the abdomen, ultrasound, angiography, and cystoscopy.

V. **Plan.** Treatment is dependent on the etiology. It is important to remember that other than trauma, severe coagulopathy, and cyclophosphamide-induced hematuria, the causes of hematuria are rarely emergencies and a thoughtful and careful evaluation can be pursued over a period of several days.

A. **Urinary tract infection** (See Dysuria, Section V, p 97.) The infection must be eradicated and then a repeat urinalysis performed to rule out continued hematuria. If hematuria persists, further evaluation must be carried out.

B. **Urolithiasis.** If the stone is expected to pass spontaneously and there are no complicating factors (infection, obstruction), expectant therapy with analgesics and hydration is appropriate. The urine should be strained.

C. **Neoplasms.** Further workup is dictated by the type and location.

D. **Tuberculosis.** Treat appropriately with antibiotics. Initial therapy is usually with isoniazid 300 mg PO every day, rifampin 600 mg PO every day, and pyrazinamide 15–30 mg/kg with a maximum dose of 2 g per day. After 2 months, the pyrazinamide is discontinued. Long-term follow-up with intravenous pyelograms is needed as strictures are late sequalae and can lead to obstruction.

E. **Collecting system abnormality.** Usually requires surgical referral and repair.

F. **Coagulopathy.** Correct clotting factor deficiencies or adjust anticoagulant dose. Frequently the coagulopathy will induce bleeding from a preexisting abnormality. A thorough evaluation is usually indicated in a patient who has hematuria and a coagulopathy.

G. **Glomerulonephritis.** Most cases require a biopsy for definitive diagnosis, with therapy as appropriate for the underlying illness.

H. **Hemorrhagic cystitis.** Treated with continuous saline irrigation and occasionally a 1% alum irrigation.

REFERENCES

Copley JB. Isolated asymptomatic hematuria in the adult. *Am J Med Sci* 1986;291:101–111.

Finney J, Baum N. Evaluation of hematuria. *Postgrad Med* 1989;85:44–53.

■ HEMOPTYSIS

I. **Problem.** A 60-year-old male smoker comes to the emergency room complaining of "spitting up blood" for 1 week.

II. **Immediate Questions**

A. **Is the patient truly experiencing hemoptysis?** Blood from a nasal, oral, or gastric source may be aspirated to the larynx and then expectorated.

B. **What is the volume of the hemoptysis?** Massive hemoptysis (> 600 mL/24 h) connotes a life-threatening problem that demands immediate ICU admission as well as a rapid diagnostic evaluation.

C. **Has this happened before? If so, how frequently?** Patients with recurrent acute bronchitis episodes or with mitral stenosis may have had multiple episodes of minor hemoptysis.

D. **What is the smoking history?** The higher the pack-years, the more likely the patient has chronic bronchitis and/or bronchogenic carcinoma.

E. **Is there a history of productive cough preceding the hemoptysis?** If the answer is yes, then the problem may be an infection such as acute bronchitis.

F. **Has there been any accompanying chest pain?** Pleuritic chest pain may be a symptom of pneumonia or a pulmonary embolism with infarction. Angina may indicate myocardial infarction. Hemoptysis may accompany pulmonary edema from any number of causes.

III. **Differential Diagnosis**

A. **Pulmonary sources**

1. **Infection**

- a. **Acute or chronic bronchitis.** Most common cause of hemoptysis.
- b. **Pneumonia.** A necrotizing gram-negative or staphylococcal pneumonia is the usual type of pneumonia to have associated hemoptysis. Symptoms are acute.
- c. **Lung abscess.** Often foul-smelling sputum.
- d. **Bronchiectasis.** Think of this in the patient who has had recurrent episodes of respiratory infections, voluminous sputum production, and intermittent hemoptysis.
- e. **Tuberculosis.** Usually apical infiltrates on chest x-ray. Symptoms often chronic or subacute.
- f. **Mycetoma (fungus ball).** A ball of Aspergillus fungus may form in a cavity formed previously. Look for the "crescent sign" on the chest x-ray.

2. **Neoplasm**
   - a. **Bronchogenic carcinoma.** Usually the CXR is abnormal but it may be normal in up to 13% of patients with early lung cancer and hemoptysis. You cannot afford to miss it!
   - b. **Bronchial adenoma**
   - c. **Metastatic disease.** A history of preceding cancers should be uncovered during the history and physical. The chest x-ray will be abnormal.
3. **Vascular**
   - a. **Pulmonary embolism (PE) with infarction.** Only 10% of PEs present with hemoptysis but pulmonary emboli are very common and must not be missed.
   - b. **Mitral stenosis.** May arise either from rupture of the pulmonary veins or from frank pulmonary edema.
   - c. **Cardiogenic pulmonary edema.** Surprisingly common, especially now that most cardiac patients are on some form of anticoagulation.
   - d. **Arteriovenous malformation**

B. Trauma

1. **Pulmonary contusion**
2. **Bronchial or vascular tear**
3. **Retained foreign body.** Teeth and fillings have a way of finding their way down into the bronchi!

C. Systemic diseases

1. **Anticoagulation**
   - a. **Drugs.** Warfarin (Coumadin), heparin, aspirin, streptokinase (Streptase), urokinase (Abbokinase), tissue plasminogen activator (TPA).
   - b. **Uremia**
   - c. **Thrombocytopenia.** Drugs, idiopathic thrombocytopenic purpura.
   - d. **Disseminated intravascular coagulation**
   - e. **Liver disease.** Severe liver disease can result in thrombocytopenia and decreased production of coagulation factors.

2. **Autoimmune diseases**
   a. **Wegener's granulomatosis.** Look for renal changes (red cell casts, hematuria, proteinuria) and/or sinus disease. The CXR often is abnormal. Bilateral nodular densities and cavitation are common.
   b. **Goodpasture's syndrome.** This disease also involves the kidney. Proteinuria, hematuria, and red cell casts may be present. Diffuse alveolar infiltrates are often present.
   c. **Systemic lupus erythematosus (SLE).** Lupus more frequently involves the pleura but patients may develop life-threatening hemoptysis from lupus pneumonitis.

IV. Database

A. Physical examination key points

1. **Vital signs.** Imperative! Look particularly for fever and signs of impending respiratory failure: breath rate above 30 per minute, abdominal paradox with inspiration, accessory muscle use.
2. **HEENT.** Look carefully for a nasal or oropharyngeal source of bleeding.
3. **Chest.** Inspect and palpate for signs of trauma such as rib or clavicle fractures. Listen carefully for a pleural rub, localized rales, or signs of consolidation.
4. **Heart.** An irregularly irregular pulse signifies atrial fibrillation and suggests mitral stenosis or a possible source of emboli. An S_3 and jugular venous distension suggest congestive heart failure as a possible etiology. Always listen carefully for the low diastolic rumble of mitral stenosis.
5. **Abdomen.** Palpate the epigastrium, liver, and spleen carefully. Peptic ulcer disease or alcoholic liver disease could certainly cause GI bleeding, which might mimic hemoptysis.
6. **Extremities.** Examine lower extremities carefully for signs of deep venous thromboses or edema. Look carefully for cyanosis and clubbing. Clubbed fingers associated with hemoptysis would generally implicate either bronchiectasis or a pulmonary neoplasm.
7. **Skin.** Inspect the skin for petechiae, ecchymoses, angiomata, and rashes.

B. Laboratory data

1. **Complete blood count.** May reveal an anemia which could be caused by the hemoptysis or, more likely, is related to the hemoptysis. A normocytic anemia with a normal or low reticulocyte count may represent anemia of chronic disease possibly related to cancer. An elevated reticulocyte count indicates a hemolytic anemia possibly secondary to SLE. An iron deficiency may indicate Goodpasture's syndrome.
2. **Platelet count, prothrombin time, and partial thromboplastin time.** All are indicated to rule out coagulopathy as a cause. (See Coagulopathy, p 60.) If platelet dysfunction is sus-

pected, a bleeding time will be prolonged in the presence of a normal platelet count.

3. **Blood urea nitrogen, creatinine, and urinalysis.** For rapid evaluation of "pulmonary-renal" syndromes (Goodpasture's syndrome, Wegener's granulomatosis, SLE, and vasculitis).
4. **Arterial blood gases.** Check for adequate ventilation and oxygenation. Most of these patients already have underlying pulmonary disease and may develop respiratory failure at the time of their hemoptysis.
5. **Sputum examination.** Gram stain, acid-fast bacillus stain and culture, and cytology are all imperative.
6. **PPD skin test.** May also need an anergy screen. To help rule out tuberculosis and evaluate immune function.

C. Radiologic and other studies

1. **Chest x-ray.** First and most important test after history and physical. The pattern and location of any infiltrate coupled with the history and physical information will dictate the remainder of your workup.
2. **Ventilation/perfusion ($\dot{V}/\dot{Q}$) lung scan.** If pulmonary embolism is highly suspected, a $\dot{V}/\dot{Q}$ scan must be done.
3. **Angiography.** If pulmonary embolism is suspected and $\dot{V}/\dot{Q}$ scans are not clearly positive or negative, then pulmonary angiography is indicated. Angiography may also be indicated for the diagnosis of pulmonary arteriovenous malformations.
4. **Chest computerized tomography scan.** This will provide a much better anatomic view of pulmonary pathology compared with chest radiographs and will also reveal lesions not seen previously; however, the CT scan is only indicated acutely when looking for an aortic dissection.
5. **Electrocardiogram.** May indicate myocardial infarction. An axis change and/or right bundle branch block may suggest a PE. Classically, a PE produces an S wave in lead I and a Q wave and inverted T wave in lead III (S_1–Q_3T_3).
6. **Bronchoscopy.** Patients with unclear sources of hemoptysis, massive hemoptysis, or the suspicion of a neoplasm require fiberoptic bronchoscopy. The earlier it is done, the more likely the source of bleeding will be identified.

V. Plan

A. Intensive care unit

1. **Massive hemoptysis**
2. **Present or pending hypoxemic or hypercarbic respiratory failure**

B. Establish intravenous access. Death comes from asphyxia rather than hemorrhage but IV medications will be needed.

C. Always protect the airway. This may require early intubation.

D. Correct any coagulapathy (See Coagulopathy, Section V, p 63.)

E. **Fiberoptic bronchoscopy.** Arrange for this early if the diagnosis is in doubt or hemoptysis continues.
F. **Consult.** Obtain a thoracic surgery consultation if the patient has massive or continuous hemoptysis. Medical management of massive hemoptysis is associated with a high mortality rate.
G. **Cough suppression.** Retard the cough reflex with codeine-based drugs and place the patient on quiet bedrest.
H. **Treat the underlying disease state**
   1. Lung cancer can be treated surgically if there are no metastases and the pulmonary reserve is adequate. Otherwise, radiation or laser therapy can rapidly control bleeding.
   2. Treat infections with antibiotics as dictated by the gram stain and clinical picture.
   3. Treat pulmonary emboli acutely with heparin.

REFERENCE

Greenberger NJ, et al. *The Medical Book of Lists: A Primer of Differential Diagnosis in Internal Medicine.* Chicago: Yearbook Medical Publishers; 1983:169.

■ HYPERCALCEMIA

I. **Problem.** A 60-year-old man is admitted for severe back pain and is found to have a calcium of 5.5 mEq/L or 2.75 mmol/L (normal: 4.2–5.1 mEq/L or 2.10–2.55 mmol/L).

II. **Immediate Questions**

A. **What other symptoms are present?** Classic history for primary hyperparathyroidism is "stones, bones, moans, and groans" from renal calculi, osteitis fibrosa, constipation, and neuropsychiatric problems, respectively. Renal calculi and osteitis fibrosa are seldom associated with hypercalcemia of malignancy because both result from long-standing hypercalcemia. Hypercalcemia causes a variety of nonspecific symptoms including polyuria, polydypsia, constipation, nausea, vomiting, anorexia, and mental status changes which can range from confusion to coma. There may also be associated bone pain.

B. **Does the patient have any condition that could be related to hypercalcemia?** Hypertension, peptic ulcer, and nephrolithiasis are associated with hyperparathyroidism.

C. **Is the patient on any medications that could cause hypercalcemia?** Thiazide diuretics, vitamin D, and exogenous sources of calcium are possible causes.

D. **Is there a family history of hypercalcemia?** An unusual cause is familial hypocalciuric hypercalcemia. Also, there are three syndromes of multiple endocrine neoplasia (MEN) that are inherited in an autosomal dominant pattern. MEN I includes primary hyperparathyroidism and hypersecretion of pancreatic islet hormones and possibly other endocrine tumors. MEN II consists of primary hyperparathyroidism and medullary carcinoma of the thyroid. MEN III includes features of MEN II along with pheochromocytoma.

E. **Has the patient been noted to have elevated calcium in the past?** Long-standing hypercalcemia suggests primary hyperparathyroidism. Recent-onset hypercalcemia would suggest another condition such as malignancy.

III. Differential Diagnosis

A. **Primary hyperparathyroidism.** About 20% of patients with hypercalcemia will have hyperparathyroidism. Usually from a single hyperfunctioning adenoma. Characteristically, an elevated calcium, a low phosphate, and elevated or relatively elevated parathyroid hormone.

B. **Malignancy.** From bony metastasis or more often from a humoral factor produced by a tumor.
   1. **Metastatic carcinoma to bone.** Breast, lung, and renal cell carcinoma.
   2. **Hematologic malignancies.** Direct bone involvement with multiple myeloma and lymphoma.
   3. **Humoral factors.** Prostaglandins, parathyroid hormone–like substance, and osteoclast-activating factor (OAF). Most commonly seen with squamous cell, renal cell, transitional cell carcinoma, and multiple myeloma.

C. **Medications**
   1. **Thiazide diuretics.** Increase renal reabsorption of calcium.
   2. **Vitamin D intoxication.** A fat-soluble vitamin that increases intestinal absorption, increases mobilization from bone, and increases renal reabsorption of calcium.
   3. **Vitamin A intoxication.** Another fat soluble vitamin that is a rare cause of hypercalcemia. Causes increased bone reabsorption.
   4. **Exogenous calcium.** Calcium carbonate such as in certain antacids.

D. **Granulomatous diseases—Sarcoidosis.** Increased sensitivity to vitamin D.

E. **Milk-alkali syndrome.** From increased intake of calcium and alkali. Results in hypercalcemia, hypocalciuria, hyperphosphatemia, renal failure, and metastatic calcifications.

F. **Immobilization.** Prolonged bedrest increases bone reabsorption resulting in hypercalcemia and osteoporosis.

G. **Recovery from acute renal failure.** Felt to be from secondary hyperparathyroidism.

H. **Endocrinopathies**
   1. **Hyperthyroidism.** Bone reabsorption induced by thyroid hormone.

2. **Acromegaly**
3. **Adrenal insufficiency**

I. **Paget's disease.** Calcium is usually normal but may increase with immobilization.

IV. **Database**

A. **Physical examination key points**

1. **Vital signs.** Hypertension may be associated.
2. **Skin.** Excoriations may occur as a result of pruritus from metastatic calcifications in the skin.
3. **Lymph nodes.** Lymphadenopathy suggests carcinoma, hematologic malignancy, or sarcoidosis.
4. **HEENT.** An enlarged thyroid gland suggests hyperthyroidism.
5. **Chest.** Look for evidence of lung carcinoma.
6. **Abdomen.** An enlarged liver or spleen suggests metastatic carcinoma, a hematologic malignancy, or sarcoidosis.
7. **Musculoskeletal exam.** Bone pain by palpation or percussion points to carcinoma or Paget's disease. Myopathy from hypercalcemia can cause proximal muscle weakness.
8. **Neurologic exam.** Impaired mentation, weakness, and hyperreflexia may result from hypercalcemia.

B. **Laboratory data**

1. **Repeat calcium along with an albumin or obtain an ionized calcium.** Always confirm an elevated calcium and the severity of the hypercalcemia before initiating therapy. Remember, a high normal total calcium may also signify hypercalcemia in the presence of marked hypoalbuminemia. A calcium value must be corrected in the presence of hypoalbuminemia. Normally, the total calcium decreases by 0.2 mmol/L or 0.4 mEg/L for every 1 g/dL decrease in the serum albumin without changing the ionized calcium level. Symptoms usually develop at 6.5 nEq/L or 3.25 mmol/L.
2. **Phosphorus.** Low in primary hyperparathyroidism; elevated in vitamin D intoxication.
3. **Arterial blood gases.** A decrease in the pH will increase the ionized calcium mostly by displacing calcium bound to albumin. An acidosis may also be seen with adrenal insufficiency, a potential cause of hypercalcemia. An increase in the pH is seen in milk-alkali syndrome and possibly with thiazide diuretics if there is associated volume depletion.
4. **Alkaline phosphatase.** Increased in primary hyperparathyroidism with bone disease and in Paget's disease, and can be increased with bony metastases.
5. **Blood urea nitrogen and creatinine.** Renal insufficiency will exacerbate hypercalcemia or can be secondary to hypercalcemia.
6. **Total protein and albumin.** An increased total protein-to-albumin ratio points to multiple myeloma. If there is an elevated total protein-to-albumin ratio, then quantitative immuno-

globulins and serum and urine protein electrophoresis should be ordered.

7. **Urinalysis.** Hematuria may arise from renal cell carcinoma or secondary to nephrolithiasis.

C. **Radiologic and other studies**

1. **Chest x-ray.** Bilateral hilar adenopathy implies sarcoidosis. Also, carcinoma or lymphoma may be detected. Osteopenia of the vertebral column may be evident on the lateral film.
2. **Abdominal x-rays.** May reveal renal calcifications as a result of hypercalcemia. Other findings may suggest carcinoma.
3. **Bone films.** Especially if there is localized bone pain. May reveal osteolytic lesions from carcinoma or multiple myeloma. If present, a bone scan would be helpful to reveal extent of the disease. A bone scan will be negative with multiple myeloma because of the absence of associated osteoblastic activity.
4. **Skull films and skeletal survey.** Obtain if multiple myeloma is suspected. Will classically see multiple punched-out lesions. May also be helpful in detecting subperiosteal resorption resulting from primary hyperparathyroidism, especially evident on hand films.
5. **Electrocardiogram.** Associated shortening of QT interval and lengthening of PR interval.

V. **Plan.** Decrease the calcium and then treat the underlying disorder. Treat more aggressively with severe hypercalcemia greater than 7.5 mEq/L or 3.75 mmol/L or when symptomatic. Treatment is directed at decreasing release from bone or increasing deposition in bone, decreasing absorption from the gastrointestinal tract, and increasing excretion renally or through chelation.

A. **Restrict calcium intake and encourage mobilization.**

B. **Treat underlying causes.**

C. **Institute saline diuresis.** Patients with moderate to severe symptomatic hypercalcemia are frequently volume depleted. It is imperative to restore the volume status and then to maintain a urine output of at least 2 L/d. Sodium increases calcium excretion by inhibiting proximal tubule reabsorption. Administration of large volumes of normal saline can be hazardous in the elderly or in patients with renal failure or with left ventricular dysfunction.

D. **Administer medications**

1. **Furosemide (Lasix) 20–80 mg IV every 2–4 hours.** Furosemide is a calciuric agent; however, calcium excretion is not promoted if volume depletion develops. It is imperative to closely follow urinary output as well as the volume of normal saline administered and daily weights. Older patients with tenuous cardiac conditions should undergo hemodynamic monitoring in an ICU if vigorous saline diuresis is attempted.
2. **Mithramycin 25 μg/kg in 1 L of normal saline over 3–6 hours.** Often inhibits bone reabsorption. Effect may not occur for 12–24 hours. Renal, hepatic, and bone marrow toxicity can

occur. Used to treat hypercalcemia associated with malignancy and vitamin D intoxication.

3. **Thyrocalcitonin.** Rapid-acting. Inhibits bone reabsorption and increases urinary excretion of calcium. Usually only a temporary measure as resistance to the calcium-lowering effect often develops.
4. **Corticosteroids.** Hydrocortisone 50–75 mg every 6 hours decreases calcium absorption from the GI tract and inhibits bone reabsorption. Effective for treating hypercalcemia associated with sarcoidosis, vitamin D intoxication, and malignancy, especially multiple myeloma, lymphoma, leukemia, and breast carcinoma.
5. **Phosphates, oral and intravenous.** Works by increasing deposition of calcium in bone and soft tissues and decreasing bone reabsorption. Oral phosphates also decrease intestinal absorption of calcium. Can result in metastatic calcification, renal failure, and death. Contraindicated in patients with renal insufficiency.
6. **Etidronate disodium (Didronel).** A diphosphonate used to treat hypercalcemia of malignancy.
7. **Indomethacin (Indocin) 25–50 mg PO three times daily.** Variable response in treating hypercalcemia of malignancy, possibly by inhibiting bone reabsorption caused by prostaglandins.
8. **Sodium ethylenediaminetetraacetic acid (NaEDTA).** A chelating agent that is immediately effective. Nephrotoxic.

E. **Dialysis.** A last resort.

REFERENCES

Agus ZS, Wasserstein A, Goldfarb S. Disorders of calcium and magnesium homeostasis. *Am J Med* 1982;72:473–488.

Burtis WJ, Broadus AE. Hypercalcemia and hypocalcemia. In: Kelly WN, ed-in-chief. *Textbook of Internal Medicine.* Philadelphia: JB Lippincott; 1989:2246–2252.

Popovtzer MM, Knochel JP. Disorders of calcium, phosphorus, vitamin D and parathyroid hormone activity. In: Schrier RW, ed. *Renal and Electrolyte Disorders.* 3rd ed. Boston: Little, Brown; 1986:251–329.

■ HYPERGLYCEMIA

I. **Problem.** A 44-year-old man is admitted in the afternoon to another service. His lab work is called to you later that night and shows a glucose of 428 mg/dL or 23.79 mmol/L.

II. **Immediate Questions**

A. **What are the patient's vital signs?** Fever may indicate sepsis, which can exacerbate hyperglycemia. Hypotension and/or tachycardia may indicate volume depletion common in diabetic ketoacidosis (DKA) and hyperosmolar states. Tachypnea may be due to Kussmaul respirations in DKA.

B. Is the patient known to be diabetic? A history of diabetes should make one consider factors such as noncompliance with medication/diet, sepsis, acute stress, glucocorticoid use, and myocardial infarction (MI), which can result in poor control of hyperglycemia. The absence of a prior history of diabetes should make one consider all of the preceding factors as unmasking latent carbohydrate intolerance and also the fact that there may be a laboratory error.

C. If the patient is diabetic, what medications is he taking and when was his last meal in relation to the time of phlebotomy? To modify the regimen it is important to know whether the patient is receiving large or small amounts of insulin or whether he is receiving oral hypoglycemic agents. In addition, it is important to know whether the blood sugar was drawn randomly (and therefore could be postprandial) or whether it represents a fasting level.

III. Differential Diagnosis

A. Diabetes mellitus

1. **Type I (previously called juvenile diabetes, insulin-dependent diabetes).** Type I diabetics require insulin even when not eating (NPO) although in lower doses. They are more likely to be thin or normal in weight, young, and "brittle," and are prone to DKA. Diabetic ketoacidosis may be defined as a blood sugar greater than 300 mg/dL (16.68 mmol/L), urine ketones that are strongly positive, and a serum bicarbonate less than 17 mmol or a pH of 7.30 or less.
2. **Type II (previously called adult-onset diabetes, non–insulin-dependent diabetes mellitus).** Type II diabetics tend to be obese and older and are more prone to hyperosmolar states than ketoacidosis. In ideal settings (on a metabolic unit), many of these patients can be managed with diet alone. Weight loss may normalize carbohydrate metabolism; however, the reality is that a majority of patients require oral hypoglycemic drugs or insulin for adequate control.
3. **Gestational diabetes.** Glucose intolerance associated with pregnancy. Close monitoring and tight control are important to improve outcome of mother and infant.

B. Acute stress. In patients with mild carbohydrate intolerance, acute events such as sepsis, MI, trauma, and surgery may cause relatively marked hyperglycemia. Some of these patients will not require therapy once the acute event has resolved.

C. Exogenous glucose load. Hyperalimentation and peritoneal dialysis.

D. Glucocorticoids. Either exogenous or endogenous (Cushing's syndrome).

E. Pancreatic disease. Severe acute pancreatitis or long-standing chronic pancreatitis with endocrine pancreatic insufficiency.

F. Spurious hyperglycemia. Drawing blood above an intravenous line that contains dextrose, mislabeling, or inadvertently switching blood on different patients. When in doubt, immediately repeat the test before treating.

IV. Database

A. Physical examination key points

1. **Vital signs.** Include orthostatic blood pressure and pulse to evaluate volume status. Fever implies sepsis. Kussmaul respirations (deep, regular respirations whether slow or fast) suggest DKA.
2. **HEENT.** Fruity odor on breath suggests ketones and DKA. Fundoscopic exam may show diabetic retinopathy, which suggests long-standing disease and increases the likelihood of other diabetic complications such as nephropathy and neuropathy.
3. **Lungs.** Evaluate for signs of pneumonia.
4. **Heart.** Listen for associated findings of ischemia/MI such as a third (S_3) or fourth (S_4) heart sound or murmur of mitral insufficiency.
5. **Peripheral vascular system.** Listen for bruits.
6. **Abdomen.** Evaluate for cause of sepsis. Rebound tenderness suggests peritonitis. A positive Murphy's sign (see Abdominal Pain, p 1.) suggests acute cholecystitis which is more common in diabetics.
7. **Extremities.** Check for diabetic foot ulcers and cellulitis.
8. **Neurologic exam.** A clouded sensorium suggests more severe disease (ketoacidosis or hyperosmolar state).

B. Laboratory data

1. **Serum glucose.** Significantly elevated fingerstick glucoses should be evaluated with a serum glucose determination.
2. **Complete blood count.** Leukocytosis with a left shift suggests the presence of infection. An elevated white blood cell count may be seen in DKA without an associated infection or sepsis, but a left shift, toxic granulation, and vacuolization should be absent.
3. **Serum electrolytes, blood urea nitrogen and creatinine, phosphorus, calcium, magnesium, amylase.**
   a. Even though serum potassium may be normal, most patients are total body potassium depleted and potassium repletion is indicated. An initially normal or elevated potassium will decrease with insulin administration and with correction of acidosis if present.
   b. Serum sodium is spuriously lowered by 1.6 mmol/L for each 100 mg/dL (5.56 mmol/L) rise in glucose concentration.
   c. Serum bicarbonate is low in isolated DKA. Anion gap is elevated in DKA.
   d. Creatinine may be falsely elevated in the presence of

serum ketones. Both BUN and creatinine may be elevated as a result of profound volume depletion or diabetic nephropathy.

e. Phosphate may fall with treatment and should be monitored, although routine prophylactic treatment with phosphate is no longer recommended.
f. Calcium may be low with acute pancreatitis.
g. Magnesium may be low especially in DKA.
h. An elevated amylase may indicate pancreatitis, but ketone bodies may factitiously elevate the serum amylase.

4. **Arterial blood gases.** To evaluate the degree of acidemia. A careful look at the pH, pCO_2, and serum bicarbonate often reveals more than one acid-base disorder. (See Acidosis, p 9, and Alkalosis, p 17.)
5. **Urine or serum for ketones.** This helps to distinguish between DKA and hyperosmolar coma. Acetoacetate is the ketone that is measured on standard tests; however, β-hydroxybutyrate is the predominant ketone in DKA. Initially, the level of ketones may not decrease or may actually increase as β-hydroxybutyrate is metabolized to acetoacetate.
6. **Cultures.** If sepsis is suspected, then appropriate cultures should be ordered.

C. **Radiologic and other studies**

1. **Chest x-ray.** To evaluate for pneumonia and congestive heart failure.
2. **Electrocardiogram.** To rule out MI. Diabetics often have "silent" MIs.
3. **Miscellaneous studies.** Depending on clinical suspicion, for example, CT of the abdomen if intra-abdominal abscess is suspected.

V. **Plan.** Management depends on the clinical setting and severity of hyperglycemia. This section is divided into three parts on the basis of severity.

A. **Type II diabetes with a serum glucose below 450 mg/dL or 25.0 mmol/L (no ketones, no acidosis, and probably asymptomatic)**

1. **Insulin.** May increase usual dose of intermediate-acting insulin plus short-acting insulin every 6 hours based on results of fingerstick glucoses. For a typical regimen, see Table 1–6.
2. **Oral hypoglycemic agents.** Some patients with type II diabetes mellitus may be managed with oral hypoglycemic agents, especially those whose glucose is below 300 mg/dL (16.68 mmol/L).
3. **Diet.** In the short term, an 1800-calorie American Diabetes Association (ADA) diet is useful although other modified diets may be appropriate in certain settings. Diet is controversial. A nutritious diet low in simple sugars and fat will usually suffice. If there is a complicating condition such as a foot ulcer that re-

TABLE 1–6. Sliding Scale Insulin for Hyperglycemia

Glucose Level	Insulin (Short-Acting/Regular)
<180 mg/dL (10.00 mmol/L)	0 U SC
180–240 mg/dL (10.00–13.34 mmol/L)	3–5 U SC
240–400 mg/dL (13.34–22.23 mmol/L)	8–10 U SC
>400 mg/dL (>22.23 mmol/L)	10–15 U SC[a]

[a] Follow with a stat serum glucose and notify the house officer of result. SC = subcutaneous.

quires positive nitrogen balance for resolution, be sure the patient receives adequate calories and protein.

B. Hyperosmolar, hyperglycemic nonketotic coma

1. **Glucose greater than 600 mg/dL or 33.35 mmol/L (no ketones, no acidosis).** More aggressive management is indicated, often in the intensive care unit.
2. **Saline**
   a. Depending on the degree of volume depletion, 500–1000 mL of normal saline is given in the first hour, after which the rate is decreased to 250–500 mL/h until signs of volume depletion resolve. Obviously, caution is indicated, particularly in smaller or older individuals or in those with limited cardiac and renal reserve. These patients need frequent (every 1–2 hours) assessment of volume status with orthostatic blood pressure and pulse, heart exam for S_3, and lung exam for rales. Some patients will need monitoring with a pulmonary artery catheter for optimal fluid management.
   b. Some authors prefer switching from normal saline to half-normal saline after the first liter or alternating the half-normal saline with normal saline. When the blood sugar reaches the range 250–300 mg/dL (13.90–16.68 mmol/L), then IV fluids are switched to D5 half-normal saline at a rate based on volume assessment.
3. **Potassium.** If serum potassium is less than 5.5 mmol/L, add 20–30 mmol/L at a rate not to exceed 10–15 mmol/h. Follow levels every 4 hours. Keep potassium at 4.0–5.0 mmol/L.
4. **Insulin.** There are many ways of giving insulin; however, in recent years, the continuous IV infusion drip of short-acting insulin has gained favor. An initial dose of 0.15 U/kg of a short-acting insulin is given as a bolus and is followed immediately by a continuous infusion drip at 0.1 U/kg/h. This should be adjusted to ensure that blood glucose is falling at least 10% per hour.
5. **Lab work.** Serum glucose measurements are needed every 1–2 hours. Magnesium should be checked initially and repeated if there are signs of magnesium deficiency. Potassium

should be checked every 4–6 hours, and phosphate should be repeated after 6–12 hours.

6. When glucose falls to the range 250–300 mg/dL (13.89–16.68 mmol/L), then the insulin drip may need to be decreased and the IV fluids changed to D5 half-normal saline with the goal of maintaining the glucose at 100–200 mg/dL (5.56–11.12 mmol/L).

C. **Diabetic ketoacidosis.** A medical emergency. Often requires management in the ICU setting. In the setting of profound ketoacidosis, patients are less responsive to insulin and larger doses are required. Volume repletion is essential.

1. **Intravenous fluids.** One liter of normal saline in the first hour followed by 200 mL to 1 L per hour until hydration improves. The same volume assessment parameters should be followed as in hyperosmolar coma described earlier. Some authors prefer switching or alternating half-normal saline with normal saline. When serum glucose levels reach 250–300 mg/dL (13.89–16.68 mmol/L), then change to D5 half-normal saline at a rate based on volume assessment. Some cases may require a pulmonary artery catheter for appropriate fluid management.
2. **Insulin.** A continuous infusion drip is initiated by a bolus of 0.2 U/kg of a short-acting insulin initially and is followed by 0.1 U/kg/h as described earlier. If the serum glucose falls by less than 10% in the first hour, then the rate is doubled and a repeat bolus of 0.2 U/kg is given. Repeat IV boluses are given every 1–2 hours if the glucose is not falling by at least 10% per hour, and the rate is doubled every 2 hours until the serum glucose concentration reaches 250 mg/dL (13.89 mmol/L).
3. **Potassium.** If serum potassium is less than 5.5 mmol/L, then potassium 20–30 mmol/L is given in IV fluids at a rate not to exceed 15 mmol/h unless the patient's rhythm is being continuously monitored. If serum potassium is less than 3.3 mmol/L, then potassium 10–15 mmol/h is given to maintain serum potassium at 3.0–5.0 mmol/L. Doses of potassium greater than 10–15 mmol/h should not be administered without cardiac monitoring.
4. **Bicarbonate.** Its use is controversial and most authors are more conservative than in the past. One approach is to use bicarbonate to correct the pH to 7.00. For pH 6.90–7.00, give 44 mmol over 1–2 hours; for pH below 6.90, give 88 mmol of sodium bicarbonate over 1–2 hours.
5. **Lab work.** Glucose should be repeated every 1–2 hours, and electrolytes every 4–6 hours. Magnesium should be checked initially, and phosphate initially and after 6–12 hours. The ABG are obtained every 2–4 hours if acidosis is severe or if the patient requires sodium bicarbonate. Serum/urine ketones may be of some use, although increasing ketones may be spurious (see Section IV.B.5).

6. **Associated conditions.** Treat any associated condition such as sepsis, myocardial infarction, or stress appropriately.

REFERENCES

Kitabchi AE, Rumbak M. The management of diabetic emergencies. *Hosp. Pract* 1989;24:129–144.

Sperling MA, et al. *Physicians' Guide to Insulin Dependent (Type I) Diabetes.* American Diabetes Association, Alexandria, Virginia; 1988.

■ HYPERKALEMIA

I. **Problem.** A 64-year-old man with diabetes admitted for a myocardial infarction is found to have a potassium of 7.1 mmol/L.

II. **Immediate Questions**

A. **What are the patient's vital signs?** Hyperkalemia can result in life-threatening ventricular arrhythmias. Obtain an electrocardiogram.

B. **What is the urine output?** Acute oliguric renal failure is the most common cause of potentially fatal elevation of plasma potassium. Evaluate urine output and renal function tests.

C. **Is the patient receiving potassium in an intravenous solution?** Often a standard IV solution contains 20–40 mEq/L potassium; hyperalimentation solutions may contain more. Stop all exogenous potassium until the problem is resolved.

D. **Is the patient on any medications that could elevate the potassium?** Potential causes include potassium-sparing diuretics such as spironolactone (Aldactone), triamterene (Dyrenium), and amiloride (Midamor); nonsteroidal anti-inflammatory drugs, and angiotensin-converting enzyme (ACE) inhibitors.

E. **Is the lab result correct?** If hyperkalemia is unexpected or inconsistent after the preceding questions are satisfactorily answered, consider pseudohyperkalemia, especially if the ECG shows no changes of hyperkalemia. There are a number of causes of factitious hyperkalemia, the most common being the tourniquet method of drawing blood. A tight tourniquet around an exercising extremity can elevate the potassium above 2.0 mmol/L. Hemolysis of a blood sample prior to the chemical determination is another frequent source of error. Extreme leukocytosis (>70,000) or thrombocytosis (>1,000,000) can also elevate the serum potassium. If there is a question, obtain a plasma potassium.

III. **Differential Diagnosis.** In general, true hyperkalemia results from one of two mechanisms: a shift of potassium from the intracellular to the extracellular space or impaired renal excretion of potassium.

A. **Acidosis.** With acidosis, potassium moves out of the cells and hydrogen ions moves into the cells. A common example is diabetic ketoacidosis. Although insulin deficiency per se is probably not a cause of hyperkalemia, it may increase the degree of hyperkalemia in response to either an endogenous or an exogenous potassium load.

B. **Tissue breakdown.** Any condition associated with rapid destruction of cells results in the release of potassium into the extracellular fluid. Examples include rhabdomyolysis, burns, massive hemolysis, and tumor lysis.

C. **Digitalis intoxication.** Massive overdose of digitalis is a rare cause. This results from inhibition of sodium/potassium-dependent ATPase pump and intracellular potassium is lost.

D. **Succinylcholine.** Mild increases in serum potassium occur in most patients treated with this commonly used muscle relaxant. In patients with tissue destruction or neuromuscular disease, life-threatening hyperkalemia may occur. Succinylcholine causes cell membrane depolarization, resulting in intracellular-to-extracellular shifts in potassium.

E. **Hyperosmolality.** Administration of hypertonic mannitol or saline results in major increases in serum osmolality and thus may cause hyperkalemia.

F. **Arginine hydrochloride.** Intravenous administration of arginine hydrochloride, whether used diagnostically to assess growth hormone reserves or therapeutically in the treatment of metabolic alkalosis, may lead to hyperkalemia. This is probably due to an arginine-potassium exchange.

G. **Hyperkalemic periodic paralysis.** This rare, inherited disorder is characterized by spontaneous episodes of hyperkalemia and muscle weakness.

H. **Chronic renal failure.** Most patients with chronic renal failure maintain normal potassium balance until function is severely impaired; however, when these patients are challenged with a potassium load or are treated with potassium-sparing diuretics (spironolactone, triamterene, amiloride), ACE inhibitors (captopril, enalopril), or NSAIDs (indomethacin, ibuprofen), the patient's adaptive mechanisms are inadequate and hyperkalemia occurs.

I. **Acute renal failure.** Hyperkalemia is most likely to complicate oliguric renal failure because of the flow dependence of distal tubular potassium secretion. Acute renal failure often occurs in the setting of increased potassium load (trauma, blood transfusions, or postoperative hypercatabolic state).

J. **Adrenal insufficiency.** Adrenal insufficiency, in particular hypoaldosteronism, results in reduced renal ability to excrete potassium.

K. **Hyporeninemic hypoaldosteronism.** Patients with this condition have hyperkalemia as well as hyperchloremic metabolic acidosis (type IV renal tubular acidosis). They often have mild renal insufficiency secondary to diabetic nephropathy or interstitial nephropathy. This syndrome may be aggravated by administration of NSAIDs or potassium-sparing diuretics.

L. **Heparin.** Long-term anticoagulation with heparin may lead to hyperkalemia, probably through the inhibition of aldosterone synthesis.

M. **Potassium-sparing diuretics.** Hyperkalemia secondary to triamterene or spironolactone is usually seen in patients with underlying renal insufficiency. But there have been cases, especially in diabetics, where patients with normal renal function developed hyperkalemia on these drugs.

N. **Nonsteroidal anti-inflammatory agents** (See Section III.H).

O. **Angiotensin-converting enzyme inhibitors** (See Section III.H).

P. **Systemic lupus erythematosus, renal transplant, sickle cell disease.** Patients with these disorders may demonstrate an isolated defect in renal potassium excretion, thought to result from aldosterone resistance.

Q. **Increased exogenous intake.** High-potassium foods, potassium salts (salt "substitutes"), or large doses of potassium penicillin are examples of exogenous sources of potassium. Often these patients are also on potassium-sparing diuretics, an ACE inhibitor, or a NSAID.

IV. Database

A. Physical examination key points

1. **Cardiovascular exam.** The conduction system of the heart is most vulnerable to hyperkalemia, which may result in bradycardia, ventricular fibrillation, or asystole.
2. **Neuromuscular exam.** Skeletal muscle paralysis may occasionally dominate. Other findings are weakness, tingling, and hyperactive deep tendon reflexes.

B. Laboratory data

1. **Electrolytes.** A low bicarbonate may indicate a metabolic acidosis. A low sodium may result from aldosterone deficiency.
2. **Plasma potassium.** If the serum level is in doubt.
3. **Blood urea nitrogen and creatinine.** Assess renal function.
3. **Arterial blood gases.** Along with a serum bicarbonate, ABG are essential in establishing acid-base status.
4. **Platelets and white blood cell count.** Elevations may cause factitious hyperkalemia.
5. **Serum creatine phosphokinase (CPK).** To detect rhabdomyolysis.
6. **Digoxin level.** If indicated.
7. **Serum aldosterone level.** Indicated after initial workup. Lack of stimulation with volume depletion is consistent with mineralocorticoid deficiency.

C. **Radiologic and other studies.** An electrocardiogram is **a must!** The cardiac abnormalities that occur with hyperkalemia are initially a tall, peaked T wave in the precordial leads, followed by decreased amplitude of the R wave, widened QRS complex, prolonged PR interval, and then decreased amplitude and disappearance of the P wave. Finally, the QRS blends into the T wave, forming the classic sine wave of hyperkalemia. Ventricular fibrillation and asystole may follow.

V. Plan. Hyperkalemia should be treated as an emergency if the serum potassium has reached 7 mmol/L, although cardiac or neuromuscular symptoms may mandate urgent treatment at lower potassium levels.

A. Acute hyperkalemia

1. Calcium is initial treatment. Calcium antagonizes the membrane effects of hyperkalemia and restores normal excitability within 1–2 minutes. Calcium chloride 10% or gluconate 10–20 mL should be given intravenously over 3–5 minutes.
2. Potassium can be quickly shifted into cells by the administration of alkali or glucose plus insulin.
   - **a.** Sodium bicarbonate (1 ampoule [44 mmol] of bicarbonate) may be administered intravenously over several minutes.
   - **b.** A 50-g ampoule of dextrose and 15 U of intravenous regular insulin may be given (3 g glucose for every 1 U of regular insulin).

B. Subacute hyperkalemia. It should be noted that calcium, alkali, glucose, and insulin do not lower the total body potassium. Once the patient is stabilized, the total body potassium needs to be reduced.

1. Potassium-binding resins may be used when the immediate life-threatening cardiac manifestations are under control. Kayexalate may be given orally, 40 g in 25–50 mL of 70% sorbitol every 2–4 hours, or rectally, 50–100 g in 200 mL water as a retention enema for 30 minutes every 2–4 hours.
2. Hemodialysis and peritoneal dialysis are definitive measures for controlling hyperkalemia in renal failure.

REFERENCES

Gabow PA, Peterson LN. Disorders of potassium metabolism. In: Schrier RW, ed. *Renal and Electrolyte Disorders.* 3rd ed. Boston: Little, Brown; 1986:207–249.

Rose BD, Maffly R. Renal function and disorders of water, sodium and potassium balance. In: Rubenstein E, ed-in-chief; Federman DD, ed. *Scientific American.* Sect 10: *Nephrology,* vol 2, pt I. New York: Scientific American Inc; 1990:28–30.

Sterns RH, Narins RG. Disorders of potassium balance. In: Stein JH, ed-in-chief. *Internal Medicine.* 3rd ed. Boston: Little, Brown; 1990:853–864.

■ HYPERNATREMIA

I. Problem. The clinical chemistry lab calls to tell you that the 65-year-old female patient admitted with pneumonia has a serum sodium of 155 mmol/L (normal 136–145 mmol/L).

II. Immediate Questions

A. Is the patient awake, alert, and oriented or lethargic and confused? Mortality and symptoms are related to the level and the acuity of the hypernatremia. Mortality in adults is increased with sodium levels above 160 mmol/L.

B. **What medications is the patient taking?** Mannitol can cause an osmotic diuresis, resulting in hypernatremia with low total body sodium. Exogenous steroids can cause an increase in the total body sodium, resulting in hypernatremia. Salt tablets can cause hypernatremia.

C. **What are the intake/output values for the past few days?** A loss of total body water by fluid deprivation (inadequate administration of fluids) or from sweating can cause hypernatremia.

D. **Are there underlying conditions?** Certain diseases, such as central and nephrogenic diabetes insipidus, hyperaldosteronism, and Cushing's syndrome, are associated with hypernatremia.

E. **Does the patient have a condition that prevents access to water?** Dehydration can result from inadequate access to water secondary to being bedridden. This may result in hypernatremia.

F. **Is the lab value accurate?** As with any lab result that is unexpected, the error could be in the lab itself. It may be of value to repeat the test.

G. **What is the composition of fluids administered?** Check sodium content of fluids. Hypertonic solutions such as hypertonic dialysate can cause hypernatremia. Is the patient receiving adequate free water (usually 35 mL/kg/24 h in adults)? This is often a problem in patients on tube feedings.

H. **Is there a history of polyuria and polydypsia?** Diabetes mellitus and diabetes insipidus can cause hypernatremia.

III. **Differential Diagnosis.** The differential diagnosis is best considered in light of the cause of hypernatremia: a loss of water and sodium; a loss of total body water; rarely, an increase in total body sodium.

A. **Water and sodium loss.** Significant sodium loss with even greater loss of water.
   1. **Renal losses**
      a. **Osmotic diuresis**
         (1) **Mannitol**
         (2) **Hyperglycemia**
         (3) **Urea**
      b. **Diuretics.** For example, thiazides and furosemide.
      c. **Postobstructive diuresis.** Caused by relief of long-standing bilateral renal obstruction.
      d. **Acute tubular necrosis.** Polyuric phase.
   2. **Nonrenal losses**
      a. **Cutaneous losses**
         (1) **Fever.** Losses of 500 mL/24 h for each degree centigrade increase above 38.3°C.
         (2) **Burns**
         (3) **Profuse sweating**
      b. **Gastrointestinal losses**
         (1) **Vomiting**
         (2) **Nasogastric suction**

(3) **Diarrhea.** Hypotonic diarrhea in children or with the use of lactulose.

(4) **Fistulas**

B. **Water losses without loss of sodium**

1. **Renal losses**

a. **Central diabetes insipidus.** Results from failure to produce adequate amounts of antidiuretic hormone (ADH). If thirst mechanism is intact and patient has free access to water, hypernatremia may be minimal. May be idiopathic or caused by central nervous system surgery, trauma, infection, or tumor (metastatic or primary).

b. **Nephrogenic.** Antidiuretic hormone is not effective. May be congenital or caused by sickle cell disease, hypokalemia, hypercalcemia, polycystic kidney disease, or drugs such as lithium, alcohol, phenytoin, and glyburide.

2. **Nonrenal losses**

a. **Pulmonary losses.** Insensible losses, especially in intubated patients who are not receiving adequate humidification.

b. **Cutaneous losses.** Fever or sweating.

C. **Increase in total body sodium without a change in total body water**

1. **Increase in mineralocorticoids or glucocorticoids**

a. **Exogenous steroids such as prednisone**

b. **Primary aldosteronism**

c. **Cushing's syndrome.** Cushing's disease, bilateral adrenal hyperplasia, or ectopic adrenocorticotropin (ACTH) production.

2. **Administration of hypertonic sodium**

a. **Sodium chloride tablets**

b. **Hypertonic dialysate**

c. **Hypertonic sodium bicarbonate.** Given during resuscitation after cardiopulmonary arrest.

IV. Database

A. **Physical examination key points**

1. **Vital signs.** Orthostatic changes in blood pressure and heart rate and decreased weight suggest volume depletion.

2. **Skin.** Check turgor. Poor turgor suggests volume depletion; however, poor skin turgor is a normal variant in the elderly.

3. **Mouth.** Check mucous membranes. Dry mucous membranes suggest volume depletion.

4. **Neurologic exam.** Look for signs of irritability, muscle twitching, hyperreflexia, or seizures. All are signs of hypernatremia.

B. **Laboratory data**

1. **Serum sodium.** Follow closely, especially if sodium is above 160 mmol/L.

2. **Urine osmolality.** Hypertonic urine suggests extrarenal fluid loss.

3. **Spot urine sodium.** A level greater than 20 mmol/L suggests extrarenal loss. In hypernatremia with water losses without loss of sodium, the spot sodium in extrarenal losses is variable.
4. **Water deprivation/vasopressin.** If you suspect diabetes insipidus (DI). The patient is fluid-deprived until the plasma osmolality is 295 mosm/kg or greater; or on three consecutive hourly urines, the osmolality does not increase; or the patient loses 3% to 5% of their body weight. Five units of aqueous vasopressin is given either intramuscularly or subcutaneously.
   a. **Normal subjects.** Urine concentrates with fluid deprivation and no change occurs with vasopressin.
   b. **Complete central DI.** Urine does not concentrate with fluid deprivation. There is a significant increase in urine osmolality after vasopressin.
   c. **Nephrogenic DI.** Urine does not concentrate and there is no change in urine osmolality with vasopressin.
   d. **Compulsive water drinkers.** The urine concentrates with fluid deprivation but not maximally. There is no change in urine osmolality with vasopressin.

C. **Radiologic and other studies.** A CT scan of head may be helpful if central DI is suspected, to rule out a CNS lesion.

V. **Plan.** The overall plan is to slowly decrease this serum sodium toward normal. Too rapid a correction of the sodium may result in cerebral edema, seizures, and herniation leading to death. The serum osmolality should not decrease any more than 2 mosm/h (or a decrease in serum sodium of 1 mmol/L/h). Specific treatment depends on whether there is a loss of sodium and water, a loss of water, or an increase in total body sodium.

A. **Water and sodium loss.** Represents significant volume depletion. If the patient is in shock, replenish volume with normal saline. If patient is hemodynamically stable, replace volume with hypotonic saline (half-normal saline).

B. **Water loss without loss of sodium.** Calculate the free water deficit:

$$\text{weight (kg)} \times 0.60 = \text{normal total body water (NTBW)}$$

$$[140 \text{ (desired Na)} \div \text{serum Na}] \times \text{weight (kg)} \times 0.60 = \text{actual total body water (ATBW)}$$

$$\text{NTBW} - \text{ATBW} = \text{total water deficit}$$

Give one half of the calculated free water deficit in the first 12 hours and the remainder in the next 24 hours.

C. **Increase in total body sodium.** Remove excess sodium. This is done by giving free water and diuretics or by dialysis with hypotonic dialysate.

D. **Underlying cause**
   1. **Central DI.** After correction of free water deficit, begin vasopressin.

2. **Diabetes mellitus.** Treat with insulin. (See Hyperglycemia, Section V, p 139.)

REFERENCES

Berl T, Schrier RW. Disorders of Water Metabolism. In: Schrier RW, ed. *Renal and Electrolyte Disorders.* 3rd ed. Boston: Little, Brown; 1986:1–77.

Demling RH, Wilson RF. *Hypernatremia in Decision Making in Surgical Critical Care.* Toronto: BC Decker; 1988:142–143.

Palevsky PM, Cox M. Approach to the patient with polyuria or nocturia. In: Kelley WN, ed. *Textbook of Internal Medicine.* Philadelphia: JB Lippincott; 1989:861–865.

Weisberg L, Szerlip HM, Davidson RL, et al. Approach to the patient with altered sodium and water homeostasis. In: Kelley WN, ed-in-chief. *Textbook of Internal Medicine.* Philadelphia: JB Lippincott; 1989:901–910.

■ HYPERTENSION

I. **Problem.** A 37-year-old patient complains of a severe occipital headache for the past 6 hours. Her blood pressure is 220/140.

II. **Immediate Questions**

A. **Is there a past history of hypertension?** You want to know if she is being treated for hypertension and sees a physician on a regular basis.

B. **What is the patient's medical regimen?** You want to know all the medications the patient is taking and if she is compliant. For example, she may have stopped taking clonidine (Catapres) or a short-acting beta blocker such as propranolol (Inderal) which can cause severe rebound hypertension. Hypertensive crisis can occur in people taking a monoamine oxidase inhibitor (MAOI) who ingest certain cheeses or wine containing tyramine. Ingestion of "street" drugs such as cocaine or amphetamines can also cause hypertensive crisis especially in patients taking an MAOI.

C. **Is the patient experiencing any other symptoms besides headache?** A patient with severe hypertension who has a headache with mental status changes may be suffering from hypertensive encephalopathy, which is a medical emergency. Hypertensive encephalopathy is more common in patients whose blood pressure suddenly rises, as seen during toxemia of pregnancy. Other manifestations of end-organ damage from malignant hypertension include angina, shortness of breath, visual loss, nausea, vomiting, seizures, focal neurologic deficits, and a decrease in urinary output.

III. **Differential Diagnosis.** The physician does not have to immediately pinpoint the underlying illness because the first concern is to lower the blood pressure. Hypertension can be classified as essential or secondary (describes the cause) and accelerated or malignant (describes urgency). Patients with malignant hypertension often have a secondary cause of hypertension.

A. Essential. Ninety to ninety-five percent of all hypertension. No underlying cause.

B. Secondary

1. **Renovascular.** From fibromuscular dysplasia (usually women 20–30 years old) and atherosclerosis (usually men older than 50).
2. **Primary aldosteronism.** Hypertension with unexplained hypokalemia.
3. **Cushing's disease.** Characteristic findings include moon facies, truncal obesity, purple striae, a buffalo hump, hirsutism, and easy bruisability. Hypernatremia and hypokalemic alkalosis are common.
4. **Pheochromocytoma.** Usually episodic hypertension. Often associated diaphoresis, palpitations, and headache.
5. **Coarctation of the aorta.** Should be expected in anyone young presenting with hypertension. Blood pressures are higher in right arm and femoral pulses are often absent.
6. **Primary renal disease.**
7. **Hyperthyroidism.** Systolic hypertension.
8. **Hypothyroidism.** Diastolic hypertension.
9. **Heavy ethanol use or withdrawal.** May cause or aggravate underlying hypertension. Hypertension associated with withdrawal is secondary to hyperadrenergic state.
10. **Drugs**
    a. **Estrogens**
    b. **Over-the-counter medications containing sympathomimetics.** For example, phenylpropanolamine or pseudoephedrine when used in excessive amounts.
    c. **Illicit drugs**
        (1) **Phenycyclidine (PCP)**
        (2) **Amphetamines**
        (3) **Cocaine withdrawal**
11. **Postoperative.** Multifactorial including hypoxia, pain, anxiety, volume overload, hypothermia, and medications.
12. **Gestational**
13. **Hyperparathyroidism**

C. Miscellaneous diseases. Other diseases can cause a marked elevation in blood pressure or may be the consequence of longstanding, poorly controlled hypertension.

1. **Cerebrovascular accident.** If the patient has suffered a stroke resulting in marked elevation of blood pressure, the physician is not quite as aggressive in lowering the blood pressure. A sudden marked drop in blood pressure can extend a stroke.
2. **Subarachnoid hemorrhage.** Patients classically complain of the worst headache of their life.
3. **Aortic dissection.** "Tearing" chest pain often with radiation to the back. Usually a previous history of hypertension.

D. Accelerated hypertension. Markedly elevated blood pressure with no current life-threatening problem secondary to the hypertension.

E. Malignant hypertension. Usually a markedly elevated blood pressure with an associated serious complication such as hypertensive encephalopathy, angina, myocardial infarction, aortic dissection, cerebrovascular accident, or proteinuria, hematuria, and red blood cell casts.

IV. Database

A. Physical exam key points

1. **Vital signs.** Take blood pressure in both arms. Feel both radial pulses and check for a radial-femoral pulse lag. Such maneuvers may point to aortic dissection or coarctation.
2. **Eyes.** Look for evidence of papilledema, hemorrhages, exudates, and severe arteriolar narrowing. Papilledema is usually present with malignant hypertension but can occur in other conditions with increased intracranial pressure.
3. **Lungs.** Presence of rales may indicate congestive heart failure.
4. **Heart.** Palpate the apical impulse for displacement. Listen for a third heart sound (S_3) indicative of left ventricular dysfunction and for a murmur of aortic insufficiency, which can occur in aortic dissection.
5. **Neurologic exam.** Assess the patient's mental status and look for any focal deficits that may indicate a cerebrovascular accident. Confusion and somnolence progressing to coma are hallmarks of hypertensive encephalopathy.

B. Laboratory data

1. **Electrolytes, blood urea nitrogen, and creatinine.** To rule out evidence of renal insufficiency, hypokalemia, or hyperglycemia. Hypokalemia occurs in renovascular hypertension and primary hyperaldosteronism. Hyperglycemia can be a manifestation of a pheochromocytoma or stress. Mild renal insufficiency points toward hypertensive nephropathy, whereas marked renal insufficiency potentially suggests a secondary cause of hypertension.
2. **Urinalysis.** To look for proteinuria, hematuria, and red cell casts for evidence of a secondary cause or hypertensive nephropathy.
3. **Complete blood count and examination of peripheral blood smear.** Red blood cell fragments and/or schistocytes occur in microangiopathic hemolytic anemia resulting from malignant hypertension.

C. Radiologic and other studies

1. **Chest x-ray.** To look for cardiomegaly, congestive heart failure, and mediastinal widening suggesting proximal aortic dissection. Rib notching and obliteration of the aortic knob suggest coarctation of the aorta.

2. **Electrocardiogram.** To look for ischemic changes and left ventricular hypertrophy.
3. **CT scan.** If patient has mental status changes or focal neurologic findings, a CT scan must be performed to exclude stroke or subarachnoid hemorrhage.

V. Plan

A. Hypertensive encephalopathy or malignant hypertension. A medical emergency. Treatment must be initiated within minutes if possible.

1. **Admission to an ICU.** Intravenous and arterial lines should be placed.
2. **Appropriate therapy.** Initiated once therapeutic goals are established. The goals of immediate therapy should be approximately a systolic pressure of 170 and diastolic pressure of 110 if the patient is known to have long-standing, severe hypertension. Overly aggressive reduction of blood pressure beyond these levels can lead to cerebral hypoperfusion and worsening neurologic deficits. This is particularly important in patients suffering from a stroke or transient ischemic attack who are susceptible to abrupt falls in blood pressure.
   - **a.** Nitroprusside is commonly used in hypertensive crises. It reduces preload and afterload in a dose of 0.5–10 μg/kg/min as a continuous IV infusion. It has the advantage of immediate onset and is easily titrated. Disadvantages include the need for constant monitoring; also, prolonged use is associated with thiocyanate toxicity.
   - **b.** Intravenous labetolol, an alpha and beta blocker, is infused at a rate of 2mg/min. Potential disadvantages include beta-blocking side effects.
   - **c.** For suspected pheochromocytoma, IV phentolamine or phenoxybenzamine can be used.
   - **d.** Hypertension associated with aortic dissection should be controlled with trimethaphan or a combination of nitroprusside and a beta blocker.
3. **Treatment of accelerated hypertension.** Can often be treated with oral medications. Nifedipine (Procardia) 10 mg sublingually or orally will decrease blood pressure in 30–60 minutes and seldom causes severe hypotension.
4. **Treatment of hypertension.** A thorough discussion of hypertension is beyond the scope of this book. Please refer to any number of references including that listed here.

REFERENCE

Kaplan NM. *Clinical Hypertension.* 4th ed. Baltimore: Williams & Wilkins; 1986.

HYPOCALCEMIA

I. **Problem.** A 54-year-old man admitted for an acute myocardial infarction (MI) has a calcium of 3.5 mEg/L or 1.75 mmol/L (normal 4.2–5.1 mEg/L or 2.10–2.55 mmol/L).

II. **Immediate Questions**

A. **Are there any symptoms relevant to the low calcium?** Asymptomatic hypocalcemia usually does not require emergency treatment. Signs and symptoms of hypocalcemia may include peripheral and perioral paresthesias, Trousseau's sign (carpopedal spasm), Chvostek's sign, confusion, muscle twitching, laryngospasm, tetany, and seizures.

B. **Does the low calcium level represent the true ionized calcium?** Most laboratories report the total serum calcium, but it is the ionized calcium level that is important physiologically. The total serum calcium level decreases by 0.2 mmol/L or 0.4 mEq/L for every 1 g/dL decrease in the serum albumin level without changing the ionized calcium level. Calculate the appropriate total calcium level or order an ionized calcium level.

C. **Is there a past history of neck surgery?** Surgical removal or infarction of the parathyroid glands is one of the more common causes of hypocalcemia. Look for a scar on the neck.

III. **Differential Diagnosis.** The causes of low ionized serum calcium can be categorized as parathyroid hormone deficits, vitamin D deficits, and loss or displacement of calcium.

A. **Parathyroid hormone (PTH) deficits**
   1. **Decreased PTH level**
      a. **Surgical excision or injury.** Including thyroid surgery.
      b. **Infiltrative diseases of the parathyroid gland.** For example, hemochromatosis and amyloid or metastatic cancer.
      c. **Idiopathic**
      d. **Irradiation.** To the neck to treat lymphoma.
   2. **Decreased PTH activity**
      a. **Congenital.** Pseudohypoparathyroidism: resistance to PTH at the tissue level.
      b. **Acquired.** Hypomagnesemia, hypermagnesemia.

B. **Vitamin D deficiency**
   1. **Malnutrition**
   2. **Malabsorption**
      a. **Pancreatitis**
      b. **Postgastrectomy**
      c. **Short gut syndrome**
      d. **Laxative abuse**
      e. **Sprue**
      f. **Hepatobiliary disease with bile salt deficiency**
   3. **Defective metabolism**

a. **Liver disease.** Failure to synthesize 25-hydroxyvitamin D.
b. **Renal disease.** Failure to synthesize 1,25-dihydroxyvitamin D.
c. **Anticonvulsant treatment with phenobarbital or phenytoin (Dilantin).** Possibly from an increase in the metabolism of vitamin D in the liver leading to a vitamin D deficiency.

C. Calcium loss or displacement

1. **Hyperphosphatemia.** Increases bone deposition of calcium.
   a. **Acute phosphate ingestion**
   b. **Acute phosphate release by rhabdomyolysis or tumor lysis**
   c. **Renal failure**
2. **Acute pancreatitis**
3. **Osteoblastic metastases.** Especially breast and prostate cancer.
4. **Medullary carcinoma of the thyroid.** Increased calcitonin.
5. **Decreased bone resorption.** Overuse of actinomycin, calcitonin, or mithramycin.
6. **Miscellaneous disorders.** Sepsis, massive transfusion, hungry bone syndrome, toxic shock syndrome, and fat embolism.

IV. Database

A. History and physical exam key points

1. **History.** Perioral paresthesias (acute), cramps, fatigue, myalgias (chronic).
2. **Skin.** Dermatitis with chronic hypocalcemia.
3. **HEENT.** Cataracts with chronic hypocalcemia. Laryngospasm is rare but life-threatening. Look for surgical scars on the neck.
4. **Neuromuscular exam.** Confusion, spasm, twitching, facial grimacing, and hyperactive deep tendon reflexes all indicate symptomatic hypocalcemia.
5. **Specific tests for tetany of hypocalcemia**
   a. **Chvostek's sign.** Present in 5% to 10% of normocalcemic patients. Tap on the facial nerve near the zygoma and observe for a twitch.
   b. **Trousseau's sign.** Inflate a blood pressure cuff above the systolic pressure for 3 minutes and observe for carpal spasm.

B. Laboratory data

1. **Serum electrolytes.** Particularly calcium, phosphate, potassium, and magnesium. Calcium must be interpreted in terms of the serum albumin (see Section II.B., p 153). Hypomagnesemia and hyperkalemia may potentiate the effects of hypocalcemia.
2. **Serum albumin.** As mentioned earlier.
3. **Blood urea nitrogen and creatinine.** To rule out renal failure.

4. **Parathyroid hormone level.** A low normal level is inappropriately low in the presence of true hypocalcemia.
5. **Vitamin D levels.** 25-Hydroxyvitamin D and 1,25-dihydroxyvitamin D.
6. **Urinary cyclic AMP.** May indicate evidence of PTH resistance.
7. **Fecal fat.** To evaluate for steatorrhea.

C. **Radiologic and other tests**
1. **Electrocardiogram.** A prolonged QT interval and T wave inversion can occur with marked hypocalcemia, as can various arrhythmias.
2. **Bone films.** May show bony changes of renal failure or osteoblastic metastases.

V. **Plan.** Assess the patient for tetany, which can potentially progress to laryngeal spasm or seizures, and requires immediate treatment. Otherwise, establish the diagnosis by testing blood for calcium, albumin, magnesium, phosphate, and PTH levels, and begin appropriate oral therapy.

A. **Emergency treatment.** Emergency treatment is usually needed for a calcium level below 1.5 mmol/L (3 mEg/L) to prevent fatal laryngospasm. Give 100–200 mg of elemental calcium IV over 10 minutes in 50–100 mL of D5W; follow with a 1–2 mg/kg/h infusion for 6–12 hours. Use caution in patients on digitalis as calcium may potentiate its effects (heart block).
1. **10% calcium gluconate.** One 10-mL ampoule contains 23.25 mmol (93 mg) of calcium. Give 10–20 mL initially; follow with the infusion.
2. **10% calcium chloride.** One 10-mL ampoule contains 68 mmol (272 mg) of calcium. Give 5–10 mL IV, being careful to avoid extravasation, which can cause skin to slough; then start an infusion.

B. **Chronic therapy.** With primary PTH deficiency the goal is to give 2–4 g of oral calcium daily in four divided doses, adding vitamin D as necessary. With vitamin D disorders, vitamin D must always be supplemented.
1. Calcium carbonate, 240 mg of calcium per 600-mg tablet.
2. Calcium lactate tablets and calcium glubionate syrup are also available.
3. Ergocalciferol (vitamin D_2) 50,000 U/day or dihydrotachysterol (vitamin D_2 analog) 100–400 µg/d or calcitriol (1,25-dihydroxyvitamin D_3) 0.25–1.0 µg/day.
4. Patients on parenteral nutrition need at least 4–7 mg/kg/d of magnesium.

C. **Magnesium deficiency** (See Hypomagnesemia, Section V, p 166.)
1. In an emergency, one can give 10–15 mL of $MgSO_4$ 20%

solution IV over 1 minute, followed by 500 mL of $MgSO_4$ 2% solution in D5W over 4–6 hours.

2. More typically, 6 g (49 mEq or 24.5 mmol) of $MgSO_4$ in 1000 mL of D5W is given IV over 4 hours, followed by 6 g every 8 hours times 2, followed by 6 g every day.

REFERENCE

Zaloga GP, Chernow B. Hypocalcemia in critical illness. *JAMA* 1986;256:1924–1929.

■ HYPOGLYCEMIA

I. **Problem.** A 33-year-old white woman was admitted for diabetic ketoacidosis (DKA) 24 hours ago. The nurse calls to report that 1 hour ago, the patient's fingerstick glucose was 50 mg/dL or 2.78 mmol/L.

II. **Immediate Questions**

A. **What are the patient's vital signs and is the patient asymptomatic now?** Assessing current status and vital signs provides the house officer with a sense of urgency; ie, is there time to wait for a repeat fingerstick and/or blood serum glucose or should therapy be instituted immediately? Patients with hypoglycemia can have multiple symptoms. Early symptoms include headache, hunger, palpitations, tremor, and diaphoresis. As hypoglycemia progresses, abnormal behavior (such as combativeness) and slurred speech mimicking ethanol intoxication are followed by loss of consciousness, seizures, and even death. Beta blockers can mask the early symptoms of hypoglycemia except diaphoresis which is a cholinergic response.

B. **What are the patient's medications?** Presumably a patient in DKA will be on insulin instead of oral hypoglycemic agents as oral agents are not indicated for the treatment of type I diabetes mellitus.

1. The dose, route, and type of insulin are important in determining the timing and severity of the hypoglycemia. Patients on intermediate-acting insulin (NPH or Lente) generally have a peak effect between 6 and 16 hours, whereas those on rapid-acting insulin (regular) given subcutaneously peak at 2–6 hours. Only regular insulin is used intravenously. Intravenous bolus insulin produces its maximum effect in 30 minutes. Patients on continuous IV infusion insulin drips and continuous subcutaneous insulin (by insulin pump) can show very rapid decreases in their serum glucose although the total dose received may be relatively small.
2. Some patients have different responses to rapid-acting and intermediate-acting insulin such that the peak effect is extended to 18–24 hours for intermediate-acting insulin and to 6–12 hours or longer for regular insulin.

3. Knowing the amount, type, and route for administration of insulin will help determine the likelihood of the patient's hypoglycemia worsening or recurring after treatment as well as the changes that need to be made in the insulin regimen. If a patient is on an oral hypoglycemic agent, it is important to know which agent. Chlorpropamide (Diabinese) has an extremely long half-life (32 hours) and may cause recurrent hypoglycemia, especially if the patient is fasting.

C. **What IV fluids are running?** This is necessary to determine that IV access is available to administer D50 if needed and to ascertain whether the patient is receiving a fluid that contains dextrose.

D. **When was the patient's last meal or snack?** If the patient has eaten a meal in the hour since the fingerstick was obtained, the sense of urgency will be slightly less since the meal may have already treated the hypoglycemia.

III. Differential Diagnosis

A. Medications

1. **Insulin.** Accidental overdose, as when insulin is given to the wrong patient; or administration of the wrong type or by the wrong route; or intentional overdose as in Munchausen's syndrome.
2. **Oral hypoglycemic agents.** Especially chlorpropamide in elderly patients.
3. **Medications and ethanol.** Ethanol intoxication, acetaminophen (Tylenol), pentamidine (Pentam), haloperidol (Haldol), *para*-aminosalicylic acid (PAS), and disopyramide (Norpace) can cause hypoglycemia.
4. **Drug interactions.** Activity of oral hypoglycemic agents is increased when taken with nonsteroidal anti-inflammatory agents, sulfonamides, or monoaminoxidase inhibitors.

B. **Reactive hypoglycemia.** Hypoglycemia that occurs after eating. Found in 5% to 10% of patients who have undergone partial to complete gastrectomies as well as de novo in the general population.

C. **Severe liver disease.** With massive liver destruction, glycogen stores are easily depleted.

D. **Insulinoma.** Pancreatic islet cell tumor. May be malignant. Serum insulin levels helpful.

E. **Endocrinopathies.** Addison's disease, pituitary insufficiency, myxedema.

F. **Renal disease.** Usually in the setting of combined uremia and malnutrition.

G. **Sepsis.** Especially in the setting of septic shock.

H. **Malnutrition/prolonged fasting.** Hypoglycemia is common in protein calorie malnutrition (kwashiorkor).

I. **Abrupt discontinuation of total parenteral nutrition (TPN).** More likely if the TPN solution contained insulin.

J. **Factitious hypoglycemia.** As a result of either a marked elevation in the white blood cell count and metabolism by leukocytes or prolongation of contact of serum with red blood cells.

K. **Neoplasms.** Retroperitoneal sarcoma, hepatocellular carcinoma, and oat cell carcinoma can cause hypoglycemia by production of insulin-like hormone, impaired glycogenolysis, or glucose consumption.

IV. Database

A. Physical examination key points

1. **Vital signs.** Hypertension and tachycardia caused by catecholamine response to hypoglycemia. This response can be eliminated with a beta blocker.
2. **Skin.** Diaphoresis common. Generally not blocked by beta blockers as it is a cholinergic response.
3. **Neurologic exam.** Sensorium/orientation often altered. (See Coma, Acute Mental Status Changes, p 65.) May note tremor at rest and with intention. Unconsciousness and seizures indicate need for urgent treatment. Occasionally hypoglycemia presents with focal neurologic findings.

B. Laboratory data

1. **Serum glucose.** This is the most critical value. In general, a glucose level below 50 mg/dL **and** the presence of symptoms are diagnostic of hypoglycemia. Fingerstick values should always be confirmed by serum glucose measurements as they are prone to error from strips that have been left exposed to air, inappropriate preparation of the finger with betadine, presence of alcohol on the finger, incorrect timing, or an uncalibrated machine. In the presence of symptoms, blood should be obtained immediately but treatment **should not** be withheld pending results or a delay in obtaining blood.
2. **Electrolytes, blood urea nitrogen and creatinine, liver function studies, complete blood count, urinalysis.** In the setting of hypoglycemia with no history available, all are indicated to evaluate for common diseases listed in the differential diagnosis.
3. **Drug screens.** Look specifically for oral hypoglycemics as well as ethanol, acetaminophen, and antipsychotics such as haloperidol.
4. **Serum insulin.** May indicate either exogenous insulin administration or insulinoma.
5. **C-peptide.** Will help differentiate insulinoma and exogenous insulin administration. C-peptide will be elevated with an insulinoma and low with the administration of exogenous insulin.

C. Radiologic and other studies.

In specific circumstances, may be indicated to rule out infection, malignancy, or pituitary lesion.

V. Plan

A. **Administer glucose.** Do not wait for the results of the serum glucose if you strongly suspect the diagnosis. Optimally, blood is drawn before giving glucose; however, if there will be a significant delay before blood can be obtained and the patient is markedly symptomatic, proceed with treatment. If the patient is awake and able and willing to take fluids, glucose should be given orally. Otherwise, glucose is administered intravenously.

1. Orange juice with added sugar is usually readily available. Specific glucose-containing liquids are being stocked on most hospital floors and may be substituted for orange juice.
2. Give 1 ampoule of 50% dextrose (D50) IV push; repeat in 5 minutes if no response. If there is no response after the second ampoule, the diagnosis should be seriously questioned and other causes for the symptoms should be considered such as hypoxia, transient ischemic attack, and ethanol or other drug intoxication or overdose.
3. If the patient is unable to take glucose PO and IV access is not immediately available, give glucagon 0.5–1 mg IM or SC (may induce vomiting).
4. Start maintenance IV fluids with D5W at 75–100 mL/h, especially if the hypoglycemia may recur such as that resulting from chlorpropamide or sepsis.
5. Follow serial glucoses frequently. Depending on the severity of the hypoglycemia, repeat glucose after treatment and again in 1–2 hours depending on the results.

B. Adjust medications. Review schedule and dosing of insulin and/or oral hypoglycemics. (See Chapter 7, pp 435 and 497.)

C. Miscellaneous. If the patient is not on hypoglycemic agents, then consider other causes listed in the differential diagnosis and evaluate accordingly.

REFERENCE

Campbell PJ: Mechanisms for prevention, development and reversal of hypoglycemia. *Advances in Internal Medicine* 1988;33:205–230.

■ HYPOKALEMIA

I. Problem. A 72-year-old woman on medication for hypertension develops profound muscle weakness after 3 days of vomiting. Her serum potassium is 2.5 mmol/L (2.5 mEq/L).

II. Immediate Questions

A. What are the patient's vital signs? Premature atrial contractions (PACs), premature ventricular contractions (PVCs), or ventricular arrhythmias may be suspected by examination of the pulse.

B. What medications is the patient talking? Medications, especially diuretics, can cause renal potassium ion wasting. Also, digitalis toxicity is potentiated by hypokalemia.

C. Has the patient had vomiting, diarrhea, or nasogastric suction? These are possible sources of potassium loss.

D. Is there a history of excessive sweating? A prolonged, elevated temperature or delirium tremens can result in hypokalemia from sweating.

III. Differential Diagnosis. Hypokalemia, in general, is caused by cellular shifts or by renal and gastrointestinal losses.

A. Hypokalemia resulting from cellular shifts

1. **Alkalosis.** Both respiratory alkalosis and metabolic alkalosis are associated with hypokalemia. Hyperventilation during surgical anesthesia can cause acute respiratory alkalosis and produce significant hypokalemia.
2. **Familial periodic paralysis.** This rare, inherited disease is characterized by intermittent attacks of varying severity, ranging from muscle weakness to flaccid paralysis.
3. **Barium poisoning.** Ingestion of soluble barium salts may cause profound hypokalemia, muscle paralysis, and cardiac arrhythmias, probably as a result of intracellular shifts, although associated vomiting and diarrhea may also contribute.
4. **Treatment of megaloblastic anemia.** Hypokalemia may occur within 48 hours of administration of folate or vitamin B_{12}. It results from sequestration of potassium ion by a marked increase in bone marrow activity.
5. **Leukemia.** Hypokalemia may be produced by sequestration of potassium ion by rapidly proliferating blast cells.
6. **Insulin.** Intravenous administration of glucose and insulin is an effective treatment of hyperkalemia. The clinical importance of insulin as a cause of hypokalemia is not well established.
7. **β_2-Adrenergic agents.** Isoproterenol, terbutaline, and other β_2-adrenergic agents can cause potassium ions to shift into cells. This is of uncertain clinical importance and is not sufficient reason to undertreat asthmatics.

B. Hypokalemia resulting from normal losses

1. **Diarrhea.** Diarrhea from virtually any cause may result in hypokalemia. But severe hypokalemia secondary to diarrhea is suggestive of colonic villous adenoma or non–insulin-secreting pancreatic islet cell tumor.
2. **Excessive sweat.** The sweat glands contain an aldosterone-dependent sodium/potassium exchange mechanism.
3. **Clay ingestion.** Said to be relatively common in the southeastern United States. Clay binds potassium and carries it into the stool.

C. Hypokalemia resulting from renal losses

1. **Diuretics.** Loop diuretics, thiazides, and acetazolamide (Diamox) may all cause hypokalemia.
2. **Vomiting**
   a. Although gastric contents contain some potassium ion, the major loss through vomiting occurs in the urine. The loss of gastric hydrogen ion generates metabolic alkalosis, which stimulates potassium ion secretion. The sodium and water

losses from vomiting cause volume depletion and stimulate aldosterone secretion.

b. In cases of surreptitious vomiting (bulimia), hypokalemia, metabolic alkalosis, volume depletion, and low urine chloride ion suggest the diagnosis.

3. Renal losses caused by excess mineralocorticoid

a. Primary aldosteronism. Should be suspected in hypertensive patients who are hypokalemic prior to institution of diuretic therapy or in those who become profoundly hypokalemic ($<$ 2.5 mmol/L) with diuretics.

b. Cushing's syndrome. Fifty percent of patients with Cushing's syndrome have hypokalemia. Hypertension and metabolic alkalosis are also common.

c. Ectopic ACTH production. Most commonly seen with small cell carcinoma of the lung.

d. Adrenogenital syndrome. 11-Hydroxylase deficiency is manifested by virilization in the female, precocious puberty in the male, hypokalemia, metabolic alkalosis, and hypertension. 17-Hydroxylase deficiency is a rare form of congenital hyperplasia associated with hypokalemia and hypertension.

e. Licorice ingestion. Natural licorice contains glycyrrhizic acid which has potent mineralocorticoid activity. These patients clinically resemble those with primary aldosteronism.

f. Hyperreninemic states. Hypokalemia is accompanied by hypertension and metabolic alkalosis in renal vascular hypertension, malignant hypertension, and renin-producing tumors. Distinguished from primary aldosteronism by elevated plasma renin.

g. Bartter's syndrome. A rare disorder characterized by hypokalemia, metabolic alkalosis, elevated renin and aldosterone levels, and normal blood pressure.

h. Liddle's syndrome. A rare disorder characterized by hypokalemia, hypertension, metabolic alkalosis, low plasma renin, and low urinary aldosterone.

i. Type I (distal) renal tubular acidosis. Characterized by hyperchloremic metabolic acidosis and hypokalemia. Results from an inability to maintain a hydrogen ion gradient.

j. Type II (proximal) renal tubular acidosis. Impaired proximal bicarbonate reabsorption results in distal delivery of bicarbonate and urinary loss of potassium ion as well as bicarbonate.

k. Antibiotics. Carbenicillin and ticarcillin, administered as sodium salts, enhance potassium ion excretion. Amphotericin B alters distal tubule permeability, resulting in hypokalemia.

l. Magnesium depletion. This may increase mineralocorticoid activity, but the pathophysiology is unknown.

m. **Ureterosigmoidostomy.** Hypokalemic hyperchloremic metabolic acidosis occurs because of an exchange mechanism in the colon. Ureteral implantation into a loop of ileum is now performed.

IV. Database

A. Physical examination key points

1. **Cardiovascular.** Irregular pulse may represent new arrhythmias (PACs or PVCs) or digitalis toxicity.
2. **Abdomen.** Look for distension and presence of bowel sounds. Ileus secondary to hypokalemia may be present. Abdominal examination may reveal a cause of vomiting.
3. **Neurologic exam.** Weakness, blunting of reflexes, paresthesias, and paralysis may be seen.

B. Laboratory data

1. **Serum electrolytes.** Hypomagnesemia may coexist.
2. **Arterial blood gases.** Look for alkalosis.
3. **Urine potassium, chloride, and sodium.** If the patient is not taking diuretics. A low urine sodium or chloride indicates volume depletion. A relatively high urine potassium in the face of hypokalemia indicates renal losses.
4. **Digoxin level.** A must if patient on digoxin. Hypokalemia may potentiate digoxin toxicity.

C. Radiologic and other studies.

An electrocardiogram may show digitalis effect or manifestations of hypokalemia ranging from PACs and PVCs to life-threatening ventricular arrhythmias. A U wave is a common finding.

V. Plan.

The degree of hypokalemia cannot be used as a rigid determinant of the total potassium ion deficit. It has been estimated that in a normal adult, a decrease in serum potassium from 4 to 3 mmol/L corresponds to a 100- to 200-mmol decrement in total body potassium. Each additional fall of 1 mmol/L in serum potassium represents an additional deficit of 200–400 mmol.

A. Parenteral replacement

1. **Indications.** Should be considered in the following situations: digoxin toxicity or significant arrhythmias, severe hypokalemia (< 3.0 mmol/L), and inability to take oral replacement (NPO, ileus, nausea and vomiting). Ideally parenteral solutions should be administered through a central venous catheter. In most other cases, hypokalemia can be safely corrected in a slow, controlled fashion with oral supplementation.
2. **Implementation.** The maximum concentration of potassium chloride used in peripheral veins should generally not exceed 40 mmol/L because of the damaging effects on the veins of high concentrations, although in an emergent situation 60 mmol/L can be attempted. Potassium chloride 20 mmol diluted in 50–100 mL D5W or normal saline can be infused over 1 hour through a central line safely, with doses repeated as needed when severe depletion or life-threatening hypokalemia is pres-

ent. Special care must be taken to ensure slow infusion of high doses. For lesser degrees of hypokalemia that require parenteral replacement, 10–15 mmol/h can be infused peripherally.

3. **Monitoring.** With large total replacement doses, check serum every 2–4 hours to avoid hyperkalemia. Cardiac monitoring in an ICU is required if arrhythmias are present or for rapid infusions of potassium chloride.

B. **Oral replacement.** Generally indicated for asymptomatic, mild potassium depletion (potassium usually > 3.0 mmol/L). Oral replacements include liquids and powder. Slow-release pills typically contain 8–10 mmol per tablet and thus are not usually appropriate for repletion therapy. The replacement rate should be 40–120 mmol/d in divided doses depending on the patient's weight and level of hypokalemia. Maintenance therapy, if needed, should be given in doses of 20–40 mmol daily using the preparation best tolerated by the patient. In patients with normal renal function, it is difficult to induce hyperkalemia through the **oral** administration of potassium. An important exception is the use of potassium supplements in patients on potassium-sparing diuretics, which should be avoided.

C. **Replacement of ongoing losses.** Large amounts of nasogastric aspirate should be replaced milliliter for milliliter with D5 half-normal saline with 20 mmol/L potassium chloride every 4–6 hours.

D. **Refractory cases.** Rarely, hypokalemia may not be correctable because of concomitant hypomagnesemia.

REFERENCES

Gabow PA, Peterson LN. Disorders of potassium metabolism. In: Schrier RW, ed. *Renal and Electrolyte Disorders.* 3rd ed. Boston: Little, Brown; 1986:207–249.

Rose BD, Maffly R. Renal function and disorders of water, sodium and potassium balance. In: Rubenstein E, ed-in-chief; Federman DD, ed. *Scientific American.* sect 10: *Nephrology,* vol 2, pt I. New York: Scientific American Inc; 1990:27–28.

Sterns RH, Narins RG. Disorders of potassium balance. In: Stein JH, ed-in-chief. *Internal Medicine.* 3rd ed. Boston: Little, Brown; 1990:853–864.

■ HYPOMAGNESEMIA

I. **Problem.** A 34-year-old white male alcoholic is admitted for new onset of seizures. A stat magnesium level returns at 0.5 mEq/L (normal 1.5–2.1 mEq/L).

II. **Immediate Questions**

A. **What are the patient's vital signs?** Magnesium deficiency is associated with cardiac arrhythmias including atrial fibrillation, supraventricular tachycardia, ventricular tachycardia, and ventricular fibrillation. Determining that the patient is not in any immediate distress and does not have hypotension or a tachyarrhythmia is important.

B. **Is the patient tremulous or currently having a seizure?** Tremor, tetany, muscle fasciculations, and seizures are all associated with magnesium deficiency. Determining the presence of these neurologic problems will help guide the urgency of treatment.

III. **Differential Diagnosis.** The diagnosis of magnesium deficiency, in general, rests on a high degree of suspicion, clinical assessment, and measurement of serum magnesium. It is important to recognize that serum magnesium levels do not always correlate well with intracellular magnesium levels. Thus, it is possible to have total body and/or intracellular magnesium depletion with normal (or even high) serum magnesium levels. For this reason, several groups have suggested that an initial 24-hour urine collection for magnesium and/or a 24-hour urine magnesium retention test after parenteral administration of magnesium be done to determine whether magnesium depletion is really present. Although such tests may be useful in specific settings, the acutely ill patient is generally treated on the basis of serum level and good clinical judgment.

A. **Hypocalcemia.** The signs and symptoms of hypocalcemia are similar to those of hypomagnesemia and often both problems are present in a single patient. Hypocalcemia that does not correct with intravenous supplementation suggests the presence of magnesium deficiency.

B. **Hypokalemia.** Potassium depletion often coexists with hypomagnesemia and can cause arrhythmias and muscle weakness, similar to hypomagnesemia. Hypokalemia that does not correct appropriately with potassium repletion also suggests magnesium depletion.

C. **Lab error.** More likely if a colorimetric assay is used. When in doubt, ask the lab to repeat the test and controls.

D. **Causes of hypomagnesemia**

1. **Increased excretion**
   a. **Medications.** Medications, especially diuretics, antibiotics (ticarcillin, amphotericin B), aminoglycosides, *cis*-platinum and cyclosporin, often cause hypomagnesemia.
   b. **Alcoholism.** Very common cause as a result of decreased intake and renal magnesium wasting.
   c. **Diabetes mellitus.** Commonly seen in patients treated for diabetic ketoacidosis.
   d. **Renal tubular disorders.** With magnesium wasting.
   e. **Hypercalcemia/hypercalcuria**
   f. **Hyperaldosteronism/Bartter's syndrome**
   g. **Excessive lactation**
   h. **Marked diaphoresis**
2. **Reduced intake/malabsorption**
   a. **Starvation.** A common cause.
   b. **Bowel bypass or resection**

c. **Total parenteral nutrition without adequate magnesium supplementation**
d. **Chronic malabsorption syndrome.** Such as pancreatic insufficiency.
e. **Chronic diarrhea**

3. **Miscellaneous**
   a. **Acute pancreatitis**
   b. **Hypoalbuminemia**
   c. **Vitamin D therapy.** Resulting in hypercalcuria.

IV. Database

A. Physical examination key points

1. **Vital signs.** Blood pressure and pulse to evaluate for the presence of hypotension and tachyarrhythmias. While taking blood pressure, leave cuff inflated for 3 minutes to check for carpal spasm (Trousseau's sign).
2. **HEENT.** Check for Chvostek's sign (tapping over the facial nerve produces twitching of the mouth and eye). Nystagmus may be present.
3. **Heart.** Check for regularity of rhythm.
4. **Abdomen.** Evaluate for evidence of pancreatitis, absent bowel sounds, and tenderness. Stigmata of chronic liver disease such as hepatosplenomegaly, caput medusae, ascites, spider angiomas, and palmar erythema suggest chronic alcohol abuse.
5. **Neurologic exam.** Hyperactive reflexes, muscle fasciculations, seizures, tetany can result from hypomagnesemia. Hyperactive reflexes may also be seen with alcohol withdrawal.
6. **Mental status.** Psychosis, depression, and agitation may be present.

B. Laboratory data

1. **Serum electrolytes, glucose, calcium, and phosphorus.** Hypomagnesemia frequently accompanies other electrolyte abnormalities, especially hypocalcemia, hypokalemia, and alkalosis. If the patient is an alcoholic, then hypophosphatemia is also likely. Diabetics are prone to develop hypomagnesemia (especially in the setting of diabetic ketoacidosis).
2. **24-hour urine for magnesium.** May be helpful if the diagnosis is in question or if there is a suspicion of renal magnesium wasting.
3. **Magnesium retention test.** Using either parenteral or oral magnesium. May be helpful in certain subsets of patients in whom either the diagnosis is in question or malabsorption is suspected.
4. **Miscellaneous.** As indicated by clinical situation. Liver function studies in alcoholics, serum amylase if pancreatitis is suspected, and so forth.

C. Radiologic and other studies. Electrocardiographic findings may include prolongation of the PR, QT, and QRS intervals as well as ST depression and T waves. Rhythm disturbances include supraventricular arrhythmias as well as ventricular tachycardia and ventricular fibrillation.

V. **Plan.** The urgency of treatment depends on the clinical setting. The patient who is having neurologic or cardiac manifestations should be treated urgently with parenteral intravenous therapy. Asymptomatic individuals may be treated with oral magnesium although many clinicians treat magnesium levels less than 1.0 mEq/L with parenteral magnesium regardless of the fact that there is not always a good correlation between serum levels and intracellular levels as noted earlier.

A. **Intravenous magnesium sulfate.** Magnesium sulfate 1 g (2 mL of a 50% solution of $MgSO_4$) equals 98 mg of elemental magnesium, which is equal to 8 mEq $MgSO_4$ or 4 mmol Mg^{2+}. If the patient is in tetany or status epilepticus or is having significant cardiac arrhythmias, then 2 g of magnesium sulfate can be given IV over 10–20 minutes. For slightly less urgent situations, 1 g/h may be given with close monitoring of deep tendon reflexes every 3–4 hours. Magnesium should be administered only in life threatening situations in patients with renal insufficiency and monitoring of deep tendon reflexes is required every hour. As long as signs and symptoms of hypomagnesemia are improving, the infusion can then be slowed so that the patient receives approximately 10 g of magnesium sulfate in the first 24 hours. Selected patients may require more or less based on clinical findings. Subsequently, 5–6 g of magnesium sulfate may be given over each 24 hours to replenish body reserves for the next 3–4 days.

B. **Intramuscular magnesium sulfate.** One to two grams IM every 4 hours for five doses during the first 24 hours (following the patient's clinical status and serum levels as described earlier). This can then be followed by 1 g IM every 6 hours for 2–3 days. Many patients complain about pain with the injections.

C. **Oral magnesium oxide (20 mEq of magnesium per 400 mg tablet).** One to two tablets per day for chronic maintenance therapy (may cause diarrhea, especially at higher doses).

D. **Miscellaneous.** Treat other electrolyte disorders, especially hypocalcemia (see Hypocalcemia, Section V, p 155), hypokalemia (see Hypokalemia, Section V, p 162) and hypophosphatemia (see Hypophosphatemia, Section V, p 173) as well as other underlying illnesses.

REFERENCES

Elin RJ. Magnesium metabolism in health and disease. *Disease-a-Month* 1988; 34:161–218.

Massry S. Magnesium homeostasis and its clinical pathophysiology. *Resident Staff Physician* 1981;27:106–109.

HYPONATREMIA

I. **Problem.** A 50-year-old white man is admitted for evaluation of a right pulmonary hilar mass. Shortly after admission, you are called by the lab with a "panic" lab value. The serum sodium is 118 mmol/L (normal 136–145 mmol/L).

II. **Immediate Questions**

A. **Is the patient symptomatic from the hyponatremia?** Patients with hyponatremia may be asymptomatic or there may be central nervous system changes ranging from lethargy to marked disorientation, seizures, and death.

B. **Are there any recent prior sodium levels to document the chronicity of the hyponatremia?** The rate of development of hyponatremia correlates directly with the severity of the symptoms it produces. Acute changes in sodium are more likely to produce severe symptoms.

C. **Is there any evidence of volume depletion?** Orthostatic changes in blood pressure and heart rate suggest volume depletion.

D. **Is there any history of vomiting or diarrhea?** Vomiting and diarrhea can cause wasting of sodium and extracellular fluid resulting in hyponatremia, especially if the patient replaces the deficit by drinking free water.

E. **Is there any history of renal disease, congestive heart failure, cirrhosis, or nephrotic syndrome?** Any of these edematous states suggests an excess of sodium accompanied by an even greater excess of total body water.

F. **Is there any history of hypothyroidism or adrenal insufficiency?** Hypothyroidism and hypoadrenalism cause renal wasting of sodium even in the face of hyponatremia.

G. **Is the patient on any medications that could cause the hyponatremia?** Diuretics can cause hyponatremia by inducing sodium deficits in excess of water deficits. Chlorpropamide, nicotine, cyclophosphamide, and nonsteroidal anti-inflammatory drugs as well as antipsychotic medications such as haloperidol and thioridazine may cause hyponatremia. Mannitol used to treat elevated intracranial pressure or glaucoma can cause a low serum sodium because of water moving from the intracellular space to the hypertonic extracellular space.

H. **Is there any pulmonary disease?** Pneumonia, tuberculosis, lung carcinoma, and other pulmonary pathology can cause the syndrome of inappropriate antidiuretic hormone secretion (SIADH).

I. **Is there any central nervous system disease?** Meningitis, encephalitis, brain abscess, tumors, trauma, and a variety of other diseases can cause SIADH.

J. **Is there a history suggesting neoplasm?** Weight loss, cough, hemoptysis, night sweats. Bronchogenic carcinoma as well as other cancers has been associated with SIADH.

K. **Is there any history of hyperlipidemia or hyperproteinemia?** Either can cause a low serum sodium without extracellular fluid hypertonicity. Also called pseudohyponatremia.

L. **Is there a history of diabetes?** A markedly elevated glucose can lower the serum sodium. The serum sodium is diluted by water moving from the intracellular space to the hypertonic extracellular space.

III. **Differential Diagnosis.** The initial differentiation is between true hyponatremia and laboratory artifact. True hyponatremia may be classified according to the volume status of the patient: **hypovolemic, euvolemic,** or **hypervolemic** (See Section IV.A). Hypovolemic hyponatremia may be further classified by serum and urine chemistries.

A. **Space-occupying compounds.** Lipids are the most common. The lab can ultracentrifuge the specimen to find the correct plasma sodium level. Waldenstrom's macroglobulinemia and multiple myeloma also cause pseudohyponatremia.

B. **Diabetes mellitus.** Results in a hypertonic hyponatremia from the intracellular-to-extracellular movement of water. Not a true pseudohyponatremia. The expected decrease in serum sodium is 1.6 mmol/dL for each 100 mg/dL of glucose over 100 mg/dL.

C. **Hypovolemic hyponatremia**

1. **Spot urinary sodium less than 10 mmol/L**
   a. **Gastrointestinal fluid losses.** Vomiting or diarrhea. In surreptitious vomiting or bulemia, the urinary chloride is usually less than 10 mmol/L.
   b. **Third-space fluid loss.** Such as pancreatitis or peritonitis.
   c. **Burns**
2. **Spot urinary sodium greater than 20 mmol/L**
   a. **Diuretic usage.** Caused by thiazides (eg, hydrochlorothiazide) and loop diuretics (furosemide) and often associated with hypokalemia and alkalosis; with surreptitious diuretic use, urinary chloride is greater than 20 mEq/L.
   b. **Renal disorders.** Renal tubular acidosis, medullary cystic disease, polycystic disease, and chronic interstitial nephritis can result in hyponatremia.
   c. **Addison's disease.** Hyperkalemia, low urinary potassium, and metabolic acidosis are also found.
   d. **Osmotic diuresis.** Most commonly caused by glucose, hyperglycemia, or mannitol.

D. **Euvolemic hyponatremia**

1. **SIADH.** The diagnosis of SIADH is based on the finding of low serum osmolality, elevated urine sodium (> 20 mmol/L), and concentrated urine (osmolality near normal).
   a. **Tumors.** Small lung cell cancer is most common.
   b. **Pulmonary disease.** Tuberculosis, pneumonia, lung cancer, pneumothorax.
   c. **CNS disorders.** Trauma, tumors, and infections such as meningitis and encephalitis.

d. **Stress.** Including perioperative stress.
e. **Drugs.** Oral hypoglycemics (chlorpropamide), chemotherapeutics (cyclophosphamide, vincristine), psychiatric drugs (haloperidol, thioridazine, tricyclic antidepressants), and clofibrate.
f. **Postoperative.** Anesthesia and surgical procedures cause an increase in antidiuretic hormone.

2. **Hypothyroidism**
3. **Glucocorticoid deficiency**
4. **Hypopituitarism**

E. **Hypervolemic hyponatremia**

1. **Congestive heart failure.** Urine sodium less than 10 mmol/L.
2. **Cirrhosis.** Urine sodium less than 10 mmol/L.
3. **Renal disease**
   a. **Chronic renal failure.** Urine sodium greater than 20 mmol/L.
   b. **Nephrotic syndrome.** Urine sodium less than 10 mmol/L.

IV. Database

A. **Physical exam key points.** Close attention should be paid to the assessment of the volume status.

1. **Vital signs.** Evaluate for orthostatic blood pressure changes and heart rate changes. Measure supine and standing blood pressures and heart rate. A drop in systolic blood pressure greater than 10 mm Hg or a pulse increase greater than 20 BPM is highly suggestive of volume depletion. Tachypnea may suggest volume overload and pulmonary edema.
2. **Skin.** Tissue turgor will be diminished and mucous membranes dry with volume depletion. Edema suggests volume overload. Jaundice, spider angiomas, and caput medusae suggest cirrhosis.
3. **HEENT.** Evaluate the internal jugular vein with the bed up at 45° (veins flat with volume depletion and markedly engorged with volume overload).
4. **Lungs.** Rales may be heard with congestive heart failure.
5. **Heart.** An S_3 gallop suggests congestive heart failure.
6. **Abdomen.** Hepatosplenomegaly and ascites suggest cirrhosis. A hepatojugular reflux may be present in congestive heart failure.
7. **Neurologic exam.** Hyperactive deep tendon reflexes, altered mental status, confusion, coma, or seizures may be present after a rapid fall in the serum sodium or from a chronically low serum sodium. If the hyponatremia is chronic, the neurologic and mental status exams may be normal even with levels less than 120 mmol/dL.

B. **Laboratory data**

1. **Electrolytes.** Other abnormalities may coexist. Hypokalemia can potentiate hyponatremia.

2. **Spot urine electrolytes and creatinine.** Obtain prior to any diuretic treatment.
3. **Urine and serum osmolality.** Serum osmolality will be normal in cases of laboratory artifact but decreased in true hyponatremia. Serum osmolality will be increased in hypertonic hyponatremia secondary to mannitol.
4. **Liver function tests.** To detect liver disease.
5. **Thyroid function.** Hypothyroidism must be ruled out prior to diagnosing SIADH.
6. **Cortisol levels, ACTH stimulation test also before diagnosing SIADH.** Glucocorticoid deficiency must be ruled out.
7. **Cultures (blood and sputum).** If indicated.

C. **Radiologic and other studies**
1. **Chest x-ray.** Look for congestive heart failure, lung cancer, pneumonia, or tuberculosis.
2. **Head CT scan.** If indicated.

V. **Plan.** The etiology of the hyponatremia and the presence and severity of symptoms guide therapy. Aggressive therapy for severe symptoms such as coma is discussed as are specific therapies for certain diagnoses.

A. **Emergency therapy.** Usually for severe CNS (seizure, coma) symptoms.
1. **Furosemide 1 mg/kg IV and/or normal saline.** Use the combination of normal saline and diuretics to achieve a net negative free water deficit balance in hyponatremia associated with euvolemic or hypervolemic conditions. Use normal saline alone if the hyponatremia is associated with volume depletion. Carefully document volume in and out. Supplement fluids with potassium as needed. Rapid correction of sodium to normal can be deleterious, resulting in central pontine myelinolysis. Rapidly correct to 125 mmol/L; then in the next 24 hours correct to normal. In euvolemic or hypervolemic states, the excess total body water can be calculated from

$$\text{weight (kg)} \times 0.60 = \text{normal total body water (NTBW)}$$

$$[\text{serum Na} \div 140(\text{desired Na})] \times \text{weight (kg)} \times 0.60 = \text{actual total body water (ATBW)}$$

$$\text{NTBW} - \text{ATBW} = \text{total excess body water}$$

2. **Hypertonic saline (3%).** Rarely, if ever, needed. Some institutions have banned its use entirely because of possible serious complications such as pulmonary edema and too rapid a correction of hyponatremia resulting in central pontine myelinolysis.

B. **Hypovolemic hyponatremia**
1. For almost all causes, treat by repletion of volume and sodium. Normal saline is given intravenously.

2. For diuretic abuse, repletion of lost body potassium is also needed.

C. Euvolemic hyponatremia. (Patient is not edematous.) SIADH—water restriction to 800–1000 mL daily. Demeclocycline (300–600 mg BID orally) for chronic SIADH, such as that resulting from neoplasia, but onset of action may take up to a week.

D. Hypervolemic hyponatremia. (Patient is edematous.) Restrict intravenous and oral fluids.

1. **Congestive heart failure.** Treat with digoxin (Lanoxin), diuretics such as furosemide (Lasix), angiotensin-converting enzyme (ACE) inhibitors such as captopril (Capoten) or enalapril (Vasotec), and sodium restriction.
2. **Nephrotic syndrome.** Steroids (if steroid-responsive cause), sodium and water restriction, increased protein intake. Furosemide commonly used.
3. **Cirrhosis.** Sodium and water restriction, diuretics. Initially spironolactone 25 mg PO every 6 hours, increasing dose every 2–3 days up to 100–200 mg every 6 hours. Portosystemic shunt needed in only 5% to 10% of patients to control ascites.
4. **Renal failure.** Sodium and water restriction, loop diuretics (furosemide), and dialysis if indicated.

REFERENCES

Bell T, Schrier RW. Disorders of water metabolism. In: Schrier RW, ed. *Renal and Electrolyte Disorders.* 3rd ed. Boston: Little, Brown; 1986:1–77.

Watson AJ. Hyponatremia. *Primary Care Emerg Decisions* 1987;3(9):48–58.

Weisberg LS. Pseudohyponatremia: A reappraisal. *Am J Med* 1989;86:315–318.

■ HYPOPHOSPHATEMIA

I. Problem. A 26-year-old type I diabetic male who was admitted 6 hours ago for treatment of diabetic ketoacidosis has a serum phosphate level of 1.0 mg/dL.

II. Immediate Questions

A. Are there any symptoms related to the low phosphate? Serum phosphate levels below 1.0 mg/dL require prompt treatment regardless of symptoms. Above that level, one should check for symptoms that could indicate significant adverse tissue effects related to low phosphate level such as numbness or tingling, muscle weakness, anorexia, confusion, irritability, seizures, and skeletal pain. Muscle weakness, mental status changes, and hematologic abnormalities are the most common findings.

B. What treatment is the patient receiving? Hypophosphatemia usually results from phosphate shifts within the body. This is most often a consequence of medical treatment, such as hyperalimentation, correction of diabetic ketoacidosis, or refeeding of malnourished or alcoholic patients. Antacids also can cause hypophosphatemia by binding to phosphate in the gut.

C. **Does the patient consume alcohol?** Chronic alcoholism is a common cause of hypophosphatemia secondary to poor intake and possible increased renal excretion if hypomagnesemia is also present.

III. **Differential Diagnosis.** A low serum phosphate level usually results from some combination of increased renal phosphate loss, increased intestinal loss, and/or intracellular shift of phosphate, the latter being the most common.

A. **Intracellular shift of phosphate.** Alkalosis from any etiology (see Alkalosis, p 17).

B. **Increased intestinal loss**
   1. **Phosphate-binding antacids**
   2. **Malabsorption, vomiting, diarrhea, malnutrition**

C. **Increased renal phosphate loss**
   1. **Acidosis.** Including untreated diabetic ketoacidosis (DKA).
   2. **Hyperparathyroidism, renal tubular disease, hypokalemia, hypomagnesemia, diuretics**

D. **Multifactoral**
   1. **Alcoholism and liver disease.** All three mechanisms.
   2. **Vitamin D deficiency or resistance.** Renal and intestinal loss.
   3. **Treatment of DKA and severe burns.** Renal and intracellular shift.

IV. **Database**

A. **Physical examination key points**
   1. **Vital signs**
      a. **Temperature.** Heat stroke can cause hypophosphatemia from intracellular shifts.
      b. **Sepsis.** Occurs with greater frequency in patients who are hypophosphatemic because of leukocyte dysfunction.
      c. **Respiratory rate.** Hyperventilation is a cause of extracellular-to-intracellular shifts of phosphate.
   2. **HEENT.** Look for thyromegaly. Thyrotoxicosis can cause extracellular to intracellular shifts.
   3. **Heart.** A reversible congestive cardiomyopathy may result from hypophosphatemia. Look for a laterally displaced apical pulse and a third heart sound (S_3).
   4. **Lungs.** Listen for rales as evidence for cardiomyopathy. Acute hypophosphatemia can also result in acute respiratory failure.
   5. **Neurologic exam.** Confusion and coma may be present. Sensory examination may be abnormal secondary to related paresthesias.

6. **Musculoskeletal exam.** Look for diffuse muscle weakness. Tenderness suggests rhabdomyolysis; however, the phosphate may increase to extremely high levels with rhabdomyolysis.

B. **Laboratory data**
   1. **Serum electrolytes.** Especially bicarbonate and potassium. An elevated bicarbonate may suggest a metabolic alkalosis; a low bicarbonate may represent compensation for a chronic respiratory alkalosis. Alkalosis results in extracellular-to-intracellular shifts of phosphate. Hypokalemia can cause hypophosphatemia.
   2. **Arterial blood gases and pH.** Alkalosis (either metabolic or respiratory) results in intracellular shifts of phosphate. A metabolic acidosis with an increased anion gap and an elevated glucose suggests diabetic ketoacidosis, which can have associated hypophosphatemia. An elevated pCO_2 also suggests respiratory failure.
   3. **Calcium, magnesium, and glucose levels.** A low calcium may suggest vitamin D deficiency or osteomalacia. A high calcium suggests hyperparathyroidism or thiazide diuretic use, which results in associated hypophosphatemia. Hypomagnesemia results in increased phosphate excretion.
   4. **Glucose.** There is increased urinary excretion of phosphate in diabetic ketoacidosis.
   5. **Uric acid.** Hypophosphatemia can be seen with acute gout; however, the uric acid level may be normal in acute gout.
   6. **Liver enzymes, albumin, bilirubin, and creatine phosphokinase (CPK).** Hypophosphatemia may cause liver dysfunction. A CPK should be checked to rule out rhabdomyolysis with severe hypophosphatemia, especially if muscle tenderness is present or develops.
   7. **Complete blood count with differential.** An elevated white blood cell count with a left shift suggests a bacterial infection. As a result of white cell dysfunction, patients with hypophosphatemia are susceptible to bacterial infections.
   8. **Peripheral smear.** Severe hypophosphatemia can cause hemolysis.
   9. **Platelet count.** Thrombocytopenia and platelet dysfunction can result.

C. **Radiologic and other studies**
   1. **Bone films.** May show pseudofractures.
   2. **Chest x-ray.** Possible complications of hypophosphatemia such as congestive cardiomyopathy and respiratory failure are indications for a CXR.
   3. **Electroencephalogram.** May be needed to evaluate seizures or encephalopathy, which are possible complications of hypophosphatemia.

V. **Plan.** If the phosphate level is less than 1.0 mg/dL, start intravenous replacement therapy immediately. If the level is close to 1.0 mg/dL and the patient is symptomatic, start intravenous replacement therapy. Otherwise, oral treatment will be best.

A. Intravenous treatment

1. If the hypophosphatemia is recent and uncomplicated, give 0.08 mmol/kg body weight (2.5 mg/kg) intravenously over 6 hours. Sodium phosphate and potassium phosphate intravenous solutions both contain 3 mmol of phosphate per milliliter.
2. If the hypophosphatemia is long-standing or complicated, give 0.16 mmol/kg body weight (5.0 mg/kg) intravenously over 6 hours.
3. In either case, consider using 25% to 50% higher doses if the patient is symptomatic, but do not exceed 0.24 mmol/kg (7.5 mg/kg) or 16.9 mmol (525 mg) for a 70-kg patient.
4. Recheck the phosphate level promptly after the 6-hour infusion, and reassess the need for further replacement.

B. Oral replacement

1. Neutra Phos contains 0.1 mmol of phosphate per milliliter. Phospho-soda contains 4.15 mmol of phosphate per milliliter. Both are quite unpalatable.
2. Milk contains modest amounts of phosphate (0.03 mmol/mL).

C. Precautions

1. It may be necessary to give calcium supplements to hypocalcemic patients who are being given phosphate.
2. Do not give calcium and phosphate through the same intravenous line.
3. Beware of causing hyperphosphatemia, hypotension, hyperkalemia, osmotic diuresis, and hypernatremia.

REFERENCES

Kreisberg RA. Phosphorus deficiency and hypophosphatemia. *Hosp Pract* 1977;Mar:121–128.

Lentz RD, Brown DM, Kjellstrand CM. Treatment of severe hypophosphatemia. *Ann Intern Med* 1978;89:941–944.

Popovtzer MM, Knochel JP. Disorders of calcium, phosphorus, vitamin D and parathyroid hormone activity. In: Schrier RW, ed. *Renal and Electrolyte Disorders*. 3rd ed. Boston: Little, Brown; 1986:251–329.

■ HYPOTENSION (SHOCK)

I. Problem. A 70-year-old man admitted for nausea and weight loss develops a blood pressure of 70/50.

II. Immediate Questions

A. What are all of the patient's vital signs? Repeat the blood pressure, in both arms, to verify its accuracy. An extremely slow pulse may indicate a cardiogenic etiology and tachycardia may indicate hypovolemia, hemorrhage, or sepsis, or point to a primary cardiac arrhythmia such as atrial fibrillation or ventricular tachycardia. Fever would suggest an infectious etiology, whereas hypothermia can be seen in myxedema or sepsis. Fever or hypothermia can be associated with Addisonian crisis. Tachypnea can be seen with cardiogenic shock, pulmonary embolism (PE), and sepsis.

B. **What is the patient's mental status?** This is an indicator of adequate perfusion of vital organs.

C. **What are the patient's medications and when were they last given? Have any new medications been started?** Many medications such as vasodilators (captopril [Captopen], minoxidil [Loniten]) and central-acting antihypertensive agents such as clonidine (Catapres) lower blood pressure and may do so to an extreme. Other intravenous medications with similar effects include nitroprusside, nitroglycerin, and phenytoin (Dilantin). Anaphylaxis should be considered especially if there is respiratory distress. Diuretics can rarely cause a significant enough volume depletion to cause hypotension.

D. **Does the patient have any other symptoms?** The patient's symptoms may indicate where to begin your evaluation such as any history of bleeding, diarrhea, diaphoresis, polyuria, or emesis. If the patient notes sharp, pleuritic chest pain and dyspnea, a massive pulmonary embolus should be suspected. Dull substernal chest pain with associated shortness of breath and diaphoresis suggest myocardial infarction/ischemia resulting in myocardial dysfunction and cardiogenic shock.

III. **Differential Diagnosis.** The term *hypotension* is a relative term. For elderly patients with long-standing hypertension, a systolic blood pressure of 100 mm Hg may be inadequate. But in others, a systolic pressure of 90 mm Hg may be a normal baseline. Hypotension/shock is defined as a state where the blood pressure is inadequate to provide tissue perfusion. Subcategories of hypotension/shock include the following.

A. **Hemorrhagic**
   1. **Traumatic.** Trauma patients may lose a large volume of blood into body cavities that is not readily apparent such as the chest, abdomen, and pelvis.
   2. **Postoperative or after procedures** such as liver biopsy or central venous line placement.
   3. **Miscellaneous.** Gastrointestinal bleeding, ruptured aneurysm, ruptured ovarian cyst, ectopic pregnancy.

B. **Fluid losses.** Severe vomiting, diarrhea, perspiration, extensive burns, diuresis, and "third-space losses" (peritonitis or pancreatitis).

C. **Vasogenic.** Inappropriate loss of vascular tone may develop as a result of sepsis, anaphylaxis, adrenal insufficiency, acidosis, or central nervous system insult.

D. **Cardiogenic.** Acute pump failure may develop as a result of myocardial infarction (MI) or decompensated congestive heart failure (CHF). Cardiac arrhythmia (supraventricular, ventricular, or various degrees of heart block) can cause hypotension. Tension pneumothorax, pericardial tamponade, and PE impede ventricular filling and cause hypotension.

IV. Database

A. Physical examination key points

1. **Vital signs.** Temperature, blood pressure, pulse, respiratory rate, including orthostatic blood pressure and heart rate. A decrease in systolic blood pressure of 10 mm Hg and/or an increase in heart rate of 20 BPM on movement from the supine to the standing position for 1 minute is indicative of volume depletion.
2. **Skin.** Poor skin turgor suggests volume depletion but may be a normal variant in the elderly. Cool, clammy skin indicates cardiogenic or hypovolemic shock, whereas warm, moist skin signifies vasodilation (sepsis).
3. **Neck.** Jugular venous distension (JVD) and pulsations may be helpful in determining volume status and cardiac rhythm, as well as in providing clues for diagnosis of cardiac tamponade or tension pneumothorax. Jugular venous distension with the latter two does not decrease with inspiration.
4. **Chest.** Tracheal deviation suggests tension pneumothorax. Wheezing or stridor may indicate anaphylaxis. Rales and wheezes point to cardiac failure. Abnormalities during chest percussion may indicate pneumothorax, pleural effusion, hemothorax, or pneumonia.
5. **Heart.** Palpate for a thrill or change in the point of maximal impulse. A new thrill may point to a ventricular septal defect (VSD) or papillary muscle dysfunction complicating an acute MI. Loss of a palpable apical pulse suggests a pericardial effusion. Auscultate for new murmurs suggesting acute mitral regurgitation or a VSD. A third heart sound (S_3) is heard in left ventricular failure. A new fourth heart sound (S_4) suggests an acute MI. A friction rub is present in pericarditis and possibly cardiac tamponade.
6. **Abdomen.** Rebound tenderness or positive Murphy's sign and absence of bowel sounds suggest sepsis from an abdominal source. (See Abdominal Pain, p 1.) Absent bowel sounds and tenderness may be present with a large GI bleed. A pulsatile mass suggests a leaking aortic aneurysm. Ecchymoses may be seen in retroperitoneal bleeds from a variety of causes such as hemorrhagic pancreatitis.
7. **Rectum.** Presence of hematochezia or occult blood may indicate GI blood loss.
8. **Female genitalia.** Gynecologic exam in young females is mandatory to rule out a ruptured ectopic pregnancy.

9. **Extremities.** Instability of pelvis or femurs suggests a fracture, which can result in significant bleeding into either the pelvis or the thigh. Edema may indicate volume overload or venous/lymphatic obstruction. Inspect for inflammation of vascular access sites suggesting iatrogenic infection/sepsis.
10. **Neurologic exam.** Altered mental status may indicate inadequate cerebral hypoperfusion as well as suggest possible etiologies such as a cerebrovascular accident.

B. Laboratory data

1. **Complete blood count.** Serial hematocrits may indicate blood loss. Acute blood loss may not be reflected by an immediate drop in the hematocrit, but will fall as intravascular volume equilibrates. The white blood count and differential may indicate infection. The platelet count will be low in disseminated intravascular coagulation (DIC), suggesting sepsis.
2. **Serum electrolytes.** A low serum bicarbonate could be caused by a lactic acidosis secondary to decreased perfusion. Severe acidosis or hypokalemia may cause an arrhythmia.
3. **Prothrombin time, partial thromboplastin time.** A coagulopathy may indicate DIC, hepatic dysfunction, or excessive anticoagulation.
4. **Arterial blood gases.** Early sepsis may produce a respiratory alkalosis, but usually a metabolic acidosis develops. Metabolic acidosis also develops in shock as a result of poor perfusion. Severe acidosis ($pH < 7.20$) may inhibit the effectiveness of vasopressors and cause arrhythmias and should be corrected. Hypoxemia may also be present and requires ventilatory support.
5. **Lactic dehydrogenase (LDH) and creatine phosphokinase (CPK) with isoenzymes.** Monitor if MI is suspected as well as to rule out injury secondary to the hypotension.
6. **Type and cross-match.** Blood should be set up for patients in whom hemorrhage is suspected.
7. **Pregnancy test.** To rule out ectopic pregnancy in young females.
8. **Blood, sputum, urine, and wound cultures.** For suspected sepsis.

C. Radiologic and other studies

1. **Chest x-ray.** May indicate source of sepsis or congestive heart failure. May be diagnostic for pneumothorax or hemothorax.
2. **Electrocardiogram.** Myocardial infarct or ischemia may be evident and arrhythmias can be evaluated.
3. **Pulmonary artery catheter (Swan-Ganz).** Very helpful in a patient with shock. Hemodynamic measurements may be used to aid the diagnosis and management of the hypotensive patient (see Table 1–7). Also useful when ruling out cardiac tamponade, which results in equalization of pressures. The right

atrial pressure equals the elevated right ventricular diastolic pressure in this condition.

4. **Angiography.** Pulmonary angiograms may reveal a PE. Abdominal angiograms are often helpful in detecting the source of GI bleeding, particularly of the lower GI tract.
5. **Nuclear scans.** A ventilation/perfusion ($\dot{V}/\dot{Q}$) lung scan may aid in diagnosing PE. Radiolabeled red blood cell scans may identify bleeding sources in the GI tract.
6. **Echocardiogram.** An easy noninvasive test to evaluate global ventricular function and valvular function and to rule out mechanical defects such as VSD or ruptured papillary muscle. Pericardial effusion resulting in tamponade can also be excluded.
7. **Paracentesis, thoracentesis, culdocentesis, pericardiocentesis.** If indicated.

V. Plan. Establish adequate tissue perfusion as soon as possible. Generally, a systolic blood pressure greater than 90 mm Hg is adequate. Signs of adequate perfusion include improved mental status and increased urine output (0.5–1.0 mL/kg/min).

A. Emergency management

1. Control external hemorrhage with direct pressure.
2. Establish venous access, preferably two large bore (14–16 gauge) peripheral intravenous lines.
3. Trendelenburg position (supine with feet elevated) or pneumatic antishock garment (PASG or MAST) may be useful in hypovolemic shock.
4. Insert Foley catheter for monitoring of urinary output.
5. Administer supplemental oxygen and ventilatory support as needed.
6. Correct severe metabolic acidosis (pH < 7.10–7.20) with intravenous sodium bicarbonate. Remember, an ampoule of sodium bicarbonate is hyperosmolar. After several ampoules, it is prudent to start an isotonic bicarbonate drip for persistent acidosis. A bicarbonate drip is made by adding 3 ampoules of sodium bicarbonate (50 mmol/50 mL) to 1 L of D5W. Respiratory acidosis can be corrected by improving minute ventilation (V_e) to reduce pCO_2.

TABLE 1–7. Parameters Useful in the Evaluation of Hypotension[a]

Type	CVP	PCWP	CO	HR	SVR
Sepsis	↑ or ↓	↓	↑ ↑	↑	↓
Hypovolemia	↓	↓	↑ or ↔	↑	↑ ↑
Cardiogenic	↑	↑	↓	↑ or ↔	↑

[a] CVP, central venous pressure; PCWP, pulmonary capillary wedge pressure; CO, cardiac output; HR, heart rate; SVR, systemic vascular resistance.

7. Central venous pressure (CVP) or Swan-Ganz catheterization will aid in the differential diagnosis of shock and fluid management.

B. Hypovolemic shock

1. Administer fluids (intravenous normal saline or lactated Ringer's) and red blood cells if indicated (HCT $\leq$ 30%) using blood pressure, urine output, and central filling pressures as a guide.
2. Use vasopressor agents such as norepinephrine and dopamine if hypotension persists despite a fluid challenge sufficient to achieve adequate filling pressures (PCWP 16–18 mm Hg). Dopamine is started at a dose of 2.5–5.0 μg/kg/min and increased up to 20 μg/kg/min. The dose of norepinephrine is 1–12 μg/min.

C. Neurogenic shock

1. Institute moderate IV fluid administration and avoid volume overload.
2. Low-dose vasopressors may be necessary.

D. Vasogenic shock

1. **Septic shock.** Identify and treat the source of the infection.
   a. Administer intravenous fluids and vasopressors as indicated.
   b. Broad-spectrum antibiotics are generally used if a specific source cannot be readily identified. A gram stain of infected fluid will guide antibiotic choice. An aminoglycoside and an antipseudomonas penicillin such as ticarcillin is a good antibiotic combination to begin with in the case of sepsis in a neutropenic patient or in a patient with a hospital-acquired infection.
2. **Anaphylactic shock.** (See Anaphylactic Reaction, p 22.)
   a. Remove precipitating agent as soon as possible.
   b. Immediately administer epinephrine 0.1 mL of 1:1000 subcutaneously.
   c. Maintain an adequate airway.
   d. An antihistamine such as diphenhydramine (Benadryl) 25 mg IM or IV and corticosteroids such as hydrocortisone 100–250 mg IV can also be given.
3. **Addisonian crisis.** Give hydrocortisone 100 mg IV bolus, then 100 mg IV every 6–8 hours in any patient in whom this diagnosis is suspected.

E. Cardiogenic shock

1. This form of shock is usually complicated and more difficult to manage; therefore, hemodynamic monitoring with a Swan-Ganz catheter should always be used to guide therapy.
2. Initial priority should be given to supporting adequate perfusion pressure (systolic blood pressure $\geq$ 90 mm Hg) while hemodynamic monitoring catheters are placed.
3. Once cardiac hemodynamics has been evaluated, appropriate use of diuretics (IV furosemide), cardiac inotropes (dopamine,

dobutamine), vasopressors (dopamine, norepinephrine, see above), antiarrhythmics, and intra-aortic balloon counterpulsation can be instituted.

4. Pericardiocentesis is indicated if there is hemodynamic compromise secondary to pericardial tamponade.
5. If a tension pneumothorax is present, a 14- to 16-gauge needle should be placed in the second or third intercostal space just superior to the rib in the midclavicular line until a chest tube can be placed.

■ HYPOTHERMIA

I. **Problem.** You are called to see a patient in the emergency room with a temperature of 32.0°C (89.6°F).

II. **Immediate Questions**

A. **Does the patient have any possible source of infection?** Septic patients can be hypothermic. Look for evidence of pneumonia, urinary tract infection, or any other cause of bacteremia. In a review by Lewin and colleagues, 41% of patients admitted because of hypothermia had a serious infection.

B. **Is there a history of other medical problems?** Hypothyroidism, hypoglycemia, hypopituitarism, and hypoadrenalism can all present with hypothermia. Alcohol also predisposes someone to environment-induced hypothermia.

C. **What is the clinical setting? Is there a history of exposure to cold weather or inadequate heating or clothing?** The very young and old are susceptible to environmental exposure as a cause of hypothermia.

D. **Is the patient on any medications?** Barbiturates and phenothiazines impair hypothalamic thermoregulation. Alcohol is a vasodilator and central nervous system depressant and increases the risk for environmental exposure. The use of insulin, thyroid medication, or steroids may point to an etiology.

III. **Differential Diagnosis**

A. **Sepsis.** Bacteremia must be ruled out.

B. **Environmental exposure.** Was the patient found outside or in an unheated building?

C. **Metabolic abnormalities**

1. **Myxedema.** Thermoderegulation resulting in hypothermia associated with hypothyroidism often has associated mental status changes (coma). There is often a precipitating event.
2. **Hypoglycemia.** Many potential etiologies (See Hypoglycemia, p 156). Hypoglycemia may also be associated with overwhelming sepsis or, in alcoholics, with depleted glycogen stores.
3. **Addison's disease.** Can be acute or chronic. Often there is a history of steroid ingestion. May be from metastatic carcinoma or idiopathic.

4. **Uremia.** Easily ruled out by checking BUN and creatinine.
5. **Hypopituitarism.** Can result in hypoadrenalism and hypothyroidism. Can also cause hypoglycemia.

D. **Central nervous system dysfunction**
1. **Cerebrovascular accident.** Look for focal neurologic findings such as motor weakness or sensory deficit, unilateral hyperreflexia or plantar extension with Babinski.
2. **Head trauma.** History and careful examination of head, eyes, ears, nose, and neck should reveal any recent head trauma.
3. **Spinal cord transection.** Paraplegia or quadraplegia on examination.
4. **Wernicke's encephalopathy.** Triad of ophthalmoplegia, mental status changes, and ataxia. Secondary to thiamine deficiency from decreased nutritional intake associated most often with chronic alcohol ingestion.
5. **Drug ingestion.** (See Section II.D.)
6. **Miscellaneous.** Other diagnoses to consider are myocardial infarction, generalized erythroderma, and anorexia nervosa.

IV. Database

A. Physical examination key points
1. **Vital signs.** Accurately record the core temperature with a rectal thermometer and be sure it is a low-recording thermometer. Standard thermometers may record to only 34.4°C (93.8°F). Hypotension and bradycardia frequently occur in hypothermia.
2. **Skin.** Look for evidence of frostbite, diffuse erythroderma, burns, or insulin injection sites.
3. **Heart.** Heart sounds may be distant, slow, or absent.
4. **Lungs.** Respirations may be slow and shallow. Look for signs of pneumonia.
5. **Abdomen.** Ileus may occur with hypothermia.
6. **Neurologic exam.** Look for signs of head trauma. Check pupil reactivity. Pupils may be nonreactive but are often sluggish and slowly react. Mental status may vary from mental slowing to confusion and coma. Check deep tendon reflexes, which may be absent with severe hypothermia. A slow relaxation phase points to hypothyroidism.

B. Laboratory data
1. **Complete blood count.** Hypothermia can cause hemoconcentration and leukocytosis. Leukocytosis or leukopenia with a left shift suggests sepsis.
2. **Platelet count.** A low platelet count suggests disseminated intravascular coagulation either caused by the hypothermia or associated with sepsis. (See Thrombocytopenia, p 246.)
3. **Prothrombin time, partial thromboplastin time.** Elevation of the PT and PTT is consistent with disseminated intravascular coagulation, which can be a complication of hypothermia or associated with sepsis. (See Coagulopathy, p 60.)

4. **Blood urea nitrogen and creatinine.** To rule out uremia.
5. **Glucose.** Hypoglycemia may be the cause of the hypothermia or associated with underlying cause.
6. **Thyroxine (T4) and thyroid-stimulating hormone (TSH).** Need to rule out hypothyroidism. The T4 can be low in the euthyroid sick state but the TSH will be normal.
7. **Cortrosyn stimulation test.** (See Chapter 2, ACTH Stimulation Test, p 261.) To rule out adrenal insufficiency since a single cortisol level can be misleading. Also, be sure to check adrenal reserve in all patients with severe hypothyroidism.
8. **Arterial blood gases.** Correct pH and pCO_2 for body temperature. For each 1° below 97.6°F, add 0.01 to the pH. To correct the pCO_2, subtract 4% of the pCO_2 at 97°F and an additional 2% for each 1° below 97°F. Your clinical lab will make these corrections for you as long as the temperature is known. The pO_2 should also be corrected; however, this is a nonlinear relationship. Refer to the listed reference for the equation.
9. **Blood cultures.** Rule out sepsis.
10. **Serum and urine drug screen**

C. **Radiologic and other studies**
1. **Chest x-ray.** Obtain to rule out a source of infection. Pneumonia is the most common sequela of hypothermia after the recovery period.
2. **Electrocardiogram.** Hypothermia can promote myocardial irritability and cause conduction abnormalities. The ECG may show T-wave inversion and PR, QRS, and QT prolongation as well as the unique J wave or Osborn wave, which closely follows the QRS complex. Continuous ECG monitoring is important with a temperature below 32°C (89.6°F) because of the risk of cardiac arrhythmias.

V. Plan

A. **General support**
1. Make sure the patient is hemodynamically stable. If ventricular fibrillation occurs, cardiopulmonary resuscitation should be instituted and continued until the core temperature rises. In this clinical setting, the statement "A patient is not dead until he or she is warm and dead" applies.
2. If you suspect hypothermia secondary to environmental exposure, place an intravenous line to replace fluids as chronic hypothermia leads to volume depletion.
3. Other therapeutic measures depend on the clinical setting. If sepsis is a possibility, then immediately begin antibiotics.
4. Give intravenous steroids if you suspect Addison's disease or intravenous thyroxine for possible myxedema coma.
5. Some authors advocate administration of 100 mg of thiamine IM or IV, an ampoule of D50, and 2 mg of naloxone (Narcan) to all hypothermic, comatose patients.

B. Rewarming techniques

1. In environmental exposure, first remove the patient from the cold environment and use some insulating material such as blankets.
2. More aggressive rewarming techniques are controversial. There is the concern that active **external** rewarming with an electric blanket may produce hypovolemic shock by peripheral vasodilation or cause "afterdrop" of core temperature through a shifting of the cold blood to the core.
3. Such concerns have led to the use of active **core** rewarming for patients with core temperatures below 32°C (89.6°F), especially in the setting of chronic hypothermia secondary to environmental exposure. Active core rewarming techniques include gastrointestinal rewarming, peritoneal dialysis, and inhalation of warmed oxygen. Gastrointestinal rewarming involves the instillation of warmed normal saline via nasogastric and rectal tubes, removal of the fluid, and repetition of the process.

REFERENCES

Carden DL, Nowak RM. Disseminated intravascular coagulation in hypothermia. *JAMA* 1982;247:2099.

Goldfrank L, Kirstein R. Emergency management of hypothermia. *Hosp Physician* 1979;Jan:47–52.

Lewin S, Brettman LR, Holzman RS. Infections in hypothermic patients. *Arch Intern Med* 1981;141:920–925.

Reuler JB. Hypothermia: Pathophysiology, clinical settings and management. *Ann Intern Med* 1978;89:519–527.

Welton DE, Mattox KL, Miller RR, et al. Treatment of profound hypothermia. *JAMA* 1978;240:2291–2292.

■ INSOMNIA

I. Problem. A patient hospitalized for a course of intravenous antibiotics for lower-extremity cellulitis complains of lying awake for hours at night.

II. Immediate Questions

A. What is the patient's mental status? Delirium and dementia can both present with sleep disturbance. Delirium frequently results in a reversal of the normal sleep/wake cycle. It is important to avoid treatment with sedative/hypnotics as they may actually worsen the symptomatology. As some causes of delirium can be life-threatening, aggressive evaluation of these patients is warranted. (See Coma, Acute Mental Status Changes, p 65.)

B. Is the patient bothered by pain? Painful stimuli result in an increased arousal state, which interferes with sleep and escalates the cycle of sleep disturbance and pain. Common examples include rheumatoid arthritis, where a worsening of morning stiffness is associated with the sleep disturbance, and fibrositis, the symptoms of which can be reproduced by disturbing delta sleep in normal subjects.

C. **What is the patient's sleep pattern during the day?** Certainly, a patient who sleeps for extended periods during the day will not be able to drop off to sleep at night. Sleep hygiene interventions can be of use here.

D. **Does the patient take sleeping medications regularly? What are his or her current medications?** Virtually all sleep medications show a tolerance effect and a disruption of the sleep patterns that can interfere with normal sleep with chronic usage. Abrupt withdrawal of these agents almost invariably results in sleep disturbance, often termed *rebound insomnia.* It is also important to remember that withdrawal from barbiturates can be associated with convulsions and death. Remember to ask specifically about over-the-counter preparations. Many of the medications prescribed in the hospital can interfere with normal sleep and a thorough review of the patient's medication record is warranted.

E. **What are the patient's habits?** Ingestion of stimulant-containing beverages (coffee, tea) and foods (some cheeses) can interfere with sleep. Cigarette smoking and alcohol consumption both have deleterious effects on the normal sleep patterns. Alcohol withdrawal is also associated with sleep disturbance and is frequently not reported by the patient.

F. **Does the patient have difficulty lying flat?** Most often this is related to a cardiorespiratory condition and is associated with a sensation of dyspnea.

G. **What is the patient's sleep pattern?** Many clues to the etiology of the patient's sleep disturbance can be derived from a careful history of the sleep/wake cycle, including duration of periods of arousal and associated symptoms. Prolonged sleep latency is frequently associated with chronic or situational anxiety. Early-morning awakening is often seen with major depression, but may be related to alcohol use. Frequent awakening with the need to void can be secondary to prostatic hypertrophy with bladder outlet obstruction, hyperglycemia with polyuria, or mobilization of fluid in a patient with congestive failure or chronic venous stasis and insufficiency. Awakening after a period of sleep with shortness of breath requiring a prolonged upright posture before resumption of sleep would suggest cardiac dysfunction.

III. Differential Diagnosis

A. Medical causes

1. **Delirium.** Evaluate for systemic illnesses, sepsis, and liver dysfunction, and consider drug toxicities.

2. **Pain.** Control of this symptom frequently relieves the sleep disturbance.
3. **Cardiac disorders.** Ventricular dysfunction with congestive symptoms, arrhythmias, and ischemia can all result in sleep disturbances. Frequent symptoms include orthopnea, paroxysmal nocturnal dyspnea, palpitations, and angina.
4. **Respiratory disorders.** Asthma, chronic obstructive airway disease, cystic fibrosis, sarcoidosis, pneumonia, and sleep apnea are among the many respiratory disorders that can result in sleep disturbance. Sleep apnea is most frequently seen in the morbidly obese. Central apnea syndrome is not related to body habitus. These patients are frequently unaware of their frequent arousals and instead complain of excessive daytime drowsiness.
5. **Hyperthyroidism.** Associated symptoms include tachycardia, heat intolerance, anxiety, and tremulousness.

B. Drugs/Toxins

1. **Tolerance to sleep medications from chronic usage**
2. **Abrupt withdrawal of sedative/hypnotics or antidepressant medications**
3. **Alcohol abuse.** Secondary disruption of appropriate sleep patterns as a result of chronic consumption. Sudden withdrawal also causes disruption.
4. **Tobacco use**
5. **Caffeine ingestion**
6. **Stimulant use or abuse**

C. Psychiatric causes

1. **Depressive illness.** Either bipolar or unipolar. Hallmarks are decreased sleep with no perception of sleep deficiency and early-morning awakening, respectively.
2. **Anxiety disorders.** Generally manifested as a prolonged sleep latency.

D. Situational causes. Often related to hospitalization.

1. **Noise.** The ICU environment and unruly roommates are commonly cited.
2. **Frequent disruptions.** Nursing duties such as administration of medications, vital signs, and hygienic activities cause frequent disruptions for inpatients.
3. **Anger.** Unexpressed anger over illness or toward staff or family.
4. **Anxiety.** Short-term and usually related to medical condition or strange environment.

IV. Database. The most important parts of the database in evaluating insomnia are the history and an evaluation of the patient's mental status.

A. Physical examination key points

1. **Cardiopulmonary exam.** Evidence of rales, elevated jugular

venous pressure, displaced point of maximal impulse, S_3 gallop, and peripheral edema all suggest congestive heart failure.

2. **Respiratory exam.** Wheezes suggest obstructive airway disease.
3. **Neurologic exam.** Mental status examination for evidence of anxiety or depression.

B. **Laboratory data.** Most often, the cause of insomnia is determined without the use of laboratory tests.

1. **Screening chemistries.** Include hepatic and renal function tests. Most useful as part of the evaluation of possible delirium.
2. **Thyroid hormone levels.** If indicated by clinical presentation. (See Section III.B.5.)
3. **Urine drug screen.** In cases where drug use is strongly suspected but denied.

C. **Radiologic and other studies.** A chest x-ray if indicated to evaluate for congestive heart failure or pneumonia.

V. **Plan.** It is most important to determine why the patient cannot sleep—medical, psychologic, or situational causes. Most cases are secondary to a situational cause and do not represent a pathologic situation. In cases where there is no contraindication to their use, it is therefore reasonable to include a sleeping medication order to be taken as needed with the admission orders. When a specific cause is determined, it should be remedied if possible rather than treating the sleeplessness symptomatically.

A. **Nonmedical treatments.** These are often as effective as medical treatment and obviously lack side effects. They include minimizing disturbances, trying to maintain the patient's normal waking and sleeping times, eliminating roommate conflicts when possible, eliminating caffeine and tobacco, and minimizing noise from monitors.

B. **Symptomatic treatment**

1. **Oral sleeping medication.** Choices include the benzodiazepines, chloral hydrate, and antihistamines. Barbiturates are not recommended.
   a. **Benzodiazepines.** Most frequently used for the short-term treatment of insomnia. Rapidly absorbed, short-half-life agents such as triazolam (Halcion) 0.125–0.25 mg PO every night are preferable. Other commonly used benzodiazepines include temazepam (Restoril) 15–30 mg PO every night and flurazepam (Dalmane) 15–30 mg PO every night. Lower doses should be used in the elderly.
   b. **Chloral hydrate.** Available in both oral and rectal forms. The dose is 500–1000 mg by either route. Do not use in hepatic or renal failure.
   c. **Antihistamines.** Be conscious of anticholinergic side effects, particularly in the elderly.

(1) **Diphenhydramine (Benadryl) 25–50 mg PO or IM**

(2) **Hydroxzine (Vistaril) 25–50 mg PO or IM**

d. **Antidepressants.** Many have significant anticholinergic side effects and should be used with caution in the elderly. Also be aware of cardiac side effects.

(1) **Amitriptyline (Elavil) 25–50 mg PO every night.** Significant anticholinergic side effects. Most useful when chronic pain syndromes accompany sleep disturbance.

(2) **Imipramine (Tofranil) 75 mg PO every night.** Same precautions as with amitriptyline but less useful in chronic pain.

(3) **Desipramine (Norpramin) 50 mg PO every night.** May have fewer anticholinergic side effects.

REFERENCES

Erman MK. Sleep disorders, insomnia. *Psychiat Clin North Am* 1987;4:525–539.

Schmidt PJ. Evaluation and treatment of sleep disorders in the medical setting. *Gen Hosp Psychiatry* 1988;10:10–15.

■ IRREGULAR PULSE

(See also Tachycardia, p 241, and Bradycardia, p 35.)

I. **Problem.** An 80-year-old man being admitted with mental status changes is noted to have an irregular pulse.

II. **Immediate Questions**

A. **What is the heart rate?** The heart rate, as well as the degree of irregularity, can assist the physician in determining a differential diagnosis of an irregular heart rhythm. For instance, an irregularly irregular rhythm with an apical pulse of 130 suggests atrial fibrillation.

B. **What are the other vital signs?** Hypotension signifies an urgent situation. (See Hypotension, p 174.)

C. **Has the patient been noted to have an irregular pulse before?** A history of skipped beats suggests a chronic problem. The occurrence of premature atrial contractions (PACs) or premature ventricular contractions (PVCs) may be chronic and is often a common benign condition.

D. **Is there any history of previous cardiac disease?** A history of mitral stenosis points to atrial fibrillation.

E. **What medications is the patient taking?** Ask specifically about cardiac medications such as digitalis, antiarrhythmics, and diuretics. Digitalis can cause various degrees of heart block. Diuretic-induced hypokalemia and antiarrhythmics can induce PACs and PVCs, which, if frequent, can result in an irregular rhythm.

III. Differential Diagnosis

A. Premature contractions

1. **Premature atrial contractions.** Seen with stress, infections, inflammation, myocardial ischemia, or tobacco, alcohol, or caffeine use. Premature atrial contractions may lead to other supraventricular tachycardias (SVTs) but usually do not require specific therapy in the absence of SVT.
2. **Premature ventricular contractions.** The prevalence of PVCs increases with age, but PVCs are also seen in infection, myocardial ischemia, with anesthesia or stress, or during excessive use of tobacco, alcohol, or caffeine. They may also be seen with hypoxia, acidosis, hypokalemia, and hypomagnesemia. Patients with hypertrophic cardiomyopathy and mitral valve prolapse may have PVCs, as may patients with myocardial infarction (MI). In the absence of underlying organic heart disease, the presence of PVCs does not alter lifespan and therefore does not require therapy.

B. Sinus arrhythmia. Occurs in any age group and is a normal variant. Treatment is rarely indicated.

C. Sinoatrial exit block. Defined by the absence of a normally timed P wave resulting in a pause that is a multiple of the P-to-P interval. Seen during vagal stimulation, acute myocarditis, MI, or fibrosis of the conduction system and with drugs such as quinidine, procainamide, and digitalis. Syncope is a rare event.

D. Atrial fibrillation. Defined as chaotic atrial depolarizations and a grossly irregular ventricular response. Atrial fibrillation can be seen in patients with apparently normal hearts or in patients with rheumatic heart disease, cardiomyopathy, hypertensive heart disease, pulmonary embolism (PE), pericarditis, coronary artery disease, or thyrotoxicosis.

E. Atrial flutter. May be irregular if the atrioventricular conduction varies but is usually regular. Associated with same diseases as atrial fibrillation.

F. Second-degree atrioventricular block. Both Mobitz type I (Wenckebach) and Mobitz type II. May be seen with acute MI, degenerative disease of the conduction system, viral myocarditis, acute rheumatic fever, and Lyme disease. Mobitz type I can be a normal variant.

IV. Database

A. Physical examination key points

1. **Vital signs.** Palpate the brachial or carotid pulses; note the rhythm and any pattern of irregularity. Be careful to separate an irregular pulse from a variation in pulse amplitude. Changes in pulse amplitude can be seen during pulmonary bronchospasm, severe MI, and aortic regurgitation. Urgent action needs to be initiated if hypotension is present. A temperature

suggests an infection, which can cause PVCs and PACs; several specific infections such as acute rheumatic fever and Lyme disease can cause atrioventricular block.

2. **Heart.** A thorough cardiac examination is essential. Atrioventricular block with an associated murmur might suggest acute rheumatic fever. A fourth heart sound (S_4) might suggest MI, and a variety of arrhythmias may be associated including PVCs, PACs, varying degrees of atroventricular block, atrial fibrillation, and flutter. If atrial fibrillation is present, listen for the murmur of mitral stenosis. Listen at the apex with the bell, with the patient in the left lateral decubitus position for the characteristic diastolic rumble.

B. Laboratory data

1. **Electrolytes.** Rule out hypokalemia. Also, a low serum bicarbonate suggests metabolic acidosis.
2. **Magnesium.** Rule out hypomagnesemia if PVCs are present.
3. **Arterial blood gases.** If PVCs are present, rule out hypoxemia. A severe acidosis or alkalosis can also induce PVCs.
4. **Drug levels.** A digoxin level is imperative if the patient is on medication. Digitalis intoxication can cause PVCs, sinoatrial exit block, or second-degree heart block.

C. Radiologic and other studies. With the electrocardiogram, be sure to include a long rhythm strip. During examination of the ECG and rhythm strip, identify all the P waves that are present and then note their relationship to the QRS complex. P waves are best seen in leads I, II, aVR, aVF, and V1. You may need to examine a rhythm strip from several leads to identify the rhythm. Also look carefully for evidence of ischemia (ST depression or ST elevation and T-wave changes), drug effect (prolongation of the QT interval), PE (S1-Q3-T3, right bundle branch block, right-axis deviation), and pericarditis (diffuse ST elevation with upward concavity and PR depression).

V. Plan. Most of the arrhythmias that result in an irregular pulse do not need specific therapy; however, they should be identified and the predisposing condition treated appropriately. Possible exceptions include the following:

A. Frequent or complex premature ventricular contractions in a post-MI patient or a patient with impaired left ventricular function. Initially be sure to rule out hypokalemia, hypoxia, hypomagnesemia, acidosis, and recurrent ischemia. Treat with either lidocaine 2 mg/min as a continuous drip or procainamide 25–50 mg over at least 1 minute every 5 minutes up to a total dose of 1 g or disappearance of the arrhythmia, then 1–4 mg/min as a continuous drip.

B. Mobitz type II second-degree atrioventricular block. This condition frequently progresses to complete heart block so permanent cardiac pacing should be considered, especially in the presence of symptoms.

C. **Atrial fibrillation and flutter.** (See Tachycardia, Section V, p 244.)

REFERENCE

Zipes DP. Specific arrhythmias, diagnosis and treatment. In: Braunwald E, ed. *Heart Disease: A Text Book of Cardiovascular Medicine.* 3rd ed. Philadelphia: WB Saunders;1988:658–716.

■ JAUNDICE

I. **Problem.** You are asked by the emergency room physician to see a 45-year-old man with jaundice.

II. **Immediate Questions**

A. **What are the vital signs?** Fever and tachycardia with or without hypotension could indicate sepsis associated with ascending cholangitis. This is a medical emergency and needs immediate attention.

B. **Does the patient have diabetes?** Diabetics are much more commonly afflicted with ascending cholangitis. Cholecystitis or ascending cholangitis in a diabetic is a medical emergency.

C. **Is there a history of alcoholism or chronic alcohol use?** Cirrhosis could be the source of jaundice.

D. **Is there a history of intravenous drug abuse, homosexuality, or exposure to hepatitis?** Viral hepatitis could be the source of the jaundice.

E. **Is there any history of abdominal pain?** A history of postprandial right upper quadrant or epigastric pain, especially with radiation to the back, may represent biliary colic.

F. **Is there a history of previous biliary surgery?** Jaundice can occur as a result of a retained common duct stone or biliary stricture.

III. **Differential Diagnosis.** Disease processes causing jaundice include hemolysis, hepatocellular disease, and cholestasis. If cholestatic jaundice is suspected, determine whether extrahepatic or intrahepatic disease is present.

A. **Acute biliary obstruction.** Includes carcinoma and common bile duct stones.

B. **Alcoholic liver disease.** Alcoholic hepatitis or cirrhosis. Alcoholic cirrhosis is usually seen after at least 10 years of heavy ethanol ingestion. Think of this in patients with physical findings suggestive of alcoholic liver disease. (See Section IV.A.)

C. **Viral hepatitis.** Consider this diagnosis with a history of intravenous drug abuse, exposure to other persons with jaundice, in homosexual males, or people from endemic areas.

D. **Other causes of hepatitis.** Autoimmunity or drugs such as isoniazid and halothane.

E. **Hemolysis.** This rarely raises the bilirubin over 5 mg/dL.

F. **Primary biliary cirrhosis.** Usually middle-aged women who present with jaundice, fatigue, and pruritus.

G. **Pregnancy.** Uncommon. Generally not serious but can be life-threatening.

H. **Drugs.** Can cause hepatitis, cholestasis, or hemolysis. Cholestasis is most commonly associated with phenothiazines and estrogens.

I. **Total peripheral nutrition (TPN).** Associated with high carbohydrate loads. Usually long-term TPN.

J. **Postoperative cholestasis.** Diagnosis of exclusion.

K. **Sepsis.** Very uncommon. Diagnosis of exclusion.

IV. **Database.** An experienced clinician can, by history, physical examination, and simple laboratory tests, decide whether the patient has extrahepatic cholestasis with an accuracy of approximately 85%.

A. **Physical examination key points**

1. **Vital signs.** A fever may suggest ascending cholangitis and/or sepsis.
2. **Skin.** Palmar erythema and telangiectasia points toward chronic liver disease.
3. **Breasts.** Gynecomastia in males is consistent with chronic liver disease.
4. **Abdomen.** The physical exam should be centered on the abdomen. Look for hepatomegaly or palpable gallbladder (Courvoisier's sign) which may indicate malignant obstruction. The presence or absence of abdominal tenderness, particularly right upper quadrant tenderness and Murphy's sign (tenderness in the right upper quadrant with palpation with inspiration), should be documented. Ascites may be present in patients with cirrhosis.
5. **Rectum/genitourinary system.** A rectal exam should be done looking for occult blood. Testicular atrophy may be present in patients with chronic liver disease.

B. **Laboratory data**

1. **Liver function studies.** Including transaminases (AST [SGOT] and ALT [SGPT]), bilirubin total and fractionated, alkaline phosphatase, and γ-glutamyl transpeptidase (GGT). Abnormalities in the laboratory profile should be categorized as either hepatocellular (predominantly an elevation in AST and ALT) or hepatocannulicular (predominantly an elevation in bilirubin, alkaline phosphatase, and GGT). Elevations in AST and ALT above 300 virtually never occur in alcoholic liver disease without the combined effect of some other toxin such as Tylenol. Bilirubins above 20 are very suggestive of extrahepatic cho-

lestasis. An elevated indirect bilirubin suggests hemolysis and a total bilirubin secondary to hemolysis seldom exceeds 5 mg/dL.

2. **Amylase.** Elevations in amylase, particularly above 1000, are associated with extrahepatic biliary obstruction.
3. **Hepatitis serology.** Hepatitis B surface antigen, hepatitis B IgM core antibody, and hepatitis A IgM antibody. (See Chapter 2, Laboratory Tests: Hepatitis, p 278.)
4. **Other serology.** Antinuclear (ANA), antimitochondrial, and anti–smooth muscle antibodies may be helpful. The triad of antimitochondrial antibody, elevated alkaline phosphatase, and elevated class M immunoglobulin is consistent with primary biliary cirrhosis. A high ANA titer suggests autoimmune hepatitis. High titers of anti–smooth muscle antibodies are seen in chronic active hepatitis.

C. Radiologic and other studies

1. **Ultrasound and computerized tomography.** These studies are done when extrahepatic cholestasis is suspected. The selection of either ultrasound or CT is dependent on many factors. There are arguments for both studies, but both should not be done together. Generally, select one or the other and do it on a routine basis. Mainly, ultrasound and CT are good for detecting dilated ducts, pancreatic masses, and stones in the gallbladder. The sensitivity and specificity for dilated ducts and stones in the gallbladder are quite good and are approximately the same for ultrasound and CT. Detection of stones in the common bile duct is uniformly poor with both of these tests.
2. **Endoscopic retrograde cholangiopancreatography (ERCP).** Test of choice in patients with nondilated ducts and extrahepatic cholestasis. It is particularly recommended in patients with ascites, coagulation abnormalities, a previous history of percutaneous transhepatic cholangiography that has failed, a suspected case of sclerosing cholangitis, and a planned sphincterotomy. It is also the test of choice when carcinoma of the pancreas is suspected as a biopsy can be done.
3. **Percutaneous transhepatic cholangiogram (PTC).** Test of choice when the patient has dilated ducts, previous gastric surgery with Bilroth II anastomosis, a previous failed ERCP, or a mass involving the proximal bile duct.
4. **Liver biopsy.** Generally not useful in the diagnosis of jaundice. Occasionally reveals an unsuspected medical cause such as metastatic tumor.
5. **Nuclear scans (HIDA).** This scan is generally of low utility in the diagnosis of jaundice. It is very helpful when the diagnosis of acute cholecystitis is suspected.

V. Plan. The tempo of diagnostic evaluation is dictated by whether or not the patient is suspected of having ascending cholangitis. Patients who present with fever, jaundice, toxemia, and other findings suggestive of sepsis are medical emergencies and require rapid diagnostic evaluation.

A. **Hepatocellular cholestasis**
   1. **Viral hepatitis.** Patients who are dehydrated, are vomiting, or have significant coagulopathy will need admission for treatment with intravenous fluids and fresh-frozen plasma.
   2. **Alcoholic liver disease.** Supportive care. This entails dietary restriction of protein, full evaluation of any coagulopathy (see Coagulopathy, p 60), and treatment of associated electrolyte deficiencies that are often encountered in alcoholics such as hypocalcemia, hypomagnesemia, and hypophosphatemia. Thiamine, folate, and multivitamins may be needed.

B. **Extrahepatic cholestasis**
   1. If there is a strong clinical suspicion of extrahepatic obstruction, proceed straight to ERCP or PTC.
   2. If extrahepatic obstruction is possible but not definite, obtain a biliary ultrasound or CT scan first. If obstruction is confirmed, then proceed with ERCP or surgery. If ascending cholangitis is suspected and confirmed by ultrasound or CT scan, begin antibiotics (ampicillin and gentamicin) and request immediate surgical consultation.

C. **Hemolysis.** Treat underlying cause.

REFERENCES

Frank BB. Clinical evaluation of jaundice. *JAMA* 1989;262:3031–3034.

Sherlock S. Jaundice. In: *Disease of the Liver and Biliary System.* 8th ed. Oxford: Blackwell Scientific; 1989:230–247.

Vennes JA, Board JH. Approach to the jaundiced patient. *Gastroenterology* 1983;84:1615–1618.

■ JOINT SWELLING

I. **Problem.** A 35-year-old woman is admitted with right knee swelling and pain.

II. **Immediate Questions**

A. **Is there a previous history of joint swelling?** A history of multiple joint involvement will suggest an etiology that results in polyarthritis rather than monoarthritis. Remember that many diseases causing a polyarthritis can present initially as a monoarthritis. The pattern of joint involvement may suggest the cause, for example, the first metatarsophalangeal (MTP) in gout or metacarpophalangeal (MCP) and proximal interphalangeal (PIP) of the hands in rheumatoid arthritis. The history of onset, such as acute, chronic, or migratory, may be helpful in diagnosis.

B. **Is there a history of trauma?** Trauma to the joint would lead one to consider fracture, ligamentous tear, loose body, or dislocation. A sport and occupational history is essential.

C. **Does the patient have any constitutional problems?** The presence of fever requires one to rule out septic arthritis, although it must be considered in any case of monoarticular arthritis even in the absence of fever. Malaise, fatigue, and weight loss suggest a systemic arthritis. Morning stiffness of significant duration (more than 1 hour) suggests inflammatory arthritis.

D. **Are there any systemic symptoms?** It is important to obtain a full rheumatic disease systems review. A photosensitive rash suggests systemic lupus erythematosus, whereas diarrhea leads one to consider inflammatory bowel disease or reactive arthritis. A partial list of systemic systems would include rash, alopecia, Raynaud's phenomenon, oral or genital ulcers, urethritis or cervicitis, diarrhea, eye inflammation, sicca symptoms, weakness and CNS disturbances.

E. **What is the patient's past medical and family history?** Inquire into the past few weeks to months for febrile illnesses, tick bites, and other events, as the patient may not associate these symptoms with the onset of arthritis. A drug history may provide a clue to diagnosis such as hemarthrosis associated with warfarin therapy, or a positive family history may suggest arthritis associated with psoriasis, hemoglobinopathies, or coagulopathies.

III. **Differential Diagnosis.** Arthritis is classified as being either monoarticular or polyarticular. Subclassification is often based on the joint fluid analysis (see Section IV). Remember that an arthritis that is generally polyarticular can present as a monoarticular arthritis.

A. **Monoarticular arthritis**

1. **Infection.** May be bacterial, viral, fungal, or tubercular.
2. **Trauma.** Etiologies include loose foreign bodies, fracture, plant thorn synovitis, and internal derangement.
3. **Hemarthrosis.** Causes include hemoglobinopathy, coagulopathy, warfarin therapy, and pigmented villonodular synovitis.
4. **Tumors.** Consider osteogenic sarcoma, metastatic tumor, synovial osteochondromatosis, and paraneoplastic syndromes.
5. **Crystal.** Types of crystal associated with arthritis include gout (first MTP involvement characteristic), pseudogout (may be secondary to hyperparathyroidism and hemochromatosis), and hydroxyapatite.
6. **Noninflammatory disease.** Includes avascular necrosis, which is often associated with a history of trauma, steroid use, alcohol use, or sickle cell anemia; osteoarthritis; endocrine disorders; amyloid; osteochondritis dissecans; and neuropathy.
7. **Inflammatory-connective tissue diseases.** Rheumatoid arthritis or Reiter's syndrome.

B. Polyarticular arthritis

1. **Infection or associated with infection**
   a. **Gonococcal infection.** Frequently associated with a migratory arthritis, tenosynovitis, and a pustular rash.
   b. **Lyme disease.** Associated with both an acute arthritis and a late chronic destructive arthritis.
   c. **Rheumatic fever.** Primarily lower-extremity large joints. In the adult, arthritis is rarely migratory.
   d. **Acquired immunodeficiency syndrome.** Septic arthritis, Reiter's syndrome, and a lupus-like presentation with nondestructive polyarthritis, rash, pleuritis, and CNS symptoms have all been described.
   e. **Subacute bacterial endocarditis**
   f. **Chronic active hepatitis.** Chronic hepatitis B infection is associated with arthritis alone or in association with polyarteritis nodosa and mixed essential cryoglobulinemia.
2. **Crystal.** For example, gout, pseudogout, and hydroxyapatite.
3. **Metabolic disorders.** Etiologies include hypothyroidism, acromegaly, hemochromatosis, ochronosis, (alkaptonuria—associated with osteoarthritis primarily of the spine and hips), hemophilia, and hyperparathyroidism. Hyperparathyroidism and hemochromatosis are associated with pseudogout.
4. **Noninflammatory disease**
   a. **Osteoarthritis.** Consider when distal interphalangeal (DIP) and carpal-metacarpal joints of hands are involved.
   b. **Intestinal bypass surgery**
5. **Spondyloarthropathies.** Associated with axial involvement. Peripheral arthritis is often asymmetric. Tendonitis is common. Includes ankylosing spondylitis, Reiter's syndrome (genitourinary or postdysentery forms), enteropathic arthritis (ulcerative colitis or Crohn's disease), psoriatic arthritis, and Behcet's disease.
6. **Inflammatory disease**
   a. **Juvenile rheumatoid arthritis.** Also called adult Still's disease. Fever, often systemic complaints (sore throat), and myalgias are present. Rheumatoid factor (RF) is negative.
   b. **Rheumatoid arthritis.** A symmetric arthritis characteristically involving the MCP and PIP joints of the hands.
   c. **Systemic lupus erythematosus (SLE).** Resembles rheumatoid arthritis but is rarely an erosive arthritis.
   d. **Scleroderma.** Significant joint swelling is uncommon.
   e. **Polychondritis**
   f. **Mixed connective tissue disease.** Defined by a positive antiribonuclear protein (anti-RNP) antibody. Includes features of rheumatoid arthritis, scleroderma, polymyositis, and SLE.

g. **Sarcoidosis.** An acute migratory arthritis frequently associated with tenosynovitis and erythema nodosum and a chronic pauciarticular form involving the knees and ankles.

IV. Database

A. **Physical examination key points.** Physical exam must be complete. As systemic disease must be ruled out as the cause of the arthritis, there can be no shortcuts.

1. **Skin.** A rash may indicate etiology. For evidence of psoriasis, frequently overlooked areas include under the hairline or rectum. Telangiectasia, nailfold infarcts, palmar erythema, and livedo reticularis suggest connective tissue disease or vasculitis. Nodules are seen in rheumatoid arthritis and gout.
2. **Eyes.** Retinal abnormalities may suggest an infectious etiology such as subacute bacterial endocarditis.
3. **Mouth.** Oral and nasal ulcers point to SLE or Behcet's syndrome.
4. **Musculoskeletal system.** All major joints should be examined for range of motion, tenderness, deformity, and swelling. One must ensure that there is true swelling (arthritis) rather than bone pain, muscle pain, or pain from bursitis, tendonitis, or torn ligaments or menisci.

B. **Laboratory data**

1. **Complete blood count with differential.** To rule out infection and to identify anemia or thrombocytopenia if a systemic arthritis is considered.
2. **Joint fluid analysis**
   a. Any initial presentation of arthritis should be worked up with a joint aspiration if possible. (See Chapter 3, Arthrocentesis, p 307.) Fluid should be sent for gram stain and bacterial, acid-fast bacillus, and fungal cultures if indicated, crystal exam, and cell count with differential. A WBC count of 0–300 is normal, 300–2000 is noninflammatory, 2000–75,000 is inflammatory, and greater than 100,000 indicates septic arthritis; however, cell counts from a bacterial source may be as low as 5000 WBC/mL. A differential count with a predominance of neutrophils suggests septic arthritis, whereas lymphocytosis suggests leukemia or tuberculosis. These values are only guidelines as there is considerable overlap in all of these diseases.
   b. Gram stain smears are positive in only 66% of subsequent culture-proven cases of septic arthritis. A negative result does not therefore exclude the possibility of infection. The monosodium urate crystals of gout are rod-shaped, negatively birefringent crystals (3–10 μm) seen within white cells during active disease and often extend beyond the cell wall. The crystal is yellow when parallel to the slow ray of the compensator. Calcium pyrophosphate dihydrate

(CPPD) crystals are rhomboid-shaped, positively birefringent crystals that are blue when parallel to the slow ray of the compensator. The crystal is usually contained within the white cell. Calcium hydroxyapatite crystals are small (< 1 μm), minimally birefringent, irregularly shaped cytoplasmic inclusions that appear under light microscopy as "shiny coins" when extracellular. Calcium hydroxyapatite crystals are more commonly associated with acute episodes of bursitis, tendonitis, or periarthritis seen in chronic renal failure patients or older women with the progressive destructive arthritis of Milwaukee shoulder syndrome.

3. **Other cultures.** Cultures of urine and blood should be obtained if septic arthritis is considered. If gonorrhea is considered, obtain cervical/urethral, rectal, and pharyngeal specimens.
4. **Creatinine.** Often obtained because many drugs, especially nonsteroidal anti-inflammatory drugs (NSAIDs), used in treatment are contraindicated if creatinine is elevated.
5. **Urinalysis.** Proteinuria, red cells, and casts may indicate a systemic cause such as SLE.
6. **Rheumatic disease workup.** If a collagen vascular disease is suspected, obtain a Westergren erythrocyte sedimentation rate (ESR), antinuclear antibodies (ANA), and RF. An anti–double-stranded deoxyribonucleic acid (anti-DS DNA) should be obtained if SLE is considered. Tests for complement (CH50, C3, C4), cryoglobulin, and other serologies such as the extractable nuclear antigens (anti-RNP and anti-Smith) are usually not obtained initially. HLA-B27 is rarely helpful.

C. **Radiologic and other studies.** Plain films of the involved joints are often helpful, especially if the arthritis is chronic. If normal, they can serve as a baseline as the arthritis progresses. Films of the hands and feet are particularly helpful when RA is considered.

V. **Plan.** Treatment is dependent on the type of arthritis diagnosed. An individual discussion of each is beyond the scope of this book.

A. **Drug therapy.** Ensure from the patient's history and laboratory tests that there are no contraindications to the medication chosen. The patient must be informed of side effects. The most commonly prescribed medication, NSAIDs, is contraindicated in patients with elevated creatinine, a history of hypersensitivity reaction to aspirin or NSAIDs, platelet abnormalities, and possibly peptic ulcer disease. In the elderly, one must be aware of the CNS side effects.

B. **Supportive measures.** Dependent on the diagnosis, heat or ice therapy, specific exercises, splinting, and physical therapy may be indicated.

C. **Septic arthritis**

1. Daily drainage of joint fluid is absolutely necessary. If the joint is not easily drained, open drainage may be necessary. The

gram stain will help direct the initial choice of antibiotic pending cultures.

2. If gonococcal arthritis is suspected, penicillin is effective unless the patient is at risk of having a penicillinase-producing strain, for example in intravenous drug abusers. A third-generation cephalosporin is then indicated. (See Chapter 7, p 494.)
3. In nongonococcal bacterial arthritis, gram-positive cocci on gram stain should be treated with a penicillinase-resistant penicillin or vancomycin if methicillin-resistant *Staphylococcus aureus* are prevalent or if *Staphylococcus epidermis* is suspected. An aminoglycoside and an antipseudomonal penicillin or third-generation cephalosporin would be used for gram-negative bacilli. If the gram strain is negative in a compromised host, use broad-spectrum coverage for both gram-positive and gram-negative organisms.

REFERENCES

Kelly WN, Harris ED, Ruddy S, et al. *Textbook of Rheumatology.* 3rd ed. Philadelphia: WB Saunders; 1989.

McCarty DJ: *Arthritis and Allied Conditions.* 11th ed. Philadelphia: Lea and Febiger; 1989.

■ LEUKOCYTOSIS

I. **Problem.** A 63-year-old woman is admitted for hypoxemia, diffuse bilateral pulmonary infiltrates and fever. She is placed on broad-spectrum intravenous antibiotics after appropriate cultures are obtained. Her white blood cell count remains about 25,000–30,000/μL.

II. **Immediate Questions**

A. **What is the current clinical status of the patient?** Elevated WBC counts may be associated with obvious evidence of infection including recurrent fevers, rigors, hypotension, or tachycardia.

B. **Has the patient improved or deteriorated since the leukocytosis was first noted?** A definite clinical improvement since admission would argue in favor of a chronic process or a sustained response to the present clinical illness; however, questionable improvement or deterioration should obviously alert you to the need to completely reassess the patient.

C. **Have any intervening clinically relevant episodes of physical stress taken place since admission?** Hypotension and other signs of shock can certainly be associated with a leukocytosis. The use of mechanical ventilation or resuscitative measures can stimulate a leukocytosis.

D. **Is there a history suggestive of prior underlying systemic**

illness? Symptoms such as weight loss, prior sustained fevers, night sweats, chronic cough or dyspnea, hemoptysis, myalgias, and bone pain are all suggestive of chronic illnesses, mycobacterial or fungal infections, connective tissue diseases, or possibly a neoplastic disorder. A history of the acute development of presenting symptoms argues against a chronic or subacute illness.

E. **Are there any prior complete blood counts with which to compare this admission's counts?** Again, the presence or absence of prior leukocytosis critically aids the evaluation. Sustained leukocytosis over weeks or months strongly implies a chronic or subacute process, be it an infection such as an abscess or tuberculosis (TB) or a neoplasm or some other process.

F. **Is there evidence of infection that has not been addressed, such as intra-abdominal infection (abscess), genitourinary infection, or central nervous system infection?** In this patient, pulmonary infiltrates may represent adult respiratory distress syndrome (ARDS) occurring as a reaction to underlying sepsis, especially from an abdominal infection. Because acute infections are treatable, acute infectious causes of leukocytosis must be excluded.

G. **Is the patient currently on any medications such as vasopressors or steroids that are associated with sustained elevated WBC counts?** Corticosteroids and pressor agents are often associated with demargination and subsequent leukocytosis.

H. **Does the patient have a history of an underlying hematologic disorder?** Symptoms such as paresthesias, cyanosis in response to changes in ambient temperature, and easy bruising or bleeding are all suggestive of a primary bone marrow pathology.

I. **Does the patient have a history of prior abdominal trauma or surgery or, specifically, splenectomy?** The postsplenectomy state is often associated with a baseline WBC count that is above normal. In addition, the splenectomized patient is at greater risk of developing sepsis, especially from encapsulated organisms.

III. **Differential Diagnosis.** There are numerous causes of leukocytosis. It is a normal response to many noxious emotional and physical stimuli. Leukocytosis is defined as a WBC count greater than 10,000/μL. A broad division of causes separates leukocytosis into acute and chronic.

A. **Acute**

1. **Acute bacterial infection.** Either localized or generalized (sepsis).
2. **Other infections.** Mycobacteria, fungi, certain viruses, rickettsia, or even spirochetes.
3. **Trauma**
4. **Myocardial infarction (MI), pulmonary embolism/infarc-**

tion, mesenteric ischemia/infarction, or peripheral vascular disease with ischemia

5. **Vasculitis, antigen-antibody complexes, and complement activation**
6. **Physical stimuli.** Extremes of temperature, seizure activity, and intense pain are associated with increased WBC counts.
7. **Emotional stimuli.** Occasionally can trigger acute leukocytosis.
8. **Drugs.** Can often cause or contribute to leukocytosis. Particularly pressor agents and corticosteroids.

B. Chronic

1. **Persistent infections.** Often the same infection that caused the initial presentation.
2. **Partially treated or occult infections.** Osteomyelitis, subacute bacterial endocarditis (SBE), and intra-abdominal abscess can often present as chronic leukocytosis.
3. **Mycobacterial or fungal infections.** Notorious for promoting a sustained leukocytosis, often with little other clinical pathology on initial evaluation.
4. **Chronic inflammatory states.** Rheumatic fever, connective tissue disease such as systemic lupus erythematosus (SLE), thyroiditis, myositis, drug reactions, and pancreatitis can all chronically elevate the WBC count.
5. **Neoplastic processes.** Solid tumors and lymphoproliferative disorders can have an associated chronic leukocytosis.
6. **Primary hematologic disorders.** Include myeloproliferative disorders, myelodysplasia, leukemias, chronic hemolysis, and asplenic state.
7. **Congenital disorders.** Very rarely can be associated with chronic leukocytosis, including Down syndrome.
8. **Drugs.** Less common cause. Include pressor agents, steroids, and lithium.
9. **Overproduction of ACTH or thyroxine.** Can elevate the baseline WBC count chronically.

IV. Database

A. Physical examination key points

1. **Vital signs.** Especially check for the presence of fever or hypothermia, which suggests infection or sepsis, respectively. Fever can also indicate a neoplastic process, infarction of various tissues, or a connective tissue disorder. (See Fever, p 98.) Hypotension may occur in patients who are septic.
2. **General.** Look for evidence of acute distress or a chronic disease state (cachexia, digital clubbing, bitemporal wasting).
3. **Lymph nodes.** Check for palpable lymph nodes and note their character. Soft and tender nodes are most consistent with an infectious etiology. Rubbery and generalized nodes are most often seen with lymphoreticular disorders. Hard, fixed, and localized nodes suggest carcinoma.

4. **Skin/mucosa.** Petechiae or ecchymoses suggest sepsis with disseminated intravascular coagulation (DIC), primary bone marrow pathology with altered platelet number or function and/or clotting dysfunction, or vasculitis.
5. **Lungs.** Inspiratory rales imply pneumonitis or pneumonia. Diminished breath sounds and dullness to percussion suggest the same or possibly a pleural effusion or abscess. A pleural rub may accompany infectious processes, malignant pathology, or other processes such as thromboembolism and SLE, all commonly associated with leukocytosis.
6. **Heart.** Tachycardia is consistent with acute stress. The presence of a new murmur, particularly with fever, is suggestive of SBE. Look for evidence of volume overload, sometimes triggered by infection or occasionally associated with leukemias or myeloproliferative disorders.
7. **Abdomen.** Tenderness on rebound suggests an acute abdominal process such as perforation of a viscus or infarction.
8. **Genitourinary/gynecologic exam.** Flank, pelvic, or prostate tenderness is suggestive of acute infection.
9. **Neurologic exam.** Altered mental status, confusion, seizures, and focally abnormal deep tendon reflexes can all be seen in a variety of situations associated with leukocytosis including meningitis (infectious or neoplastic), sepsis, leukemias, lymphomas, and solid malignancies.

B. Laboratory data

1. **Blood.** Personal evaluation of the peripheral blood smear is absolutely critical. Look for a coexisting anemia, polycythemia, or abnormal platelet count. Leukocytosis with a "left shift," Döhle bodies, and toxic granulation suggest an acute infection, whereas a normal differential pattern implies a nonbacterial cause. A lymphocytosis points to a viral illness, lymphoma, or leukemia. An increase in monocytes is often seen with carcinoma or TB. Eosinophilia suggests connective tissue disease, possible drug reaction, or possible parasitic infection. Promyelocytes, myelocytes, or basophilia are consistent with myeloproliferative disorders (leukemias most commonly), although severe infections, toxic insults, and inflammation can sometimes result in the release of early myeloid forms.
2. **Liver function tests.** Can be elevated in acute hepatitis, sepsis, leukemia, lymphoma, or metastatic carcinoma.
3. **Electrolytes.** Acute infection (especially pneumonia) and chronic infection (pulmonary TB, tuberculous or fungal meningitis) involving the lung or central nervous system can cause the syndrome of inappropriate antidiuretic hormone (SIADH) release and hyponatremia.
4. **Arterial blood gases.** A metabolic gap acidosis can accompany sepsis, leukemia, or solid tumors.
5. **Cultures.** Blood, urine, cerebrospinal fluid, sputum, and other

cultures and skin tests are vital to rule in or exclude an infectious etiology.

C. Radiologic and other studies

1. **Chest x-ray.** Check for evidence of acute pneumonic process as well as a mass lesion or a mediastinal abnormality.
2. **CT scan.** Can be used to localize an abscess, define the extent of any suspicious masses or adenopathy, and determine the extent or presence of organomegaly.
3. **Bone scan.** Supports or suggests a diagnosis of osteomyelitis, primary marrow disease such as leukemia, or metastatic carcinomas.
4. **Tumor markers.** Tests like terminal deoxynucleotidyl transferase (Tdt), leukocyte alkaline phosphatase (LAP), and vitamin B_{12} level, as well as tests for a host of currently available monoclonal antibodies to carcinomas, can be quite useful. Frequently in a patient with a sustained leukocytosis, the LAP score can be one of the most useful initial lab tests to distinguish between an infectious/inflammatory etiology and a myeloproliferative disorder. The LAP score is usually elevated in infectious processes, whereas it is classically low in chronic granulocytic myelogenous leukemia (CML) and variable in the other myeloproliferative disorders.
5. **Bone marrow aspiration and biopsy.** May be required to rule in or exclude primary marrow pathology, metastatic tumor, or chronic infections. Cytogenic studies can be performed to look specifically for myelodysplasia, myeloproliferative disorders, leukemias, or lymphomas. At times, this is the only way to differentiate between a reactive bone marrow and chronic myelogenous leukemia.

V. Plan. The etiology of the increased WBC count, of course, guides therapy. When obvious acute stress (infection, trauma, inflammation) is not present, chronic infections, inflammation, carcinoma, or primary marrow pathology must be considered. As mentioned, strict attention to history, clinical presentation and course, and physical examination and personal review of the peripheral blood smear are absolutely vital to initial evaluation of a leukocytosis. The overlooked and/or inappropriately treated infection can be catastrophic. For specific treatment of the various etiologies of leukocytosis, please refer to any general reference.

REFERENCES

Beck WS, ed. Leukocytes. III. Introduction to pathology. In: Beck WS, ed. *Hematology.* 4th ed. Cambridge, Mass: MIT Press; 1985:291–304.

Bunn PA, Pidway EC. Paraneoplastic syndrome. In: Devita VT, Hellman S, Rosenberg SA, et al, eds. *Cancer: Principles and Practice of Oncology.* 3rd ed. Philadelphia: Lippincott; 1989:1896–1940.

Dale DC. Neutrophilia. In: Williams WJ, Beutler E, Erslev AJ, et al, eds. *Hematology.* 4th ed. New York: McGraw-Hill; 1990:816–820.

■ LEUKOPENIA

I. Problem. An 18-year-old white woman is placed on phenytoin (Dilantin) for seizure control. Two weeks later, she returns with complaints of fever, chills, and productive cough. She is admitted with a temperature of 102°F and the white count is 2000/μL.

II. Immediate Questions

A. What is the patient's occupation and has she been exposed to any chemicals? Farmers may be exposed to insecticides (DDT, lindane, chlordane) that can cause leukopenia. A painter or chemist may be exposed to benzene (another myelosuppressive chemical).

B. Has the patient received any antineoplastic drugs or radiation therapy? Myelosuppression is often an expected result of chemotherapy. Radiation is a direct myelosuppressant.

C. What are the patient's medications? Several commonly used drugs have been documented to cause neutropenia including β-lactams, phenothiazines, sulfonamides, phenytoin, cimetidine (Tagamet), and ranitidine (Zantac).

D. Has the patient noted any tea-colored urine? Paroxysmal nocturnal hemoglobinuria (PNH) and hepatitis can be associated with aplastic anemia.

E. Has the patient had any fever, gastrointestinal complaints, or viral symptoms? Several viral (infectious hepatitis, mononucleosis) and bacterial (salmonellosis, bacillary dysentery) illnesses and rickettsialpox have been associated with neutropenia.

F. Does the patient have a history of alcohol abuse or any history of cirrhosis? Ethanol is a direct myelosuppressant and can cause leukopenia. Folate deficiency, which can occur in alcoholics, may cause leukopenia. Cirrhotics can develop hypersplenism and sequester white cells as well as platelets in the spleen.

G. Is there any psychiatric history or history of anorexia nervosa? Several medications used in the treatment of psychiatric disorders such as phenothiazines can cause leukopenia. Anorexia nervosa and starvation can cause leukopenia; the mechanism is unknown.

H. Does the patient have rheumatoid arthritis? Felty's syndrome is a constellation of splenomegaly, neutropenia, and rheumatoid arthritis.

I. What is the ethnic background? Blacks and Yemenite Jews may have a normal racial variant of leukopenia. Neutrophil count may be as low as 1500 cells/μL.

J. What is the patient's sexual and drug history? Homosexuals, bisexuals, and intravenous drug users are at increased risk for human immunodeficiency virus infection, which can cause leukopenia; the exact mechanism is unknown.

K. Has the patient experienced recurrent, cyclic fevers? Cyclic neutropenia is a rare form of neutropenia that has fluctuations of the neutrophil count at fairly regular 3-week intervals. The only clue may be unexplained recurrent fevers every 3 weeks.

III. Differential Diagnosis. Awareness of the differential is imperative because it is not the total white count that is critical but rather the **absolute neutrophil count** (ANC). **Neutropenia** is defined as an absolute neutrophil count (% of segmented and banded neutrophils × total white count = ANC) less than $1800/mm^3$. At ANCs less than $1000/m^3$, the risk of infection begins to increase. At values of $500/mm^3$ or less, there is a further dramatic increase in the likelihood of serious infection. The causes of neutropenia can be grouped in three broad categories: (1) bone marrow failure (defective neutrophil production and/or maturation); (2) accelerated neutrophil removal; and (3) neutrophil redistribution. This classification is useful because it helps direct the choice of laboratory studies.

A. Inadequate bone marrow production

1. **Leukemia (acute).** About 25% of acute leukemics present with pancytopenia.
2. **Myelodysplastic syndromes.** Such as refractory anemia. The bone marrow is normally hypercellular or normocellular.
3. **Megaloblastic syndromes.** Both vitamin B_{12} and folate deficiencies can result in neutropenia.
4. **Marrow infiltration**
   - a. **Metastatic cancer**
   - b. **Granulomatous diseases**
5. **Drugs.** Benzene, alkylating agents (melphalan), vinca alkaloids (vincristine or vinblastine), doxorubicin (Adriamycin), and antimetabolites (methotrexate).
6. **Radiation.** A direct marrow toxin.
7. **Aplastic anemia**
8. **Cyclic neutropenia**
9. **Racial or familial neutropenia**
10. **Infections.** Twenty to thirty percent of cases with infectious mononucleosis have moderate neutropenia. Other viral infections (HIV, hepatitis A or B) and bacterial illnesses can have a direct myelosuppressive effect.
11. **Starvation/anorexia nervosa**
12. **Paroxysmal nocturnal hemoglobinuria (PNH)**

B. Accelerated removal/consumption

1. **Drug induction**
   - a. **Immune.** Such as hydralazine (Apresoline), quinidine, quinine, cefoxitin (Mefoxin), and nafcillin.
   - b. **Nonimmune.** Such as phenacitin, indomethacin (Indocin), phenytoin, chloramphenicol, cimetidine, ranitidine, and phenothiazines.
2. **Hemodialysis and cardiovascular bypass.** Exposure of blood to a dialysis coil of cellophane or nylon fiber appears

to activate the complement pathway. This increases neutrophil adhesion, causing them to sequester in pulmonary capillaries.

3. **Felty's syndrome.** Neutropenia associated with seropositive rheumatoid arthritis and splenomegaly suggests this diagnosis.
4. **Infection**
   a. **Nonimmune.** At times, the peripheral requirements for neutrophils during overwhelming sepsis can exhaust the marrow reserves. This is particularly true in the debilitated patient.
   b. **Immune.** Tests for antineutrophil antibodies are not routinely available. Thus, this is a diagnosis of exclusion.

C. Redistribution of neutrophils

1. **Enhanced neutrophil margination.** Endotoxemia in gram-negative sepsis can give rise to rapid margination of neutrophils to the tissue.
2. **Hypersplenism.** Refers to the clinical situation where, in the presence of splenomegaly and a relatively normal bone marrow, there is a decrease of one or more cell lines in the peripheral blood because of sequestration in the spleen.

IV. Database

A. Physical examination key points

1. **Vital signs.** Fever suggests infection. Hypotension may be a sign of sepsis.
2. **Skin.** Petechiae is consistent with Rocky Mountain spotted fever or disseminated intravascular coagulation (DIC). Rash may be seen in connective tissue diseases or with certain bacterial infections such as *Neisseria gonorrhoeae* or *Neisseria meningitidis.*
3. **HEENT.** Temporal wasting and oral thrush may occur in acquired immunodeficiency syndrome (AIDS). Nuchal rigidity suggests meningitis.
4. **Lymph nodes.** Lymphadenopathy can be seen in both malignant and infectious processes including HIV infection.
5. **Lungs.** Pneumonia with overwhelming sepsis may cause or be secondary to neutropenia. Inspiratory crackles, increased tactile and vocal fremitus, and egophony may be present.
6. **Abdomen.** Hepatosplenomegaly can be a sign of malignancy (leukemia or lymphoma), infection, or hypersplenism.
7. **Joints.** Look for classic findings of rheumatoid arthritis such as symmetric swelling of the proximal interphalangeal (PIP) and metacarpophalangeal (MCP) joints. Rheumatoid nodules on the extensor surface of the arms near the elbows are also classic for rheumatoid arthritis.

B. Laboratory data

1. **Complete blood count with differential.** Presence of anemia and thrombocytopenia may suggest B_{12} or folate deficiency,

aplastic anemia, PNH, or leukemia. The mean corpuscular volume will be increased with B_{12} or folate deficiency.

2. **Blood and urine cultures.** If an infectious process is suspected.
3. **Liver function test and hepatitis serologies.** If hepatitis is suspected.
4. **Peripheral blood smear.** Dysplastic, degranulated neutrophils with pseudo–Pelger-Huet anomaly (a bilobed neutrophil) may suggest a myelodysplastic syndrome. Toxic granulation and Döhle bodies suggest infection. Neutrophils with five and six lobes point toward B_{12} deficiency. Blasts are consistent with leukemia.
5. **Leukocyte alkaline phosphatase (LAP) score.** Is increased in certain infectious and inflammatory diseases and polycythemia vera. In contrast, it is decreased in chronic myelogenous leukemia.
6. **Rheumatoid factor and antinuclear antibodies (ANA).** If collagen vascular disease is suggested.
7. **Carotene (serum).** Elevated in anorexia nervosa and decreased in starvation.
8. **Vitamin B_{12} and folate levels.** To rule out megaloblastic anemia.
9. **Sucrose water test/Ham test.** Useful in making the diagnosis of PNH. The sucrose water test involves mixing the patient's red blood cells in an isotonic solution of sucrose dissolved in water. The Ham test is performed by mixing the patient's red blood cells with acidified serum. Both tests promote the binding of a small amount of complement to the surface. This results in hemolysis in patients with PNH.

C. Radiologic and other studies

1. **Chest x-ray.** To rule out pneumonia if suspected.
2. **Sinus films, dental Panorex.** As indicated when looking for source of fever in a neutropenic patient.
3. **Lumbar puncture.** Indicated when meningitis (acute or chronic) is suspected.
4. **Bone marrow biopsy and aspiration.** (See Chapter 3, Bone Marrow Aspiration and Biopsy, p 312.) This can provide critical information about granulocyte aplasia, hypoplasia or dysplasia, infiltration, cellularity, and cellular maturation. A bone marrow is essential in all patients with neutropenia except when it is mild, stable, or clinically associated with a drug known to cause neutropenia. Even in the setting of a drug-induced process, it is reasonable to document suspected marrow findings.

V. Plan. The major consequence of neutropenia is vulnerability to infection. The usual clinical manifestations of infection are often absent because of the lack of granulocytes (neutrophils). Thus, pneumonia may be present without significant infiltrate on CXR; meningitis may occur without pleocytosis or meningeal signs; and pyelonephritis may be present without pyuria. A heightened awareness for infection is extremely important in the neutropenic patient, as an untreated infection can be fatal.

A. Emergent management

1. If there is evidence of infection or fever (higher than 100.5°F) with an ANC below 500/μL, the patient should be immediately pancultured (cerebrospinal and other body fluid cultures as indicated) and broad-spectrum antibiotics initiated (tobramycin and ticarcillin and/or vancomycin if the patient has a central line or prosthesis in place). Neutropenia with infection is a medical emergency requiring immediate investigation and treatment.
2. Identify any potential drugs or chemicals that may have induced the neutropenia and stop or remove them.
3. Always wash your hands prior to touching the patient. Avoid visitors with active infections, fresh fruits or vegetables, flowers, and live plants. Avoid rectal manipulation such as with digital examination or rectal temperature.

B. Definitive care. After a complete history and physical exam, the etiology of the neutropenia can usually be placed in one of the three broad categories discussed earlier and subsequent tests can be obtained to confirm a specific diagnosis. In general, regardless of the etiology, supportive care is indicated for most of these patients. This includes antibiotics for infections and blood products for associated severe anemia or thrombocytopenia.

1. **Bone marrow failure.** For drug-induced neutropenia, remove the offending agent and give supportive care until the counts return (generally within 1–2 weeks). Treatment for viral etiology or myelodysplastic syndromes is generally supportive care.
2. **Consumption.** Treat bacterial infections as indicated. Immune consumption may require steroids. Felty's syndrome generally requires no treatment unless the patient suffers recurrent infection. Then, splenectomy may be required.
3. **Redistribution.** Patients with hypersplenism generally are able to immobilize the sequestered neutrophils and thus fight off infection; subsequently, they do not require any specific therapy.

REFERENCES

Saiki JH. White blood cell abnormalities. In: Friedman HH, ed. *Problem-Oriented Medical Diagnosis.* 3rd ed. Boston: Little, Brown, 1983:209–217.

Schrier SL. Leukocyte function and nonmalignant disorders. In: Rubenstein E, ed-in-chief; Federman DD, ed. *Scientific American.* sect 5: *Hematology and Nonmalignant Disorders.* pt VII: *Leukocyte Function.* New York: Scientific American Inc; 1989:5–11.

■ NAUSEA AND VOMITING

I. **Problem.** A 39-year-old man is admitted with diffuse abdominal pain and fever. Later that evening, you are called because the patient has severe nausea and vomiting.

II. **Immediate Questions.** When evaluating a patient with nausea and/or vomiting, a careful history and a complete physical exam are important to rule out serious causes that require prompt intervention such as peritonitis and intracranial lesions.

A. **What are the patient's vital signs?** Fever suggests an inflammatory process such as gastroenteritis, peritonitis, or cholecystitis. Hypotension may be secondary to volume depletion or associated sepsis. Hypertension and/or bradycardia may reflect increased intracranial pressure.

B. **When does the nausea and vomiting occur and is it related to meals?** Vomiting during or soon after a meal suggests psychogenic causes or may be seen with pyloric channel ulcer, pancreatitis, or biliary tract disease. If abdominal pain is relieved with vomiting, an ulcer becomes more likely. Vomiting an hour or more after a meal is more characteristic of gastric outlet obstruction, pancreatitis, or motility disorders such as diabetic gastroparesis and postvagotomy. Nausea and vomiting early in the morning on arising is often associated with alcoholism, pregnancy, uremia, and increased intracranial pressure.

C. **What are the appearance and volume of the vomitus?** Large amounts of vomitus or secretions usually indicate partial or complete bowel obstruction, gastric atony, or, in rare cases, Zollinger-Ellison syndrome. Vomiting of undigested food suggests the presence of esophageal disorders, such as achalasia or a diverticulum, as well as gastric outlet obstruction. The presence of bile indicates a patent pyloric channel. A fecal smell suggests lower abdominal obstruction. Occasionally, this can be seen with bacterial overgrowth in the proximal small intestine. Blood or coffee-ground–appearing material points to an upper gastrointestinal bleed. Vomiting can also induce hematemesis secondary to a Mallory-Weiss tear. (See Hematemesis, Melena, p 117.)

D. **Does the patient consume alcohol or ingest nonsteroidal anti-inflammatory drugs (NSAIDs)?** Pancreatitis or acute gastritis can be caused by ethanol and result in nausea and vomiting. A NSAID such as ibuprofen (Motrin) can induce gastritis.

E. **Is there associated abdominal pain?** This can be seen with most abdominal causes of nausea and vomiting. The location of the abdominal pain will help in deciding the etiology of the nausea and vomiting. (See Abdominal Pain, p 1.)

III. **Differential Diagnosis.** Those disorders that are associated with nausea and vomiting and require immediate attention can be grouped as follows.

A. **Intra-abdominal or thoracic etiology**
   1. **Gastric outlet obstruction.** Occurs in patients with a history of peptic ulcer disease, prior abdominal surgery, or neoplasms.
   2. **Small or large bowel obstruction.** May be caused by fibrous bands and adhesions (usually after surgery), primary or secondary metastatic neoplasms, impacted feces, strictures from active inflammatory bowel disease, intestinal parasites, gallstones, incarcerated hernia, or a volvulus.
   3. **Pseudo-obstruction or functional (paralytic) ileus.** Results from failure of normal intestinal peristalsis. Causes include abdominal surgery, retroperitoneal or intra-abdominal hematomas, severe infections, renal disease, metabolic disturbances such as hypokalemia, or drugs, particularly anticholinergics.
   4. **Peptic ulcer disease.** Results from local irritation or edema surrounding a pyloric channel ulcer causing a mechanical obstruction.
   5. **Pancreatitis.** Usually associated with abdominal pain that frequently (more than 50%) radiates to the back. A CT scan is helpful in demonstrating inflammation and pseudocyst formation. Retroperitoneal abscess formation can complicate pancreatitis.
   6. **Biliary colic.** From distension of smooth muscle in bile ducts secondary to stones, inflammation, or neoplasms.
   7. **Intestinal ischemia.** From local vascular compromise or from reduced cardiac output. Guaiac-positive stools are common.
   8. **Pyelonephritis or nephrolithiasis**
   9. **Hepatitis.** Viral or drug-induced.
   10. **Appendicitis.** Often associated with right lower quadrant pain and fever.
   11. **Diverticulitis.** Lower abdominal pain and fever are common.
   12. **Perforated viscus.** Usually presents as an acute abdomen.
   13. **Pelvic inflammatory disease**
   14. **Acute myocardial infarction.** Infarction, especially involving the inferior wall, can present with nausea and vomiting. Chest pain may be absent.

B. **Intracranial etiology**
   1. **Tumor or mass lesions leading to increased intracranial pressure.** Consider an acute cerebral vascular accident, neoplasm, or subdural hematoma.
   2. **Bacterial and viral meningitis**
   3. **Migraine headache.** Usually unilateral headache, with photophobia and previous history of headache. May have prodrome.
   4. **Labyrinthitis**

C. Metabolic etiology

1. **Uremia.** Often associated with weight loss, lethargy, and intense pruritus. The BUN is usually greater than 100.
2. **Hepatic failure.** From a variety of causes including cirrhosis, hypoxic injury, and drug-induced states such as acetaminophen overdose.
3. **Adrenal insufficiency.** Can occur in patients receiving chronic corticosteroid therapy that is suddenly discontinued. Associated symptoms include weakness, fatigue, hypotension, and abdominal pain.
4. **Metabolic acidosis** (See Acidosis, p 9.)
5. **Electrolyte abnormalities.** Hypercalcemia and hyperkalemia as well as hypokalemia can cause nausea.
6. **Hypothyroidism secondary to decreased intestinal motility or thyroid storm.** Weight gain, constipation, mental status changes, and dry skin suggest hypothyroidism. Weight loss, hyperdefecation, moist skin, hyperthermia, and mental status changes as well as a precipitating event are consistent with thyroid storm.

D. Miscellaneous etiology

1. **Drug induced.** Major offenders are dopamine agonists such as L-dopa and bromocriptine (Parlodel), opiate analgesics such as morphine, digoxin (Lanoxin), and certain chemotherapy agents such as cisplatin (Platinol). Also consider alcohol, NSAIDs, and aspirin.
2. **Acute gastroenteritis.** Common in the outpatient setting with "food poisoning" from bacterial endotoxin. Diarrhea is often present.

IV. Database

A. Physical examination key points

1. **Vital signs.** Hypotension may result from volume depletion or sepsis. Orthostatic blood pressure changes suggest volume depletion. An orthostatic decrease in blood pressure without an increase in heart rate suggests autonomic neuropathy, which may accompany diabetes with gastroparesis. Fever points to an inflammatory component, possibly infection. Tachycardia can result from associated pain.
2. **HEENT.** Look for signs of head trauma which would point to an intracranial process. Scleral icterus suggests hepatic failure/hepatitis. Papilledema is consistent with an intracranial process or a hypertensive emergency. An enlarged thyroid gland points toward hypothyroidism or hyperthyroidism.
3. **Skin.** Look at skin turgor and mucous membranes to estimate volume status. Yellowing of the skin may signify jaundice. Hyperpigmentation may be caused by adrenal insufficiency (Addison's disease).

4. **Chest.** Inspiratory crackles secondary to atelectasis can be associated with any intraabdominal process limiting deep inspiration because of pain, and could also suggest left ventricular dysfunction associated with myocardial infarction.
5. **Abdomen** (See Abdominal Pain, Section IV.A., pp 4 and 5.)
6. **Rectum.** Check for fecal impaction, rectal masses, and occult blood. Tenderness on the right is consistent with appendicitis. Blood can be secondary to diverticulitis, inflammatory bowel disease, peptic ulcer disease, and gastritis or may result from vomiting (Mallory-Weiss tear).
7. **Female genitalia.** Helpful in diagnosing pelvic inflammatory disease. A discharge is often present.
8. **Neurologic exam**
   a. Mental status changes may signify central nervous system lesions, encephalopathy, or severe electrolyte disturbances.
   b. Focal neurologic findings such as weakness, unilateral hyperreflexia, or a positive Babinski on one side suggest an intracranial process.
   c. Pain with flexion of the neck is consistent with meningeal inflammation secondary to either a subarachnoid bleed or meningitis. A positive Kernig's sign also indicates meningeal irritation and is performed by flexing the hip and knee to 90°. Attempts to extend the leg at the knee will result in hamstring pain and resistance to movement.

B. **Laboratory data**
1. **Electrolytes.** With severe vomiting, various electrolyte abnormalities, such as hypokalemia, hypochloremia, and metabolic alkalosis, can occur.
2. **Complete blood count with differential.** A leukocytosis with an increase in banded neutrophils suggests an infection. An elevated hematocrit can represent volume depletion. Anemia suggests chronic GI blood loss or massive acute bleeding.
3. **Blood urea nitrogen and creatinine.** To rule out renal failure.
4. **Urinalysis.** Look for white blood cells and casts suggesting pyelonephritis. Red blood cells, especially with flank pain, point to nephrolithiasis.
5. **Liver function tests, transaminases (AST [SGOT] and ALT [SGPT]), total bilirubin, and alkaline phosphatase.** To rule out hepatic failure and hepatitis.
6. **Amylase and/or lipase.** If pancreatitis is suspected.
7. **Arterial blood gases.** Needed to evaluate the presence of an acid-base disturbance as a cause or consequence of vomiting.
8. **Serum intact human chorionic gonadotropin serum.** If pregnancy is suspected.

C. **Radiologic and other studies**

1. **Acute abdominal series (KUB).** Air-fluid levels are seen in obstruction, and free air under the diaphragm indicates perforation. If pregnancy is possible, would defer KUB until result of HCG is known.
2. **Electrocardiogram.** Helpful in evaluating for acute myocardial infarction. ST segment depression or elevation or T wave inversion or Q waves suggest myocardial ischemia or infarction.
3. **Abdominal ultrasound or HIDA scan.** An aid in the diagnosis of cholecystitis, biliary duct obstruction, or abscesses. Biliary colic cannot be ruled out with a normal ultrasound. A HIDA scan is important as a means of assessing cystic duct function.
4. **Endoscopy.** Important in the diagnosis of peptic ulcer disease or esophageal diverticuli.
5. **Gastric emptying scan.** Useful in suspected gastroparesis, especially in patients with long-standing diabetes who have nausea and vomiting.

V. **Plan.** Treatment of the underlying etiology is essential in the management. A nasogastric tube should be used for decompression if obstruction is present. Treatment of each cause is beyond the scope of this section. Commonly used medications are listed here.

A. **Phenothiazines.** Most commonly used antiemetics. Principal mode of action is via depression of dopamine receptors in the central nervous system. Prochlorperazine (Compazine) 10 mg PO every 4–6 hours or 25 mg rectally, chlorpromazine (Thorazine) 25 mg PO every 8 hours, and promethazine (Phenergan) 12.5–25 mg PO, rectally, or IM every 6–12 hours prn are effective. Extrapyramidal side effects can be treated with diphenhydramine (Benadryl) 25 mg IV or IM every 4–6 hours.

B. **Butyrophenones.** Also block the dopamine receptors in the central nervous system. Administer haloperidol (Haldol) 2 mg PO or IM every 4–6 hours or droperidol (Inapsine) 2–5 mg IV or IM every 4–6 hours.

C. **Miscellaneous drugs.** High doses of metoclopramide (Reglan), 1–2 mg/kg every 4–6 hours, constitute a useful and very effective adjunct with cancer chemotherapy to prevent nausea and vomiting. Benztropine (Cogentin) 2 mg PO or IV or diphenhydramine 25–50 mg PO or IM should be given prophylactically to prevent extrapyramidal reactions with high-dose metoclopramide.

REFERENCES

Feldman M. Nausea and vomiting. In: Sleisenger MH, Fordtran JS, eds. *Gastrointestinal Disease—Pathophysiology, Diagnosis, Management.* 4th ed. Philadelphia, WB Saunders Co, 1989, pp 222–238.

Malagelada JR, Camilleri M. Unexplained vomiting: A diagnostic challenge. *Ann Intern Med* 1984;101:211–218.

OLIGURIA/ANURIA

I. **Problem.** A 72-year-old man admitted 24 hours earlier for pneumonia and altered mental status has had steadily declining urinary output overnight. On morning rounds, his nurse reports that he did not void during the previous shift.

II. **Immediate Questions**

A. **Does the patient have any symptoms or predisposing conditions that suggest hypovolemia?** Hypovolemia is a common cause of oliguria. Diarrhea, vomiting, bleeding, high fever, and poor oral intake are possible causes. Positional dizziness suggests hypovolemia.

B. **Is there any previous history of symptoms to suggest bladder outlet obstruction from prostatic hypertrophy?** A history of hesitancy, difficulty initiating voiding, and dribbling suggests prostatic hypertrophy, which can result in postrenal obstruction.

C. **Is there a history of hematuria?** Bilateral nephrolithiasis or carcinoma can cause obstruction resulting in anuria or oliguria.

D. **Is the patient likely to be suffering from acute renal insufficiency?** Acute renal insufficiency can result in oliguria, although it is an uncommon cause of complete anuria. Clues to the presence of acute renal insufficiency include baseline renal insufficiency (which amplifies the effects of ischemic or toxic insult), documented episodes of hypotension, medications known to affect renal function adversely such as aminoglycoside antibiotics and nonsteroidal anti-inflammatory agents (NSAIDs), and exposure to nephrotoxic agents, especially contrast dyes.

E. **Are there any underlying diseases that could result in oliguria/anuria?** Congestive heart failure and cirrhosis can cause oliguria/anuria by reducing effective arterial blood volume.

F. **Does the patient have any symptoms suggestive of uremia?** Nausea, vomiting, anorexia, insomnia, and mental status changes are seen with increasing renal insufficiency. Uremic symptoms are an indication for immediate dialysis.

III. **Differential Diagnosis.** Oliguria is defined as a urine output less than 500 mL/d and anuria as an output less than 100 mL/d. The differential diagnosis for acute oliguria is identical to that for acute renal failure and may be divided into prerenal, renal, and postrenal causes.

A. **Prerenal causes.** Relating to renal hypoperfusion.

1. **Shock/hypovolemia**
   a. **Hemorrhage.** From gastrointestinal bleeding or trauma or as a postoperative complication.
   b. **Inadequate fluid administration.** Fever, diarrhea, vomiting, poor oral intake without adequate fluid administration.
   c. **Sepsis.** Causing decreased renal perfusion as a result of decreased systemic vascular resistance.

2. **Apparent intravascular hypovolemia.** A relative decrease in the effective circulating volume.
   a. **"Third-space" losses.** Very common in pancreatitis, major burns and after major operations.
   b. **Congestive heart failure**
   c. **Cirrhosis.** May have associated hepatorenal syndrome.
   d. **Nephrotic syndrome**
3. **Vascular**
   a. **Renal artery occlusion (acute or chronic)**
   b. **Aortic dissection**
   c. **Emboli (such as cholesterol)**

B. Renal causes

1. **Acute tubular necrosis**
   a. **Ischemia.** Secondary to shock from any cause including sepsis.
   b. **Toxins.** Medications (aminoglycosides, amphotericin B), contrast media, heavy metals.
   c. **Transfusion reaction**
   d. **Myoglobinuria.** Secondary to rhabdomyolysis. Often seen in alcoholics. Muscle tenderness, elevated creatine phophokinase, and pigmented casts point to myoglobinuria.
2. **Acute interstitial nephritis**
   a. **Drugs.** β-Lactamase–resistant penicillins such as methicillin, sulfonamides, and NSAIDs.
   b. **Hypercalcemia.** Can cause nephrocalcinosis.
   c. **Uric acid.** Gouty nephropathy or tumor lysis (chemotherapy for leukemia or lymphoma).
3. **Acute glomerular disease**
   a. **Malignant hypertension**
   b. **Emboli, thrombosis, disseminated intravascular coagulation**
   c. **Rapidly progressive glomerulonephritis**
   d. **Systemic diseases.** Wegener's granulomatosis, thrombotic thrombocytopenic purpura, systemic lupus erythematosus, scleroderma.
   e. **Goodpasture's syndrome**

C. Postrenal causes

1. **Urethral obstruction.** Prostatic hypertrophy, catheter obstruction. Prostatic carcinoma is an unusual cause of postrenal obstruction.
2. **Bilateral ureteral obstruction.** Most often as a result of carcinoma or retroperitoneal fibrosis. Common cause of death in women with cervical carcinoma.

IV Database

A. Physical examination key points

1. **Vital signs**
   a. A decrease in weight suggests volume depletion.

- **b.** Hypertension can result from volume overload associated with anuria.
- **c.** Fever points to an infection and possibly sepsis.
- **d.** Most importantly, assess the patient for orthostatic blood pressure and pulse changes (a decrease in systolic blood pressure of 10 mm Hg and/or an increase in heart rate by 20 BPM 1 minute after movement from the supine to the standing position). Although orthostatic hypotension without a change in heart rate can be found in elderly patients secondary to autonomic insufficiency, a significant drop in blood pressure associated with a rise in pulse suggests hypovolemia, particularly if it is associated with an imbalance in intake and output (I&O) or weight loss.
- **e.** An irregularly irregular pulse is consistent with atrial fibrillation, a common cause of emboli.

2. **Skin.** Decreased tissue turgor and dry mucous membranes occur with volume depletion.
3. **HEENT.** Flat neck veins with the patient supine suggest volume depletion. There may be an increase in jugular venous pressure secondary to volume overload from oliguria/anuria.
4. **Chest.** Rales suggest congestive heart failure possibly from volume overload.
5. **Abdomen.** Determine if there is ascites or a distended bladder. An enlarged bladder suggests bladder outlet obstruction such as from prostatic hypertrophy.
6. **Genitourinary system.** Examine males for an enlarged prostate. Remember, however, that bladder outlet obstruction can occur even when the gland feels normal in size. Rule out a pelvic mass in females.
7. **Extremities.** Assess perfusion by color and temperature of skin.

B. Laboratory data (See Table 2–6, p 301, for urinary indices useful in the evaluation of renal failure.)

1. **Urinalysis.** This is useful because it can be performed immediately in a housestaff laboratory.
   - **a.** Look specifically for high specific gravity suggesting volume depletion or recent dye administration.
   - **b.** Large amounts of protein or red blood cell casts suggest glomerular disease.
   - **c.** Significant hematuria points toward renal embolization or ureteral calculi and white blood cell casts suggest infection or severe inflammation. Eosinophils are seen with allergic interstitial nephritis and frequent granular casts are consistent with acute tubular necrosis.
2. **Serum chemistries.** Compare the BUN and creatinine. If their ratio is greater than 20:1, a prerenal cause is likely, although obstruction may also cause a high ratio, as can GI bleeding

and severe catabolic states. If the ratio is less than 15:1 and the BUN and creatinine are elevated, a renal cause is likely. Note the presence of hyponatremia or hypernatremia and hyperkalemia, any of which may complicate acute renal insufficiency.

3. **Urine electrolytes and creatinine.** A urinary sodium below 15 mmol/L suggests a prerenal cause; a urinary sodium above 20 mmol/L suggests renal causes. The fractional excretion of sodium (FE_{Na}) is calculated as [urinary sodium × serum creatinine/urine creatinine × serum sodium] × 100. A FE_{Na} less than 1 suggests volume depletion; a FE_{Na} greater than 1 suggests renal causes. Acute urinary tract obstruction and dye nephrotoxicity may also reduce the FE_{Na} to less than 1.

C. **Radiologic and other studies**

1. **Ultrasound.** An accurate means of examining the collecting system for signs of obstruction, particularly ureteral obstruction that cannot be relieved by simple insertion of a urinary catheter.
2. **Central venous pressure line or pulmonary artery catheter.** Will give a more accurate assessment of volume status.
3. **Intravenous pyelogram.** For practical purposes, ultrasound is as accurate for detecting obstruction and avoids the nephrotoxicity and volume-expanding properties of radiographic dye. Avoid if creatinine >2 mg/dL.
4. **Retrograde pyelogram (RPG).** If obstruction is suspected, a RPG can reveal the cause and specific location of the obstruction. In addition, the urologist can place ureteral stints at the time of the procedure to bypass the obstruction.
5. **Renal scan.** Technetium-labeled diethylenetriaminepentacetate (DTPA) nuclear medicine study can assess blood flow to the kidneys if renal artery embolization or thrombosis is suspected.
6. **Angiogram.** Provides better detail of renal anatomy but is rarely acutely needed.
7. **Renal biopsy.** Useful in determining specific causes of renal insufficiency, particularly allergic interstitial nephritis, although not needed acutely.

V. **Plan.** As a general rule, the minimal acceptable urine output is 0.5–1.0 mL/kg/h. Accurate records of intake and output are essential. Review the patient's medications and stop all nephrotoxic drugs. Doses of renally excreted drugs should be adjusted and potassium removed from all intravenous fluids.

A. **Foley catheter drainage.** Place a Foley catheter. If an immediate flow of urine is obtained, the diagnosis of urethral obstruction is very likely and a catheter can be placed at least temporarily. If no urine is obtained, there may still be bilateral ureteral obstruction (or obstruction of a congenital or surgical single ureter). If the patient is already catheterized, assess the patency of the current catheter, and, if in doubt, replace it. (See Foley Catheter Problems, p 104.) Make sure the Foley catheter is working by irrigating with 50 mL normal saline using a catheter tip syringe. The fluid should pass easily and the entire amount should be aspirated. If a catheter problem is noted, correct it or consult urology.

B. Management of prerenal causes

1. In almost every case, it is appropriate to give the patient a potassium-free volume challenge such as 500 mL of normal saline. In patients with fragile cardiorespiratory status, smaller boluses should be given and central venous catheters used to monitor volume status. Then adjust the baseline intravenous rate accordingly.
2. Monitor volume replacement. Give crystalloid to increase central venous pressure above 10 mm Hg or pulmonary capillary wedge pressure above 12–14 mm Hg. A hematocrit greater than 25% to 30% is adequate.
3. Follow hourly urine output. Give specific criteria so as to keep apprised of the patient's condition, for example, calling houseofficer for urine output less than 25 mL/h. A typical limit is 0.5 mL/kg/h.
4. Remove potassium and magnesium from intravenous solutions unless abnormally low.
5. Consider additional measures to increase urine output once volume status is corrected, although this is rarely useful unless the renal insult has been recent (within several hours). Methods of increasing urine output carry with them the risk of hypovolemia and ototoxicity as in the case of high doses of furosemide (Lasix).
   a. **Furosemide.** Use escalating doses in an attempt to obtain increased urine output. One method is to start with 80 mg IV, then increase to 160 mg IV and then 320 mg IV. Check urine output over 1–2 hours before proceeding to the higher dose.
   b. **Mannitol.** A dose of 12.5–25 g (50–100 mL of a 25% solution) IV may induce an osmotic diuresis.
6. Review medications. Adjust doses or stop nephrotoxic drugs.

C. Management of renal causes

1. Consider increasing the urine output as in Section V.B.5. It is easier to manage a patient with nonoliguric renal insufficiency than one with oliguric or anuric renal failure.
2. Emergent dialysis should be considered in the following circumstances: severe hypervolemia unresponsive to diuretics, intractable acidosis, severe hyperkalemia, pericarditis thought secondary to uremia, and severe uremic symptoms or encephalopathy.

D. Postrenal management. Usually requires urologic consultation. Most causes can be acutely managed with a Foley catheter, ureteral catheters, or percutaneous nephrostomy tubes.

PAIN MANAGEMENT

I. **Problem.** A 72-year-old man admitted to the oncology service for metastatic prostate cancer cannot sleep because of persistent back pain.

II. **Immediate Questions**

A. **Has the patient experienced this pain before?** The initial temptation is to assume that his pain is from metastatic disease; however, if the pain is of recent onset, the patient will require a full evaluation to ensure that a cause other than cancer is not responsible. For example, the pain may be from herpes zoster, pyelonephritis, renal colic, or an epidural abscess. Clearly, these causes of low back pain require different management than metastatic disease.

B. **Is the patient currently receiving pain medication, and if so, what is the drug, dosage, and dosing interval?** If the patient has previously been on narcotics, his pain may represent the development of tolerance and therefore an inadequate dosage of medication. Likewise, a frequent mistake of physicians is to use an inappropriately long interval for administration of narcotics. Determine the interval since the last administration of medication.

III. **Differential Diagnosis.** Clearly, it is not within the scope of this problem to provide a comprehensive differential diagnosis for all causes of pain. The following discussion pertains mainly to the management of pain in the terminally ill cancer patient. The management of chronic pain (pain that has been present for months to years) is not discussed here. Pain occurring in a patient with cancer may be caused by the malignancy itself, may occur as a complication of treatment, or may be the result of a psychologic disorder.

A. **Tumor causes of pain**

1. **Tumor invasion of bone and pathologic fracture**
2. **Infiltration/compression of nerves**
3. **Obstruction of a hollow viscus**
4. **Expansion of a viscus or its capsule.** Such as with liver metastases.
5. **Tissue ischemia after tumor invasion of lymphatics and blood vessels**
6. **Paraneoplastic syndromes.** Such as arthritis and neuropathy.

B. **Iatrogenic causes of cancer pain**

1. **Surgery.** Incision, phantom limb pain.
2. **Chemotherapy.** Can cause a variety of infectious, gastrointestinal and neurologic causes of pain.
3. **Radiation.** In the short term, radiation may cause inflammation (colitis, esophagitis). Over the long term, radiation can result in fibrosis.

C. Psychologic pain. Anxiety and depression are frequently associated with malignancy and can unfavorably affect the patient's perception of pain.

IV. Database

A. Physical examination key points

1. **Vital signs.** Tachycardia occurs with a variety of causes of acute pain and therefore is too nonspecific to suggest a specific etiology. Fever, however, points in the direction of infectious etiology.
2. **Skin.** Chemotherapy and hematologic malignancies can predispose to herpes zoster infections; therefore, ascertain if the pain is in the distribution of a specific dermatome. Look for vesicular lesions that would also suggest shingles. Pain may precede the development of the typical vesicular rash by 2 days.
3. **HEENT.** In a patient with cancer complaining of a headache, be sure to examine for papilledema, which would suggest increased intracranial pressure from cerebral metastases.
4. **Neck.** A stiff neck could indicate bacterial meningitis or carcinomatous meningitis causing back or neck pain.
5. **Chest.** In addition to auscultating the lungs for evidence of pneumonia, palpate the ribs and sternum for evidence of bony pain suggesting metastases.
5. **Abdomen.** In a patient with abdominal pain, examine for hepatomegaly, which could indicate liver metastases. Bowel obstruction could result from the underlying malignant process itself or could occur as a result of decreased bowel motility from the administration of narcotics.
6. **Extremities.** Examine for evidence of bony pain or arthropathy, which may occur with underlying malignancy.
7. **Neurologic exam.** In a patient complaining of headaches, perform a careful neurologic exam looking for localizing findings that could indicate the presence of a cerebral metastasis. Stocking-glove distribution of pain may result from a peripheral neuropathy caused by underlying cancer or chemotherapeutic agents such as vincristine.

B. Laboratory data

1. **Complete blood count.** Obtain if infection is suspected.
2. **Alkaline phosphatase and serum calcium.** Order if bony metastases are suspected. Remember to correct the total calcium in the face of hypoalbuminemia or check an ionized calcium. (See Hypocalcemia, Section II, p 153.)
3. **Alkaline phosphatase, transaminases (AST [SGOT] and ALT [SGPT]), and γ-glutamyl transpeptidase (GGT).** Obtain liver function tests on patients with suspected hepatic metastases.

C. **Radiologic and other studies.** Specific radiographs will be directed by the findings on history and physical examination. Remember that bone scintigraphy is more sensitive for bony metastases than plain films. Bone scintigraphy may be falsely negative if there is bone destruction without accompanying osteoblastic response such as in multiple myeloma.

V. **Plan.** A fear of uncontrolled pain is one of the greatest concerns of a patient with malignancy. Attempts by the physician to allay the patient's anxiety regarding the pain and assurance that everything will be done to alleviate that pain may help significantly in achieving the goal of pain control. A frequent mistake made by physicians is reluctance to administer narcotics for fear of subsequent addiction. This is an unfounded fear in patients with acute pain, especially those patients with pain related to malignancy, as the great majority of these patients will not develop addiction or psychologic dependence. Physical dependence and tolerance may occur in patients who are administered narcotics for long periods. After the initial history and physical examination and once a potentially reversible cause of pain has been excluded, the management of presumed cancer pain can proceed as follows.

A. **Mild pain.** Nonnarcotic analgesics may be tried initially.
   1. **Aspirin 650 mg by mouth (PO) every 4 hours**
   2. **Acetaminophen (Tylenol) 650 mg PO every 4 hours**
   3. **Nonsteroidal anti-inflammatory drugs such as ibuprofen (Motrin) 400–600 mg PO every 4–6 hours.** Use cautiously in patients with underlying renal insufficiency.

B. **Moderate pain.** For patients whose pain persists despite the preceding measures, a weak narcotic-analgesic may be administered. Usually, these are administered in combination with either acetaminophen or aspirin as the analgesic effect is greatly heightened by adding these agents.
   1. **Tylenol with codeine No. 3 (acetaminophen 300 mg with codeine phosphate 30 mg) PO every 4 hours**
   2. **Percodan (aspirin 325 mg with oxycodone 5 mg) PO every 4 hours**
   3. **Percocet (acetaminophen 325 mg with oxycodone 5 mg) PO every 4 hours**

C. **Severe pain.** Although a variety of drugs may be used for more severe pain, morphine sulfate still remains the gold standard for management. It is important to emphasize that narcotics should be administered on an around-the-clock basis rather than on an as-needed basis. This provides a more sustained effect, reduces the overall narcotic requirement, and lessens overall patient suffering, as the goal is to circumvent the development of pain rather than to allow the patient to develop pain first and then request narcotics.

1. **Morphine sulfate initially 20 mg PO every 4 hours.** After initial titration with the immediate-release form of morphine, one of the newer longer-acting preparations such as MS Contin may be administered on an every-8-hour schedule. This preparation comes in 30- and 60-mg tablets. For patients unable to take morphine orally, morphine sulfate 8–12 mg SC every 4 hours can be used.
2. **Demerol.** Its use is to be strongly discouraged in the management of acute pain because of its short half-life requiring every-3-hour dosing and also because of the accumulation of toxic metabolites that can cause central nervous system agitation and confusion.

D. Adjunctive measures. Eighty-five to ninety percent of cancer patients obtain relief with one of the preceding regimens. For those whose pain persists, a variety of measures can be used.

1. **Epidural anesthesia**
2. **Nerve blocks or self-controlled infusions of morphine through an intravenous pump.** Other drugs may be used for relief of pain in cancer patients depending on clinical circumstances.
3. **Corticosteroids.** May be effective for intracranial metastases or neurologic compression syndromes.
4. **Prochlorperazine (Compazine) 5 mg PO every 4 hours.** Frequently necessary for nausea that is sometimes induced by narcotic analgesics.
5. **Antidepressants.** Amitriptyline (Elavil) may have some analgesic effect. Antidepressants are often ineffective, however, in treating the depression associated with malignancy.

REFERENCE

Driscoll CE. Pain management. *Primary Care* 1987;14(2):337–353.

■ PHLEBITIS

I. Problem. A 60-year-old man is being treated for pneumonia. An intravenous catheter in the arm has not been changed for 5 days and the site is now red and painful.

II. Immediate Questions

A. What are the vital signs? Fever can develop from both superficial thrombophlebitis and deep venous thrombosis.

B. Can pus be expressed from the site? Pus indicates a local infection. Sepsis and pus may indicate suppurative thrombophlebitis.

C. What medications are being administered into the intravenous line? Many antibiotics, chemotherapeutic agents, potassium, and calcium can cause irritation, especially with extravasation.

III. Differential Diagnosis. Acute venous inflammation or occlusion can occur in superficial or deep veins. Deep venous thrombosis is usually not infected. In this problem inflammation and infection of superficial veins are discussed.

- **A. Superficial thrombophlebitis.** Acute inflammation without infection is the most common presentation.
  1. The site of an intravenous catheter, especially in an upper extremity, is often involved.
  2. Extravasation of irritant medications, such as chemotherapeutic agents, may cause superficial thrombophlebitis.
  3. The etiology may be unknown, especially in the lower extremities.
- **B. Superficial suppurative thrombophlebitis.** Persistent fever, sepsis, expressible pus, and positive blood cultures indicate significant infection of the affected vein. Septic pulmonary embolization with pneumonia and abscess formation are rare complications.
- **C. Other causes**
  1. **Deep venous thrombosis**
  2. **Septic thrombophlebitis of subclavian vein**
  3. **Migratory thrombophlebitis.** May be the first sign of an occult malignancy.

IV. Database

- **A. Physical examination key points**
  1. **Vital signs.** Fever may indicate sepsis or thrombosis.
  2. **Lungs.** Examine for crackles or consolidation of a pneumonia resulting from septic embolization.
  3. **Heart.** Listen for regurgitant murmurs that could predispose to acute bacterial endocarditis in patients with bacteremia.
  4. **Extremities.** Examine intravenous sites for erythema, warmth, or tenderness in all febrile patients. Attempt to express pus if the site is erythematous. Palpate the calves for tenderness.
- **B. Laboratory data**
  1. Leukocytosis is present in suppurative superficial thrombophlebitis.
  2. Order culture and sensitivity and gram stain of purulence to identify specific bacterial agent.
  3. Remove catheter and culture the tip.
- **C. Radiologic and other studies**
  1. **Chest x-ray.** To exclude septic pulmonary embolization.
  2. **Venography.** Usually not indicated. If central vein infection or deep thrombosis is suspected in a septic patient, then venography may be necessary.
  3. **Echocardiogram.** To exclude presence of valvular vegetations if blood cultures are positive.

V. Plan. Thrombophlebitis can be prevented by rotation of intravenous sites every 48 hours. Any intravenous site that appears infected must be changed.

- **A. Superficial thrombophlebitis**
  1. **Dry or moist local heat**
  2. **Limb elevation**
  3. **Nonsteroidal anti-inflammatory agents.** For example, ibuprofen (Motrin) 600 mg PO every 6 hours or 800 mg PO every 8 hours.
- **B. Suppurative thrombophlebitis**
  1. **Intravenous antibiotics.** Must have good antistaphylococcal coverage as well as gram-negative bacteria including **Pseudomonas.** Nafcillin and gentamicin provide adequate initial coverage pending cultures.
  2. **Local wound care.** Such as wet-to-dry dressings.
  3. **Analgesics or nonsteroidal anti-inflammatory agents**
  4. **Exploratory venotomy or venectomy of involved vein.**
- **C. Other measures.** Suppurative thrombophlebitis of the subclavian vein requires resection and intravenous antibiotics as above.

REFERENCE

Scheld WM, Sande MA. Endocarditis and intravascular infections. In: Mandell GL, Douglas RG, Bennett JE, eds. *Principles and Practices of Infectious Diseases.* 3rd ed. New York: Churchill Livingstone; 1990:670–706.

■ POLYCYTHEMIA

I. Problem. A 65-year-old male is admitted to your service with a hematocrit of 62%.

II. Immediate Question. Are there any medical conditions that require the prompt institution of therapy directed at the elevated hematocrit? Usually the finding of an elevated hematocrit is an incidental finding or is discovered during the evaluation of a nonacute problem. It should be determined that there is no evidence of decompensated congestive heart failure (CHF) and cardiac or cerebral ischemia that might benefit acutely from phlebotomy. Evidence of profound intravascular volume depletion requiring fluid replacement should be noted.

III. Differential Diagnosis. When confronted with an elevated hematocrit (>50% for men, >45% for women), the differential diagnosis is relatively simple if polycythemia is divided into three broad diagnostic categories.

- **A. Relative polycythemia.** Generally asymptomatic, although patients can present with venous thrombosis, which can occur in any individual who becomes severely volume depleted for whatever reason, such as profuse diarrhea or vomiting.

B. Polycythemia vera. Onset is usually insidious, often found on routine blood counts for other reasons. Can present with major venous thrombosis or hemorrhage. Symptoms may include headache, dizziness, vertigo, tinnitus, diplopia, blurred vision, claudication, angina, symptoms of peptic ulcer disease, pruritus, mucosal bleeding, epistaxis, ecchymoses, symptoms of deep venous thrombosis, pulmonary embolism, or symptoms of cerebral vascular thrombosis. Usually a disease of middle and later years of life with a peak incidence in fifties and sixties. Slight male predominance.

1. Diagnosis is by three major criteria or the first two major criteria and two minor criteria.
   a. **Major criteria**
      (1) **Elevated red blood cell mass ($\geq$ 36 μL/kg in a male; $\geq$ 32 μL/kg in a female)**
      (2) **Arterial oxygen saturation greater than 92%**
      (3) **Splenomegaly**
   b. **Minor criteria**
      (1) **Platelet count greater than 400,000/μL**
      (2) **Elevated leukocyte alkaline phosphatase (LAP) score**
      (3) **Elevated vitamin B_{12}**
      (4) **Leukocytosis greater than 12,000/μL**

C. Secondary polycythemia. Numerous causes. Can be looked at from the standpoint of whether polycythemia is physiologically appropriate (response to tissue hypoxia) or physiologically inappropriate (inappropriate stimulation or secretion of erythropoietin).

1. **Physiologically appropriate polycythemia**
   a. **High-altitude acclimatization**
   b. **Chronic obstructive pulmonary disease (COPD).** Caused by a pO_2 below 90% saturation. May occur as a result of desaturation at night or with exercise.
   c. **Cardiovascular disease (right-to-left shunts).** Most commonly as a result of congenital heart disease.
   d. **Alveolar hypoventilation.** Sleep apnea.
   e. **High-oxygen-affinity hemoglobins.** May have a positive family history.
   f. **Congenital deficiency of 2,3-diphosphoglyceric acid**
   g. **Carboxyhemoglobinemia**
2. **Physiologically inappropriate polycythemia**
   a. **Renal vascular disease**
   b. **Hepatic tumors**
   c. **Uterine leiomyomas**
   d. **Cerebellar hemangioblastomas**

e. **Renal transplantation**
f. **Renal cell carcinoma**
g. **Ovarian carcinoma**
h. **Renal cysts.** Flank pain or hematuria may be present.
i. **Pheochromocytoma**

IV. Database

A. Physical examination key points

1. **Vital signs.** Hypertension is indicative of possible renal vascular disease or pheochromocytoma. Respiratory rate helps to assess presence of cardiac or pulmonary disease. Temperature/fever may indicate underlying systemic illness that may have caused volume depletion or underlying malignancy.
2. **General appearance.** Plethora is not helpful in the distinction of polycythemia vera from secondary polycythemia. Clubbing should be noted as a sign of underlying pulmonary or cardiac disease. Cyanosis is usually an indicator of hypoxemia and might be more suggestive of a secondary polycythemia.
3. **HEENT.** Look for conjunctival injection and, on fundoscopic exam, hemorrhages and engorged vessels. Congested mucous membranes are often present and are nonspecific. All would be more in favor of a true polycythemia.
4. **Heart.** Presence of any murmurs or S_3 might either suggest a cardiac etiology or be a sign of cardiac dysfunction caused by polycythemia.
5. **Lungs.** Rales, barrel chest, or diminished breath sounds suggest COPD.
6. **Abdomen.** Hepatomegaly and abdominal masses suggest a secondary cause, whereas splenomegaly is expected with polycythemia vera.
7. **Extremities.** Clubbing, cyanosis, and edema point to secondary physiologically appropriate causes. Evidence of deep vein thrombosis may be a complication of polycythemia.
8. **Neurologic exam.** Look for evidence of focal findings consistent with cerebrovascular accident or tumor. Global findings consistent with hypoxic encephalopathy suggest a secondary cause of polycythemia.

B. Laboratory data.

If there are obvious clues from the history and/or physical exam, an extensive lab evaluation may not be indicated. For example, a patient with a history of vomiting and diarrhea, poor oral intake, and marked orthostasis and tachycardia with a hematocrit of 55% would be appropriately treated with fluid resuscitation and evaluation of the etiology of the volume loss. Unfortunately in most cases, the diagnosis is not obvious and evaluation is indicated.

1. **Hematocrit.** Generally, a hematocrit above 60% predicts a true increase in the red cell mass; hematocrits below 60% can

be the result of either true or relative increases in the red cell mass.

2. **Platelet count.** A count greater than 400,000/μL suggests polycythemia vera.
3. **White count.** Leukocytosis greater than 12,000/μL suggests polycythemia vera.
4. **Arterial blood gases.** Oxygen saturation less than 90% points to a physiologically appropriate secondary cause.
5. **LAP score.** An elevated LAP score is consistent with polycythemia vera.
6. **Vitamin B_{12}.** Elevated B_{12} or unbound B_{12} binding capacity is seen with polycythemia vera.
7. **p50** (oxygen affinity of hemoglobin). To look for abnormal hemoglobins with high oxygen affinity.
8. **Carboxyhemoglobin level.** Presence of an elevated carboxyhemoglobin level points to a physiologically appropriate secondary cause.
9. **Erythropoietin level.** Elevated with physiologically inappropriate causes such as hepatoma and with physiologically appropriate causes.

C. Radiologic and other studies

1. **Red cell mass.** A nuclear medicine study to distinguish between relative and true polycythemia. A normal red cell mass with a diminished or low normal plasma volume is characteristic of relative polycythemia. If this is found, no further evaluation of the elevated hematocrit is needed. An elevated red cell mass with a normal or increased plasma volume is found in true polycythemia. If this is the case, then further evaluation is indicated to determine if this represents a primary (polycythemia vera) or secondary polycythemia.
2. **Abdominal CT scan.** To look for evidence of benign or malignant neoplasms of the liver, kidney, adrenals, and endometrium.
3. **CT scan or MRI scan of the brain.** To rule out cerebellar tumor.
4. **Echocardiogram.** Look for right-to-left shunts. May also show left ventricular dysfunction, a possible complication of polycythemia.
5. **Pulmonary function studies.** May reveal severe obstructive lung disease.

V. Plan. Treatment depends on the type of polycythemia.

A. Relative polycythemia. Requires no therapeutic intervention directed at specifically reducing the hematocrit, although the underlying disorder needs to be addressed (volume depletion or the stressed, obese, hypertensive, chain-smoking male executive). Isovolemic phlebotomy can be used but has not been shown to impact on the morbidity or mortality.

B. True polycythemia of secondary cause

1. In physiologically appropriate secondary polycythemia, it may be difficult to determine if symptoms are due to the underlying disease or the elevated hematocrit. One must realize that the elevated hematocrit is a physiologically important compensatory mechanism and must prove that the erythrocytosis is detrimental prior to phlebotomy. In physiologically inappropriate polycythemia, therapy should be directed at the underlying cause.
2. In physiologically appropriate polycythemia, therapeutic phlebotomy is performed if the patient is clearly symptomatic from the elevated hematocrit. If phlebotomy is indicated, the goal should be to maintain the hematocrit between 50% and 60%. In patients with physiologically inappropriate polycythemia, phlebotomy is reasonable and can be done safely. The goal should be to maintain a hematocrit of 45%, especially if surgery is contemplated.
3. Cytotoxic therapy is contraindicated in any type of secondary polycythemia.

C. Polycythemia vera. Therapy is directed at overproduction of red cells and the frequently accompanying platelet disorder.

1. **Phlebotomy.** Quite effective in lowering the hematocrit and essentially free of complications as long as the patient is monitored for signs of hypovolemia during the phlebotomy and treated appropriately with crystalloid infusion should hypotension occur or be replaced prophylactically if there is risk that a brief period of hypotension would be dangerous in a given patient. An expected long-term complication with frequent phlebotomy is iron deficiency. It has been debated whether or not iron repletion should be undertaken in this setting as this will increase the phlebotomy requirements. At least two reasons are commonly cited for iron replacement therapy.
   - **a.** As red cells become progressively more microcytic, there is actually an increase in the whole blood viscosity, which is the reason for doing phlebotomy therapeutically.
   - **b.** As there is a need for iron in many enzyme systems as a cofactor, the effects of iron depletion at this level are uncertain.
2. **Cytotoxic therapy.** In patients with a history of thrombotic and/or bleeding problems, phlebotomy may be inadequate therapy. These patients benefit from therapy with chemotherapeutic agents or radioactive phosphorus injections.
   - **a.** Hydroxyurea has been shown to be effective, appearing to have minimal, if any, risk of induction of leukemia.
   - **b.** Alkylating agents have been associated with an increased risk of secondary leukemias, especially in younger patients.

c. ^{32}P is also associated with an increased risk of secondary leukemias.

3. **Antiplatelet agents.** Cannot be recommended as they were not found to be effective in prevention of thrombosis by the Polycythemia Vera Study Group. Actually, these agents have been found to be associated with a significant risk of gastrointestinal bleeding, especially with platelet counts above 1,000,000/μL.
4. The most recent recommendations for therapy in polycythemia by the Polycythemia Vera Study Group are as follows:
   - **a.** Because of the increased risk of thrombosis associated with increasing age, patients older than 70 years are most effectively treated with radioactive phosphorus and phlebotomy.
   - **b.** Patients younger than 50 years should be treated with phlebotomy alone unless there are risk factors for thrombosis or a history of prior thrombotic event, in which case hydroxyurea would appear to be a safe alternative to radioactive phosphorus and alkylating agents.
   - **c.** In patients 50–70 years of age, the role of myelosuppressive agents is unclear. But management as in the younger than 50 age group seems appropriate.
   - **d.** Patients with other symptoms such as pruritus, bone pain, and troublesome splenomegaly are best managed by a myelosuppressive agent.

REFERENCES

Berk PD, et al. Therapeutic recommendations in polycythemia vera based on Polycythemia Vera Study Group Protocol. *Semin Hematol* 1986;23:132–143.

Erslev AJ. Relative polycythemia. In: Williams WJ, Beutler E, Erslev AJ, et al, eds. *Hematol.* 4th ed. New York: McGraw-Hill; 1990:715–717.

Erslev AJ. Secondary polycythemia. In: Williams WJ, Beutler E, Erslev AJ, et al, eds. *Hematol.* 4th ed. New York: McGraw-Hill; 1990:705–715.

Murphy S. Polycythemia vera. In: Williams WJ, Beutler E, Erslev AJ, et al, eds. *Hematol.* 4th ed. New York: McGraw-Hill; 1990:193–202.

■ PULMONARY ARTERY CATHETER PROBLEMS

(See also Central Venous Line Problems, p 47.)

I. **Problem.** A 50-year-old man is admitted to the coronary care unit (CCU) with an anterior myocardial infarction. A pulmonary artery catheter is placed and, 24 hours later, you are notified by the CCU nurse that she is having trouble interpreting the tracing.

II. **Immediate Questions**

A. **What does the waveform look like?** The pulmonary artery waveform varies with inspiration and expiration and has a characteristic systolic/diastolic waveform. (See Figure 3–11, p 339, and Chapter 3, Pulmonary Artery Catheterization, p 336.)

B. **Is there a waveform when the catheter is tapped?** The absence of a waveform or a "dampened" tracing suggests the catheter is not patent or there are technical difficulties including transducer malfunction, cracked hub, loose connections, incorrect stopcock positions, too-tight skin sutures, and too-tight plastic sleeve diaphragms.

C. **Can the catheter be flushed and can blood be withdrawn?** If the catheter cannot be flushed or blood withdrawn, the catheter may not be patent. The catheter could be kinked, or there could be a venous thrombosis. (See Central Venous Line Problems, p 48.)

D. **Is the catheter in permanent wedge?** After a period of time within the circulation, pulmonary artery catheters tend to become softer and more pliable and may migrate distally. With a decreasing pulmonary pressure, the same effect may occur as the pulmonary vascular bed shrinks relative to the catheter position. The catheter may end up wedged with the balloon deflated, a situation analogous to pulmonary embolus. Catheter position must be corrected as soon as possible. Careful evaluation is needed to ensure that the problem is really from permanent wedge and not a kink or system malfunction. If all else fails to help distinguish the various causes of a flat tracing, wedge position can be confirmed with blood gas sampling, showing saturation in the arterial range as opposed to the mixed venous range usually found when blood gases are sampled from the pulmonary artery position.

E. **Can a wedge tracing be obtained with the balloon inflated?** If not, the balloon may have ruptured or the catheter may have been partially removed.

F. **Are there any associated symptoms?** Chest pain could result from a pulmonary artery catheter in permanent wedge resulting in a pulmonary infarction. Hemoptysis can result from pulmonary infarction or from pulmonary artery rupture or erosion. This is usually associated with inflation of the balloon in a vessel smaller than the balloon, rupturing the pulmonary artery with entry of blood into the airways. Hemoptysis usually results and can sometimes be severe, but rarely life-threatening. A fever may be secondary to catheter infection or sepsis or pulmonary infarction.

G. **What is the relative necessity of the pulmonary artery catheter?** If critical measurements are being made such as hourly pulmonary artery wedge pressure, the situation is more serious than if the line has outlived its usefulness and can be removed.

III. **Differential Diagnosis.** Problems with pulmonary artery catheters (Swan-Ganz) can conveniently be divided into problems occurring inside the patient and outside the patient.

A. Outside the patient

1. **Transducer error.** Often results in a "dampened" or flattened tracing. This is probably the most common source of problems, particularly with aging, nondisposable transducers. Bubbles within the transducer and any improper mounting will result in a poor-quality pressure tracing.
2. **Cables.** As with most electrical systems, particularly nondisposable systems, cables are a common source of problems.
3. **Monitor-related problems.** Perhaps the most common monitor-related problems arise when the monitor is set on an improper scale or is not properly balanced.

B. Inside the patient

1. **Catheter migration.** The catheter may have moved from its original insertion position, either migrating distally or proximally. Migration distally can result in a permanent wedge.
2. **Thrombosis.** A blood clot in the pressure-monitoring lumen may preclude good-quality pressure recordings.
3. **Kinks.** The most common sites are at the skin, under the clavicle, and at the proximal and distal ends of the sheath. Results in a poor-quality tracing.
4. **Malfunctioning balloon.** If the catheter will not wedge, the balloon may have ruptured or the catheter may have migrated proximally. Do not continue to inject air into the catheter system if a wedge tracing does not appear, as a ruptured balloon may be the cause.

IV. Database

A. Physical examination key points

1. **General exam.** As in most technical areas of medicine, it is important to be sure that the information provided by your technology is in broad general agreement with your clinical assessment.
2. **Vital signs.** The presence of a fever suggests catheter infection or sepsis, especially if the catheter has been in place more than 3 days.

B. Laboratory data

1. **Blood gases.** Helpful in determining whether a pulmonary artery catheter is in permanent wedge position. If the catheter is wedged, the oxygen saturation will approximate arterial oxygen saturation, whereas mixed venous saturation is found in pulmonary artery locations.
2. **Blood cultures.** Should be obtained in the presence of a fever or elevated white count with an increase in segmented and banded neutrophils.

C. Radiologic and other studies

1. **Chest x-ray.** Useful in determining whether the catheter is kinked or in the correct position. Permanent wedge may be

suggested by a markedly distal location of the catheter tip. After injection with air, a deflated balloon also points to balloon rupture.

2. **Culture of catheter tip.** If catheter-related sepsis or infection is suspected, the catheter **must be removed** and the catheter tip sent for culture.

V. Plan. For replacement of a pulmonary artery catheter, see Chapter 3, Pulmonary Artery Catheterization, p 336.

A. Problems outside the patient. If simply tapping the catheter does not result in a waveform, the fault clearly resides outside the patient. Transducer, cable, and monitor-related problems should be addressed first.

B. Problems inside the patient. When a good waveform is obtained by tapping the catheter, the problem most likely resides within the patient.

1. **Permanent wedge.** This problem is reported much more often than it exists. Often, a well-placed pulmonary artery catheter is pulled back when the position is fine.
   - **a.** The system must be thoroughly checked out before any catheter movement is attempted. The transducer should be evaluated for proper functioning. The system should be evaluated for leaks, loose connections, and so on, prior to any manipulation of the catheter.
   - **b.** A chest x-ray should be obtained for positioning. If the catheter is truly stuck in wedge, the chest x-ray will show the catheter to be distal in the pulmonary circulation.
   - **c.** As mentioned earlier, the oxygen saturation will be arterial when obtained from a truly wedged catheter.
   - **d.** If it is really wedged and the waveform cannot be returned to the expected waveform by manual aspiration or flushing of the catheter, the catheter should be withdrawn centimeter by centimeter while flushing between each withdrawal using a pressure-bag flush system. When an appropriate waveform returns, the balloon should be reinflated to be sure the catheter will wedge when desired. The balloon should be inflated about 1 cm^3 to obtain the wedge tracing.
   - **e.** Less commonly, the balloon will not deflate because the catheter is kinked. A chest x-ray is the best tool to assess this.
2. **A balloon that will not wedge.** Most often, the catheter has been pulled back or the balloon is not functioning. The catheter should not be advanced unless a sterile sleeve protects the catheter lying outside the patient. If the balloon is malfunctioning, the catheter should be removed.
3. **A flattened tracing.** Can be the result of a kinked catheter. A chest x-ray is used to rule out kinking of the catheter.
4. **Inaccurate or poorly reproducible cardiac outputs.**

   a. In cases of apparently inappropriate cardiac outputs, be sure that the constant on the cardiac output computer is correct for the catheter being utilized. The thermodilution technique is not accurate in patients with very low cardiac outputs or significant tricuspid regurgitation. Use the mixed venous oxygen and the Fick oxygen method to confirm a low cardiac output.
   b. If no cardiac output is obtained, the catheter may not be properly connected to the computer or the wire connecting the thermistor to the computer may be fractured. Most computers will give a code indicating that the catheter is at fault in this circumstance.

5. **Pulmonary artery rupture or erosion.** Treatment is dependent on the severity of the bleeding. It is prudent to remove the pulmonary artery catheter and, if it is crucial for managing the patient, it can be replaced. The new catheter should be directed toward the opposite lung. This requires fluoroscopy. Careful attention to the adequacy of ventilation and blood pressure, serial chest x-rays, and a low threshold for requesting cardiothoracic surgery consultation are all advisable in this situation. This complication can be avoided by always carefully inflating the balloon slowly and alertly watching the pressure waveform so that the catheter is not overwedged. For replacement of central venous catheters, see Chapter 3, Central Venous Catheterization, p 314.

REFERENCE

Grossman W, Barry WH. Cardiac catheterization. In: Braunwald E, ed. *Heart Disease: A Textbook of Cardiovascular Medicine.* 3rd ed. Philadelphia: WB Saunders; 1988:242–267.

■ SEIZURES

I. **Problem.** A 25-year-old woman is found seizing 1 day after admission for pyelonephritis.

II. **Immediate Questions**
   A. **Has the patient ever had seizures before?** A patient with a history of prior seizures is often on an anticonvulsant. In these patients, a common cause of seizures is the failure to take the prescribed medication.
   B. **Is the patient on any anticonvulsant medications?** Find out what medications the patient is taking. Is the patient receiving all the medications she was on prior to admission? If the patient is on nothing by mouth (NPO), be sure that an appropriate parenteral form is given. Check for other medications, as some of these can

affect the blood levels of anticonvulsants, particularly diphenylhydantoin (Dilantin).

C. **Does the patient have a history of alcohol abuse?** Alcoholic withdrawal seizures commonly occur 6–48 hours after cessation of drinking.

D. **Does the patient have a history of diabetes?** Hypoglycemia induced by hypoglycemics can cause seizures.

E. **Was the seizure generalized or focal in nature?** Seizures that begin focally suggest a central nervous system etiology.

F. **Are there any electrolyte abnormalities that could be causing the seizure?** Recent labs may reveal the cause of the seizure. Hyponatremia, hypernatremia, hypocalcemia, and hypomagnesemia can cause seizures.

III. **Differential Diagnosis.** Seizures result from abnormal electrical activity in the cerebral cortex. Seizures may result in abnormal motor activity or abnormal behavior or change in consciousness. Tonic-clonic seizures result in unconsciousness and stiffening of muscles followed by clonic jerking. There may be urinary incontinence and there is often postictal confusion, myalgia, lethargy, and headache.

A. **Idiopathic epilepsy.** The most common etiology of seizures but must be a diagnosis of exclusion in the acute situation.

B. **Tumors.** Either primary brain tumors or metastatic lesions. Frequent lesions metastatic to the brain include carcinoma of the breast, lung, or kidney, melanoma, or lymphoma.

C. **Infection.** In adults, intracranial infections such as meningitis, brain abscess, or encephalitis can cause seizures; in children, any infectious process with systemic reaction (fever) can cause seizures (febrile seizures). Rabies, Rocky Mountain spotted fever, Lyme disease, and a mycotic aneurysm from endocarditis can also cause seizures.

D. **Trauma.** A careful history must be obtained. Are there signs of skull fracture or other trauma?

E. **Alcohol/drug withdrawal.** Common after hospitalization, resulting in cessation of alcohol or other drugs such as barbiturates or benzodiazepines.

F. **Chronic renal failure.** With uremia.

G. **Anoxia.** Generalized hypoxemia or focal anoxia secondary to embolism or thrombosis.

H. **Electrolyte abnormalities.** Hypoglycemia, hyponatremia, hypocalcemia, hypomagnesemia, hypernatremia, and hyperosmolar states.

I. **Collagen-vascular disease.** Systemic lupus erythematosus (SLE), vasculitis (polyarteritis), sarcoidosis.

J. **Drugs.** Cocaine use and amphetamine intoxication.

K. **Porphyria.** Acute intermittent porphyria.

L. **Degenerative disease.** Tay-Sachs disease.

M. **Vascular lesions.** Infarction (thrombotic or embolic), hypertensive encephalopathy, carotid sinus disease, subarachnoid hemorrhage.

N. **Syncope.** Often what is thought to be a seizure is just a syncopal attack. Obtain a careful description from both nurses and the patient about the event. (See Syncope, p 236.)

O. **Psychogenic seizures.** May be difficult to distinguish from true tonic-clonic seizures. Often the patient remains conscious, there is no postictal confusion, and there is a psychiatric history.

P. **Toxemia of pregnancy.** Occurs in the third trimester of pregnancy. Hypertension, renal dysfunction (decreased glomerular filtration rate or proteinuria), thrombocytopenia, and coagulopathy may be present.

Q. **Hyperventilation.** Rapid, shallow breathing, paresthesia, and tremulousness.

R. **Inadequate level of prescribed anticonvulsants.** Especially phenytoin (Dilantin), where the level can be altered by many other medications such as aspirin.

IV. Database

A. Physical exam key points

1. **Vital signs.** Fever suggests an infection. Check blood pressure or palpate pulse to ensure adequate perfusion.
2. **HEENT.** Nuchal rigidity suggests meningitis or subarachnoid hemorrhage. The tongue may be lacerated from the seizure. Look for evidence of head trauma.
3. **Neurologic exam.** Perform a complete neurologic exam including all cranial nerves, full sensory and motor function, deep tendon reflexes and Babinski, and mental status. There may be transient deficits after the seizure (the postictal state). Focal findings may suggest a cerebrovascular accident or tumor. Evaluate for loss of bladder or bowel control associated with a tonic-clonic or grand mal seizure.
4. **Skin.** Rash may suggest a vasculitis.

B. Laboratory data

1. **Serum electrolytes.** Especially sodium, calcium, magnesium, and creatinine.
2. **Serum glucose.** To rule out hypoglycemia as the etiology cause.
3. **Arterial blood gases.** To rule out hypoxemia as the cause. A gap metabolic acidosis secondary to lactic acid is often encountered after a tonic-clonic seizure.
4. **Drug levels of anticonvulsants being taken.** Do this immediately as a patient seizing with adequate drug levels will need to have new therapy instituted. (See Table 7–11, p 498.)
5. **Drug screen.** Consider to rule out barbiturates or cocaine as the cause.
6. **Complete blood count with differential.** To rule out infectious causes. Also, a low white blood cell count and anemia may point to a systemic illness such as SLE.

7. **Collagen-vascular workup.** Antinuclear antibodies, sedimentation rate and complement studies if SLE or vasculitis is suspected.
8. **Cerebrospinal fluid analysis.** If indicated. (See Chapter 3, Lumbar Puncture, p 330.)

C. Radiologic and other studies

1. **Head CT scan.** If this episode represents new-onset seizures and there is no obvious etiology, then a CT scan of the head is indicated but need not be done emergently unless other evidence suggests a space-occupying lesion that may require emergent treatment or if the seizures recur without an obvious etiology.
2. **Lumbar puncture.** May help if there is evidence of meningeal irritation. If meningitis is suspected, the lumbar puncture should be done immediately. A CT scan should precede the lumbar puncture if there is papilledema or focal findings on neurologic exam suggesting increased intracranial pressure.

V. Plan. Support life functions (the ABCs of cardiopulmonary resuscitation) and prevent self-inflicted injury during the seizure. Follow with a careful workup to determine the cause and institute appropriate therapy.

A. Emergency management

1. Do not interfere if the patient is spontaneously breathing. Specifically, do **not** try to force something into the patient's mouth like a tongue depressor. This can lead to injury to the patient or yourself and is totally unnecessary.
2. Position the patient in the left lateral decubitus position with a suction device readily available to prevent aspiration.
3. Most seizures will stop within 3 minutes.

B. Seizure control. (See Chapter 7 for a discussion of drugs listed here.)

1. A single seizure will usually finish prior to the onset of action of any intravenous medication and therefore need not be specifically treated.
2. Establish intravenous access as soon as possible.
3. Empirically administer thiamine 100 mg IV and 1 ampoule (50 mL) D50 IV.
4. To treat a second seizure, or status epilepticus (repeated seizures with no regaining of consciousness between seizures), diazepam (Valium) IV may be given, usually as 5 mg IV slow push repeated at 10- to 15-minute intervals as needed, or lorazepam (Ativan) 2.5–10 mg IV slow push repeating at 15- to 20-minute intervals as needed to control seizure activity. Lorazepam is replacing diazepam as the treatment of choice in status epilepticus because of its long half-life.
5. Phenytoin (Dilantin) may be used if diazepam or lorazepam fails, or to prevent recurrence of seizures if diazepam or lorazepam has provided temporary control. It must be given

slowly, no faster than 50 mg/min, directly into the vein. Check levels daily after first starting the drug.

6. Phenobarbital may also be used. It is given slowly IV usually with a 120- to 140-mg loading dose. Maintenance doses are given IV, IM, or PO to maintain therapeutic levels.
7. Be alert for the complications of aspiration, hyperthermia, and cardiovascular collapse.
8. Long-term anticonvulsant therapy is not indicated for alcohol withdrawal seizures; chlordiazepoxide or oxazepam may be useful to control other symptoms of alcohol withdrawal.
9. Refractory seizures that do not respond to the preceding management may require general anesthesia.

C. Treat underlying condition. After the acute seizure episode is controlled, treat the underlying condition. Treat electrolyte abnormalities as outlined in the specific on call problem. Treat CNS lesions as appropriate. Definitive treatment for toxemia is delivery.

REFERENCES

Gendelman S. Grand-mal seizures. *Hosp Med* 1981;17(Oct):37.
Mikati MA, Browne TR. Tonic-clonic seizures. *Hosp Med* 1987;23(March):19.

■ SYNCOPE

I. Problem. A patient admitted for palpitations and chest pain has a syncopal episode in the hallway.

II. Immediate Questions

A. What was the patient's activity and position immediately prior to the incident? Syncope in the recumbent position is almost always cardiac in origin. Vasovagal syncope or fainting from orthostatic hypotension requires the patient to have been in the seated or upright position. Exertional syncope is frequently cardiac in origin. Other key activities to ask about include turning or twisting the head, coughing, getting up quickly, and micturition.

B. Is the patient still unconscious? Vasovagal syncope rarely lasts more than a few seconds and resolves with recumbency. Persistent unconsciousness suggests a cardiac or neurologic (brainstem stroke or seizure) cause.

C. What were the vital signs during the episode? What are the vital signs now? Vasovagal syncope is associated with bradycardia during the episode, but frequently a reflex tachycardia is noted after the episode. The blood pressure is usually normal after a vasovagal faint. Orthostatic changes in blood pressure and a tachycardia are frequently evidence of volume depletion or blood loss as the cause. Neurologic causes are generally associated with a normal or elevated blood pressure. Cardiac syncope presents with a wide variety of heart rates and rhythms ranging from profound bradycardia to an irregularly irregular tachycardia, all of which are usually associated with significant hypotension.

D. **Was there evidence of seizure activity?** Urinary and fecal incontinence is associated with seizure activity.

E. **How quickly was consciousness regained and was the patient immediately oriented?** Vasovagal episodes are brief and usually have an immediate return to full consciousness. Seizures are characterized by postictal confusion. Cardiac causes, like vasovagal episodes, are associated with a rapid return to full consciousness.

F. **How did the patient feel immediately prior to the loss of consciousness?** Vasovagal episodes are normally preceded by a symptom complex consisting of sweating, lightheadedness, and abdominal queasiness. Seizures often have an aura (frequently recurring visual or olfactory sensations). Cardiac and orthostatic syncope is often not preceded by symptoms or is associated with a sensation of the room closing in or going dark.

G. **What medical conditions does the patient have?** A number of medical conditions predispose to syncope. Diabetics are at risk for hypoglycemia as well as orthostasis secondary to autonomic dysfunction. A history of atherosclerotic vascular disease suggests cardiac causes and arrhythmias as well as cerebrovascular events. Other important illnesses to ask about include a previous history of a seizure disorder, valvular disorders, and any history of head trauma.

H. **What medications is the patient receiving?** A variety of medications predispose to orthostatic hypotension including diuretics, antihypertensives, and tricyclic antidepressants such as amitriptyline (Elavil). Varying degrees of heart block can be induced by verapamil (Calan, Isoptin), diltiazem (Cardizem), digoxin (Lanoxin), and beta blockers. Many class I antiarrhythmics can also induce ventricular arrhythmia leading to syncope ("quinidine syncope").

III. Differential Diagnosis

A. **Vasovagal syncope.** Also called the "simple faint." By far, the most common cause of syncope. Associated with the symptom complex previously described.

B. **Sudden decrease in venous return**
   1. **Micturition syncope**
   2. **Cough syncope**
   3. **Valsalva maneuver.** Increases vagal tone.

C. **Cardiac syncope**
   1. **Dysrhythmias**
      a. **Tachycardias.** (See Tachycardia, p 241.)
         (1) **Ventricular tachycardia**
         (2) **Ventricular fibrillation**

(3) **Paroxysmal atrial tachycardia**
(4) **Atrial fibrillation with rapid ventricular response**
(5) **Atrial flutter**
(6) **Wolff-Parkinson-White (WPW) syndrome.** Look for short PR interval and delta wave.

b. **Bradycardias.** (See Bradycardia, p 35.)
(1) **Sinus bradycardia**
(2) **Second- and third-degree atrioventricular block.**

c. **Asystole (cardiac arrest)**

2. **Structural causes**
   a. **Atrial myxoma.** Intermittent obstruction of a valve.
   b. **Aortic stenosis.** Associated with left ventricular outflow obstruction. Syncope is a marker of significant mortality.
   c. **Idiopathic hypertrophic subaortic stenosis.** Same etiology as aortic stenosis.
3. **Pacemaker syncope.** If the patient has a pacemaker, malfunction must be considered as a possible cause of syncope.
4. **Primary pulmonary hypertension.** Cause from decreased pulmonary flow and left-sided return.
5. **Acute myocardial infarction with cardiogenic shock**

D. **Orthostatic hypotension**

1. **Hypovolemia**
   a. **Dehydration**
   b. **Blood loss**
2. **Medications.** Diuretics; vasodilators including captopril (Capoten), enalapril (Vasotec), and minoxidil (Loniten); and tricyclic antidepressants such as amitriptyline (Elavil).
3. **Neurologic causes**
   a. **Shy-Drager syndrome.** Idiopathic autonomic dysfunction.
   b. **Diabetes.** Autonomic dysfunction with long-standing diabetes.

E. **Cerebrovascular accident.** Seldom will a cerebrovascular accident involving the anterior circulation result in syncope unless there is bilateral disruption of the reticular activating system.

1. **Basilar artery insufficiency ("drop attacks")**
2. **Carotid sinus syndrome.** Presents as syncope caused by turning head to one side.
3. **Subclavian steal syndrome**
4. **Subarachnoid hemorrhage.** May present as brief syncope followed by severe headache.

F. **Miscellaneous causes**

1. **Hypoxemia**
2. **Hyperventilation**
3. **Hypoglycemia.** Often in patients on insulin or oral hypoglycemics who miss a meal or receive the wrong dose.
4. **Seizures**
5. **Acute pulmonary embolism**
6. **Psychogenic causes**

IV. Database

A. Physical examination key points

1. **Vital signs** (see Section II.C). Vitals should be rechecked frequently during the evaluation.
2. **HEENT.** Look for evidence of trauma and palpate for bony abnormalities. Look for subhyaloid hemorrhages as evidence of subarachnoid hemorrhage. Tongue or cheek lacerations suggest seizure activity. Meningitis and subarachnoid hemorrhage have associated neck stiffness. Carotid bruits suggest diffuse atherosclerosis.
3. **Chest.** Auscultate for crackles and wheezes that may accompany aspiration during the syncopal episode. Palpate for rib injury caused by a fall.
4. **Heart.** Assess rate and rhythm, especially useful during or immediately after episode. Auscultate for new fourth heart sound (S_4) suggestive of acute myocardial infarction and murmur, listening for characteristic changes with position that would differentiate aortic stenosis and idiopathic hypertrophic subaortic stenosis from other systolic murmurs. Assess the jugular venous pulse as an indicator of volume status.
5. **Genitourinary system.** Look for urinary and/or fecal incontinence.
6. **Neurologic exam.** Slow resolution of mental status to normal points to a postictal state. Focal deficits suggest a cerebrovascular event. Persistent mental obtundation suggests hypoglycemia, hypoxemia, or other metabolic derangement.
7. **Reproduction of event.** Perform maneuvers intended to reproduce event. ***Caution:*** Do this only with appropriate monitoring and resuscitation equipment available (including venous access). Have the patient cough, turn her or his head, hyperventilate, or perform carotid massage as appropriate.

B. Laboratory data

1. **Hemogram.** Anemia can potentiate cerebral ischemia.
2. **Electrolytes and glucose.** Hypokalemia and hyperkalemia can cause ventricular arrhythmias. Hyponatremia, hypernatremia, and hypoglycemia predispose to seizures.
3. **Arterial blood gases.** Look for hypoxemia and hypocarbia.
4. **Stool for occult blood.** To evaluate for an acute bleed.

C. Radiologic and other studies

1. **Electrocardiogram with a rhythm strip.** Look for tachydysrhythmias or bradydysrhythmias. A short PR interval and delta wave suggest Wolff-Parkinson-White syndrome. Also look for evidence of ischemia or myocardial damage and new conduction abnormalities.
2. **Chest x-ray.** Evaluate the cardiac silhouette for enlargement, possible effusion, or congestive failure. Look for possible causes of hypoxia, such as infiltrates, pneumothoraces, or signs of pulmonary embolism.

3. **Echocardiogram.** Look for valvular lesion, thrombi, new wall motion abnormalities, or myxoma.
4. **Holter monitor.** Useful in the evaluation of possible dysrhythmias. In the presence of a normal ECG, the yield from a 24-hour, or even a 72-hour Holter monitor recording, is low.
5. **CT scan of head.** If seizure or subarachnoid hemorrhage is suspected.
6. **Electroencephalography.** If seizure is suspected.

V. Plan. This will be dictated by your initial impression based on the preceding evaluation. The causes of syncope range from a relatively benign vasovagal episode to life-threatening complete heart block. The treatment plan should reflect the severity of the underlying cause. Remember, injuries from the fall are a significant part of the morbidity in many patients, especially the elderly. So a thorough evaluation for injury should be a part of every plan.

A. Vasovagal syncope

1. Instruct the patient to assume a recumbent position at the onset of presyncopal symptoms. If unable to lie down, the patient should be seated with their head down.
2. The patient should be aware of situations that bring on the episodes, such as prolonged standing, and should seek to avoid these situations.

B. Orthostatic hypotension

1. Assess for signs of volume contraction and correct as indicated. Review patient's medications to eliminate those that could cause volume depletion if possible.
2. If gastrointestinal bleeding is diagnosed, see Hematemesis, Melena, p 117, and/or Hematochezia, p 121.
3. Instruct the patient to rise and change positions slowly with adequate support available.

C. Cardiac syncope

1. Treat any arrhythmias. (See Bradycardia, p 35, and Tachycardia, p 241.)
2. If no arrhythmia is noted on initial ECG, but a cardiac cause is still suspected, place the patient on telemetry and consider a 24-hour Holter monitor.
3. If ischemia is the suspected etiology, treat as possible myocardial infarction and institute a rule-out myocardial infarction protocol.

D. Miscellaneous disorders

1. **Carotid sinus syndrome (carotid sinus hypersensitivity).** Instruct the patient to avoid sudden turning of the head, tight collars, or vigorous rubbing with electric shavers.
2. **Micturition.** Instruct the patient to sit when voiding and to remain seated for several minutes after voiding.
3. **Cough and hyperventilation.** Informing the patient of the cause is frequently the only thing that can be done; however, if

hyperventilation is due to anxiety, the anxiety should be addressed and treated appropriately.

REFERENCES

Branch WT Jr. Approach to syncope. *J Gen Intern Med* 1986;1:49–58.
Noble RJ. The patient with syncope. *JAMA* 1977;237:1371–1376.

■ TACHYCARDIA

I. **Problem.** You are called to see a 50-year-old man in the medical ICU because of recent onset of tachycardia—heart rate (HR) 150 beats per minute (BPM). The patient was admitted 2 days earlier after a motor vehicle accident.

II. **Immediate Questions**

A. **What are the patient's other vital signs?** Take note of the patient's blood pressure, respiratory rate, and temperature. Hypotension accompanying the tachycardia requires immediate attention. Tachypnea can suggest a pulmonary embolism (PE), pneumonia, exacerbation of chronic obstructive lung disease (COPD), or pulmonary edema—all potential causes of a tachyarrhythmia. A fever may suggest an infection, and either sinus tachycardia or a supraventricular arrhythmia may be present. A pulsus paradoxus suggests either pericardial tamponade or exacerbation of COPD.

B. **What has the patient's heart rate been since admission?** A sudden change may signify a change in rhythm such as from sinus rhythm to atrial flutter.

C. **Does the patient have any symptoms associated with this heart rate?** Dyspnea, chest pain, somnolence, and agitation may indicate inadequate perfusion.

D. **What medication is the patient taking?** Drugs that can cause tachycardia include diuretics, theophylline preparations, sympathomimetic drugs, catecholamine infusions, digitalis, and thyroid supplementation. Diuretics may induce a significant enough volume depletion to cause a reflex tachycardia. Theophylline, even in therapeutic doses, may cause a sinus tachycardia and, in toxic doses (levels greater than 20 mg/L), can cause ventricular arrhythmias.

III. **Differential Diagnosis**

A. **Sinus tachycardia.** Sinus rhythm greater than 100 BPM. The extensive differential diagnosis includes states of emotion, pain, fever, and use of drugs such as caffeine, nicotine, atropine, amylnitrate, and quinidine. Seen in anemia, hypoxemia, hemorrhage, infection, shock of any cause, thyrotoxicosis, myocardial infarction, pneumothorax, or pericardial effusion.

B. Supraventricular tachycardia

1. **Atrial flutter.** Atrial rate of 260–300 BPM. The ventricular rate, which depends on the degree of conduction block, is usually one half or one third of the atrial rate. Atrial flutter is usually regular but may be irregular if the conduction block is variable. If the degree of conduction is variable, then the ventricular rate is variable. Atrial flutter can be seen with rheumatic or ischemic heart disease, cardiomyopathy, atrial septal defect, PE, mitral or triscuspid stenosis or regurgitation, thyrotoxicosis, alcoholism, or pericarditis.
2. **Atrial fibrillation.** Atrial rate of 350–600 BPM. Ventricular rate is irregular, averaging 100–160 BPM in the untreated state. Predisposing conditions include rheumatic heart disease, cardiomyopathy, hypertensive heart disease, PE, pericarditis, ischemic heart disease, alcoholism, and thyrotoxicosis.
3. **Atrial tachycardia with block.** Atrial rate of 150–200 BPM. May be irregular and the ventricular rate depends on the degree of conduction block. Commonly seen in digitalis toxicity (50% to 75% of cases) and therefore is usually seen in patient with organic heart disease.
4. **Nonparoxysmal or accelerated atrioventricular nodal tachycardia.** Caused by enhanced automaticity of the atrioventricular (AV) nodal tissue and is characterized by gradual onset and termination. The rate of discharge is 70–130 BPM. The atria are usually controlled by the sinus node so AV dissociation may be evident. This rhythm is another common dysrythmia of digitalis toxicity but is also seen in inferior myocardial infarction (MI), myocarditis, acute rheumatic fever, and after open-heart surgery.
5. **Atrioventricular reciprocating tachycardia.** Requires the presence of a retrograde conduction accessory pathway to maintain the tachycardia. The QRS complex is most often narrow because the accessory pathway conducts retrograde from the ventricle to the atrium. A retrograde P wave seen more than 70 milliseconds after the onset of the QRS during tachycardia should increase the suspicion of an accessory pathway. This tachycardia accounts for up to 30% of all supraventricular tachyarrhythmias. Heart rates may exceed 200 BPM.
6. **Other supraventricular tachyarrhythmias (SVTs).** Include automatic atrial tachycardia, reentry atrial tachycardia, and the most common, AV nodal reentry tachycardia. Heart rates may vary from 130 to 180 BPM. These tachycardias are commonly initiated by premature atrial contractions, and the P waves are morphologically different from sinus P waves or are hidden in the QRS complex in the case of AV node reentry tachycardia. These tachycardias are most often seen in patients without organic heart disease but can also be seen in chronic lung

disease, especially with infections, acute ethanol ingestion, metabolic derangements, digitalis use, occasionally following MI, and postoperatively. The prognosis, in general, is good with these tachyarrhythmias.

C. Ventricular tachycardia (VT). Characterized by a wide-complex rhythm with rates of 70–250 BPM and usually (but not always) compromises hemodynamics if long-lasting or sustained. The rhythm can be regular or irregular. Important criteria to separate VT from SVT include QRS duration greater than 140 milliseconds, presence of fusion and capture beats, identification of P waves suggesting AV dissociation, and a QRS morphology that appears similar to isolated premature ventricular contractions seen on other rhythm strips suggesting VT. A fusion beat is a hybrid of two beats, one originating in the atrium and one originating in the ventricle. Ventricular tachycardia is invariably associated with organic heart disease.

IV. Database

A. Physical examination key points

1. **Vital signs.** The blood pressure associated with the tachycardia is of primary importance and dictates how rapidly action will need to be taken. Palpate the carotid, brachial, or femoral pulse to determine if the rhythm is regular or irregular.
2. **Neck.** Distended jugular veins may indicate heart failure, pericardial effusion, or pneumothorax, Examination of the venous pulsations for cannon "A" waves provides confirming evidence for AV dissociation. (See Bradycardia, p 35.)
3. **Chest.** The presence of rales or wheezes may suggest an etiology or be the consequence of the tachycardia.
4. **Heart.** Listen for variation in the intensity of the first heart sound (S_1), listen for a third (S_3) or fourth (S_4) heart sound and for murmurs of mitral or triscuspid stenosis or regurgitation. Absence of a precordial impulse may suggest a pericardial effusion.
5. **Abdomen.** Localized or rebound tenderness suggests an inflammatory process or perforated viscus. A painful, pulsatile abdominal mass could suggest a leaking abdominal aortic aneurysm.
6. **Extremities.** Examine for signs of peripheral perfusion.

B. Laboratory data

1. **Serum electrolytes.** Most importantly potassium and magnesium. Hypokalemia and hypomagnesemia can cause supraventricular tachycardia as well as ventricular tachycardia.
2. **Arterial blood gases.** Hypoxemia as well as severe alkalosis or acidosis can cause ventricular arrhythmias.
3. **Hemogram.** In patients with possible hemorrhage. A severe anemia can cause various tachyarrhythmias. An elevated white blood cell count suggests an infection.

4. **Thyroid function tests.** Rule out hyperthyroidism.
5. **Drug levels.** If patient is on digoxin, theophylline, or antiarrhythmics, these levels should be checked.

C. Radiologic and other studies. A 12-lead ECG can be the most important piece of information in a patient with the acute onset of tachycardic rhythm if the patient's condition will allow extra time to determine the diagnosis.

V. Plan. Making the correct diagnosis allows you to provide the correct therapy. It is difficult to differentiate the various tachycardias using a single-lead rhythm strip. The correct diagnosis is commonly made after resolution of the tachycardia, but taking a little extra time at the beginning will pay off in the end.

A. Treat underlying etiologies. Often, identifying an underlying condition that has caused the arrhythmia will correct it. The correct treatment for sinus tachycardia, and often atrial fibrillation, is treatment of the underlying etiology. In the setting of atrial fibrillation caused by pneumonia, it will be difficult to convert to and maintain sinus rhythm without treating the pneumonia. For other causes of tachycardia, the following modalities of treatment may be used depending on the underlying rhythm.

B. Synchronized electrical cardioversion. If the tachycardia is complicated by hypotension, congestive heart failure, or myocardial ischemia, the quickest and most appropriate therapy for the termination of an acute tachycardia is electrical cardioversion, after administration of adequate sedation. Most supraventricular tachycardias can be terminated using 50–100 joules and ventricular tachycardias usually respond to 100–200 joules. ***Important:*** Electrical cardioversion is contraindicated in the setting of digitalis toxicity and will not be helpful when used for sinus tachycardia.

C. Carotid sinus massage. Can be very helpful in the differential diagnosis of many supraventricular tachycardias and can terminate some tachyarrhythmias (AV nodal reentry tachycardia). Carotid sinus massage or other vagal maneuvers (valsalva or Mueller maneuvers) are the first line of therapy for this tachycardia. After each pharmacologic agent, vagal maneuvers should be repeated if the medication alone did not achieve the desired effect. Carotid sinus massage should be done in a monitored setting because of the potential for inducing bradycardia and sinus arrest.

D. Drugs

1. **Digoxin.** 0.25 mg IV every 4–6 hours for three or four doses, followed by a maintenance dose of 0.125–0.25 mg per day. Digoxin can be used in many supraventricular tachyarrhythmias to control the ventricular rate and is most commonly used in atrial fibrillation or flutter. If digoxin alone does not control the ventricular rate adequately, addition of a calcium channel blocker (verapamil or diltiazem) will often help. Rapid

IV infusion of digoxin can increase systemic vascular resistance and worsen heart failure if present.

2. **Verapamil (Calan).** Initial bolus of 2.5–10 mg IV followed by an IV infusion of 5 mg/kg/min or an oral maintenance dose of 80–120 mg TID. Verapamil IV will convert approximately 90% of episodes of AV nodal reentry tachycardia to sinus rhythm. Verapamil is also useful with atrial flutter or fibrillation. Verapamil is contraindicated in patients with heart failure and should **never** be used as the first therapy for wide-complex tachycardias. Intravenous diltiazem should be released soon and will be helpful to control ventricular rates in selected patients with contraindications to intravenous verapamil.
3. **Propranolol (Inderal).** Loading dose of 1–10 mg IV, followed usually by an oral maintenance dose. Metoprolol (Lopressor) and esmolol (Brevibloc) are other intravenous beta blockers available for use. Beta blockers are usually helpful in controlling a rapid heart rate in patients with sinus tachycardia, atrial flutter, atrial fibrillation, atrial tachycardia with block, automatic atrial tachycardia, and supraventricular tachyarrhythmias associated with digitalis toxicity. Beta blockers should not be used in patients with heart failure or chronic obstructive or bronchospastic lung disease.
4. **Quinidine sulfate.** 200–400 mg PO every 6 hours. The vagolytic effect of quinidine can result in a faster ventricular rate with atrial flutter or fibrillation via facilitation of AV node conduction. For this reason, some experts recommend that digoxin be given in conjunction with quinidine when used for supraventricular arrhythmias. Procainamide and disopyramide (Norpace) are other antiarrhythmic drugs that can be used if quinidine causes intolerable side effects.
5. **Lidocaine.** Loading dose of 1 mg/kg IV, followed by a continuous IV infusion of 1–4 mg/min and a second loading dose of 0.5 mg/kg 5–10 minutes after the initial loading dose. Lidocaine is the first drug of choice in the therapy of a wide-complex tachycardia that is not associated with hemodynamic decompensation. Lidocaine is also helpful in arrhythmias associated with digitalis excess.
6. **Procainamide.** Loading dose of 500–1000 mg IV (15–35 mg/min), followed by a maintenance infusion of 2–6 mg/min. Procainamide is the best drug available to convert wide-complex tachyarrhythmias should lidocaine be unsuccessful. Hypotension can develop during procainamide infusions greater than 5 mg/min.

Special Note: For Wolff-Parkinson-White syndrome with AV reciprocating tachycardia, treatment of a tachycardia in the presence of an accessory atrioventricular pathway should focus on drugs that prolong the refractory period of the accessory pathway or of the AV node. An acute tachycardia suspicious for an AV reciprocating tachycardia (normal QRS width, regular RR interval, rate around 200 BPM, and retrograde P waves visible in ST segment) can be approached with drugs that prolong conduction in the AV node, such as verapamil, diltiazem, beta blockers, and digoxin. If atrial flutter or fibrillation is suspected, a drug that prolongs refractory periods of ventricular muscle must be used as well. Procainamide can be given intravenously and it prolongs the effective refractory period of accessory muscle tissue and has less anticholinergic effects than quinidine, so that AV node conduction time does not change much. Procainamide's electrophysiologic properties make this drug an excellent choice for the acute pharmacologic therapy of an AV reciprocating tachycardia. Lidocaine does not prolong refractoriness of the accessory pathway and therefore should not routinely be used in this setting. Digoxin may shorten the refractory period of the accessory pathway and increase ventricular response in some Wolff-Parkinson-White patients with atrial fibrillation.

REFERENCES

Marriott H. *Practical Electrocardiography.* 7th ed. Baltimore: Williams and Wilkins; 1983.

Wellens HJJ, Bar FWH, Lie K. The value of the electrocardiogram in the differential diagnosis of tachycardia with widened QRS complex. *Am J Med* 1978;64:27–33.

Zipes DP. Management of cardiac arrhythmias. In: Braunwald E, ed. *Heart Disease: A Textbook of Cardiovascular Medicine.* 3rd ed. Philadelphia: WB Saunders; 1988:621–657.

Zipes DP. Specific arrhythmias: Diagnosis and treatment. In: Braunwald E, ed. *Heart Disease: A Textbook of Cardiovascular Medicine.* 3rd ed. Philadelphia: WB Saunders; 1988:658–716.

■ THROMBOCYTOPENIA

I. Problem. You are called to see a 73-year-old patient admitted to the cardiology service with unstable angina. His admission laboratory data reveals a platelet count of 32,000/μL.

II. Immediate Questions

A. Is the patient bleeding? The risk of bleeding increases from trauma with a platelet count of 50,000/μL or less; the risk of spontaneous bleeding increases with a platelet count less than 20,000/μL.

B. Is there a past history of low platelet count? Does this appear to be an acute problem such as immune thrombocytopenic purpura (ITP) or is there an underlying disorder contributing to the low platelet count such as hypersplenism or chronic ITP?

C. Is the patient on any medicines that could cause thrombocytopenia? Drug-induced thrombocytopenia is one of the most common causes. The number of drugs implicated in causing thrombocytopenia are many. Quinidine and quinine together account for the largest number of cases. Other commonly associated drugs are alcohol, sulfonamides, heparin, gold, thiazide diuretics, cimetidine (Tagamet), and captopen (Captopril).

D. **Is there a history of a preceding viral infection?** A viral infection days to weeks before the onset of thrombocytopenia suggests a chronic form of ITP or acute interference with normal megakaryocyte maturation.

III. **Differential Diagnosis.** Quantitative platelet disorders can frequently be divided into two categories: decreased production and peripheral destruction or sequestration.

A. **Pseudothrombocytopenia.** Thrombocytopenia may be artifactual, particularly when relying on an automated counter. Platelet autoagglutinins may cause clumping in the presence of EDTA independently or may cause adherence to neutrophils.

B. **Decreased production**

1. **Infiltrative processes.** Acute and chronic leukemias, carcinoma, and lymphoma crowd normal marrow elements, leading to decreased numbers of megakaryocytes. Granulomatous diseases (tuberculosis) occasionally causes a similar picture.
2. **Myelodysplasia (preleukemic syndrome).** Frequently leads to morphologically abnormal megakaryocytes and results in low platelet levels.
3. **Drugs.** Some known myelosuppressive drugs are particularly toxic to platelet production, for example, cytosine arabinoside (ARA-C), cyclophosphamide (Cytoxan), busulfan (Myleran), methotrexate (MTX), carboplatinum (Paraplatin), and interferon. Thiazide diuretics have been associated with a decreased number of megakaryocytes leading to thrombocytopenia. Thiazides may also induce platelet-directed antibodies that can lead to peripheral destruction. Thrombocytopenia is common in chronic alcoholism. Alcohol has been shown to decrease the number of megakaryocytes.
4. **Radiation.** Ionizing radiation can affect all marrow elements, frequently megakaryocytes to a lesser extent. Patients who have had therapeutic radiation to large areas of marrow can have transient thrombocytopenia, and full recovery to preradiation levels may not occur.
5. **Nutrition.** Malnutritional states, such as vitamin B_{12} and folate deficiency and occasionally iron deficiency, can lead to depressed numbers of megakaryocytes.
6. **Virus.** Viral illnesses such as hepatitis B, rubella, and infectious mononucleosis may cause an acute interference with normal megakaryocyte maturation.
7. **Paroxysmal nocturnal hemoglobinuria.** Can be associated with insufficient platelet production.

C. **Peripheral destruction**

1. **Immune-mediated disorders**

a. **Immune thrombocytopenic purpura,** an autoimmune disorder, is a frequent cause of thrombocytopenia. Diagnosis can be made definitively if antiplatelet antibodies can be demonstrated; however, this test is not available in all clinical labs.

(1) **Chronic.** Usually seen in adults.

(2) **Acute.** Most frequently seen in children and is usually self-limiting.

b. Drugs can also cause immune destruction. Quinidine is the best known. In addition to exerting a toxic effect on megakaryocytes, quinidine may act as a hapten with antibody complex adhering to the platelet, followed by complement-mediated platelet destruction.

c. Autoimmune thrombocytopenia also occurs in patients with systemic lupus erythematosus.

2. **Infection.** Direct platelet toxicity may occur from viruses, gram-positive organisms, or the lipopolysaccharide of gram-negative bacteria. Complement, immunoglobulins, and fibrinogen may also play a role. Disseminated intravascular coagulation (DIC) frequently caused by infection can lead to a consumptive platelet loss. Thrombocytopenia can also be seen in the absence of DIC in septicemia, as with Rocky Mountain spotted fever and malaria.
3. **Snake bite.** May be related to DIC or direct platelet destruction.
4. **Burns.** Thrombocytopenia may be secondary to sequestration within damaged tissue and can be further aggravated by concomitant sepsis.
5. **Glomerulonephritis.** Thrombocytopenia presumably secondary to immune-mediated mechanisms.
6. **Aortic valvular stenosis.** Seen occasionally. Presumed mechanism is direct platelet injury secondary to turbulent flow.
7. **Thrombotic thrombocytopenic purpura (TTP, Moschcowitz's syndrome).** This disease is a pentad of hemolytic anemia with a microangiopathic picture on the peripheral blood smear, thrombocytopenia, fluctuating neurologic findings, fever, and renal dysfunction.
8. **Direct toxins to platelets.** Heparin appears to cause a direct antiplatelet factor causing aggregation and can induce aggregation in the absence of antibody. Heparin-induced thrombocytopenia can occur with intravenous or subcutaneous delivery and with bovine or porcine heparin but is more common with bovine. This entity infrequently is associated with thromboembolism.

D. **Sequestration.** Normally, the spleen may contain 30% of the circulating platelet pool. When the spleen is enlarged and hypersplenism ensues, up to 90% of circulating platelets may be pooled within the spleen.

IV. Database

A. Physical examination key points. The physical examination should be directed toward evaluation of evidence of bleeding and of peripheral sequestration.

1. **Vital signs.** Fever requires consideration of infectious causes as well as TTP.
2. **Skin and mucous membranes.** Are there petechiae or purpura? The lower extremities frequently reveal petechiae when a petechial rash may not be easily seen elsewhere. Multiple bruises out of proportion to the degree of trauma may give further evidence of quantitative or qualitative platelet defects. Look for gingival hyperplasia or skin nodules, which suggest leukemia.
3. **Heart.** Severe aortic stenosis can result in thrombocytopenia. New murmurs may indicate bacterial endocarditis.
4. **Abdomen.** Splenomegaly may be associated with thrombocytopenia resulting from sequestration. Chronic alcoholics may have evidence of portal hypertension with dilated abdominal and chest wall venous channels, ascites, and splenomegaly. Splenomegaly is also seen with lymphoproliferative and myeloproliferative disorders, as well as infectious causes such as infectious mononucleosis and endocarditis. The lack of splenomegaly is also important to note. The presence of palpable splenomegaly makes ITP much less likely.
5. **Neurologic exam.** Fluctuating neurologic findings are frequently seen in TTP.

B. Laboratory data

1. **Peripheral blood smear.** Extremely important to review to rule out pseudothrombocytopenia. Large platelets (megathrombocytes) are frequently seen with ITP and may indicate peripheral destruction. Morphology of red blood cells may indicate DIC or TTP with a microangiopathic picture. May indicate acute leukemia. The presence of left-shifted granulocytes, nucleated red blood cells, and tear drops may indicate marrow infiltration. Left-shifted granulocytes and toxic granulation are consistent with an infectious etiology.
2. **Coagulation studies.** Elevated prothrombin time, partial thromboplastin time, and thrombin time may be seen with DIC and liver disease.
3. **Antinuclear antibodies (ANA) and rheumatoid factor.** Need to rule out collagen vascular disease as a cause of thrombocytopenia.
4. **Blood urea nitrogen and creatinine.** Renal failure can cause marrow suppression of megakaryocytes and may coexist with other causes such as sepsis, DIC, and TTP.
5. **Bone marrow** (See Chapter 3, Bone Marrow Aspiration and Biopsy, p 312.) This is essential in the evaluation. The presence of megakaryocytes in adequate or increased numbers

implies peripheral destruction. Marrow infiltration or primary marrow disease can be identified with a bone marrow aspirate and biopsy.

6. **Liver function tests.** Total bilirubin, alkaline phosphatase, and transaminases (AST [SGOT] and ALT [SGPT]) may support viral hepatitis, an alcoholic liver disease, or sepsis as the cause.

C. Radiologic and other studies

1. **CT scan of the abdomen.** Demonstrates hepatosplenomegaly or lymphadenopathy in indicated situations.
2. **Liver/spleen scan.** Demonstrates splenomegaly in questionable cases and also indicates hepatic dysfunction and findings consistent with portal hypertension.
3. **Platelet antibodies.** Much variability exists among the techniques for various assays, and frequently these are not of great clinical utility in evaluation.

V. Plan

A. Bleeding. Initially, it is important to determine if there is life-threatening bleeding, in which case platelet transfusion would be indicated. (See Chapter 5, Blood Component Therapy, p 351.) If there is no active bleeding and the thrombocytopenia is immunologic, platelet transfusions are to be avoided. In this situation, the transfusions are frequently ineffective and may actually worsen the thrombocytopenia with further immunologic challenge.

B. Immune-mediated destruction. If suspected, **all** nonessential medicines should be stopped. Do not overlook heparin flush for catheters and Hep-Locks.

C. Treatment of underlying cause. Of key importance for leukemia, lymphomas, infection, and DIC.

D. Immune thrombocytopenic purpura

1. High-dose steroids (2 mg/kg prednisone) daily is the treatment for ITP. Intravenous immunoglobulins can also be used in steroid-unresponsive ITP or if steroids are contraindicated.
2. In chronic ITP that is unresponsive to steroids or immunoglobulins, splenectomy may be required. If the platelet count is consistently greater than 50,000/μL, close observation may be best depending on the underlying medical condition of the patient.

E. Thrombotic thrombocytopenic purpura

1. **Plasmapheresis.** Considered standard treatment though the mechanism of action is unknown. May be related to removal of an offending agent or replacement of missing factor(s).
2. **High-dose prednisone.** Frequently used treatment; however, there is no proven benefit.
3. **Dipyridamole (Persantine) and aspirin.** The value of antiplatelet drugs is unclear at present.

F. Prophylactic platelet transfusion. May be indicated for patients with myeloproliferative disorders or bone marrow suppression from myelotoxic drugs. Frequently, transfusion is given for platelet counts below 20,000/μL. Three units per meter squared, or approximately six units, should give an adequate increment in most adults. Repeated transfusion may cause alloimmunization, with resultant smaller increments after transfusion. Human leukocyte antigen matched platelets will increase platelet survival and are indicated in patients receiving multiple platelet transfusions with a suboptimal response.

REFERENCES

Aster RH, George JN. Thrombocytopenia due to enhanced platelet destruction by immunologic mechanisms. In: Williams WJ, Beutler E, Erslev AJ, et al, eds. *Hematology.* 4th ed. New York: McGraw-Hill; 1990:1370–1398.

Aster RH, George JN. Thrombocytopenia due to platelet loss. In: Williams WJ, Beutler E, Erslev AJ, et al, eds. *Hematology.* 4th ed. New York: McGraw-Hill; 1990:1401–1402.

Aster RH, George JN. Thrombocytopenia due to sequestration of platelets. In: Williams WJ, Beutler E, Erslev AJ, et al, eds. *Hematology.* 4th ed. New York: McGraw-Hill; 1990:1398–1400.

George JN, Aster RH. Thrombocytopenia due to diminished or defective platelet production. In: Williams WJ, Beutler E, Erslev AJ, et al, eds. *Hematology.* 4th ed. New York: McGraw-Hill; 1990:1343–1351.

George JN, Aster RH. Thrombocytopenia due to enhanced platelet destruction by nonimmunologic mechanisms. In: Williams WJ, Beutler E, Erslev AJ, et al, eds. *Hematology.* 4th ed. New York: McGraw-Hill; 1990:1351–1370.

■ TRANSFUSION REACTION

(See also Chapter 5, Blood Component Therapy, p 349.)

I. **Problem.** During a transfusion of packed red blood cells (PRBCs), the patient's temperature rises to 38.5°C (101.3°F).

II. **Immediate Questions.** The patient is probably having an immediate transfusion reaction. This could be secondary to a life-threatening hemolytic reaction, a reaction to contaminated blood, or a self-limiting febrile reaction. Your assessment is directed at differentiating among these different diagnoses.

   A. **What are the patient's vital signs?** The presenting signs and symptoms of fever and chills, tachycardia, and tachypnea are not specific enough to allow you to differentiate reliably between a self-limiting and a life-threatening transfusion reaction.

   B. **Does the patient have any complaints?** Bronchospasm and chest or back pain and pulmonary edema are consistent with a serious reaction.

   C. **Is there any evidence of generalized bleeding from mucous membranes, previous venipuncture sites, or the present intravenous site?** Diffuse bleeding would be consistent with disseminated intravascular coagulation (DIC) and suggests a severe, life-threatening hemolytic reaction.

D. **Has the patient ever been transfused before? If so, has she or he ever reacted to blood products in the past?** The patient may have a variety of antibodies if there is a history of previous transfusion. Previous fevers with blood products suggest a more benign process.

E. **Most importantly, does the name on the unit of packed cells match that on the patient's armband?** An error of this nature often results in a severe hemolytic reaction. Most severe hemolytic reactions occur because of administration of correctly cross-matched blood to the **wrong** patient.

III. Differential Diagnosis

A. Hemolytic transfusion reaction

1. The risk of severe sequelae from a hemolytic transfusion reaction appears to be proportional to the volume of incompatible blood transfused. Severe complications rarely follow the transfusion of less than 200 mL of PRBCs. Therefore, one of the earliest therapeutic decisions to be made is the decision whether to stop the transfusion.
2. Of all fatal transfusion reactions reported between 1976 and 1978, approximately 77% were hemolytic reactions that occurred because of administration of correctly cross-matched blood to the wrong patient. Check the label on the unit of blood against the patient's armband.
3. Transfusion of ABO-incompatible blood results in intravascular hemolysis. Disseminated intravascular coagulation may result, leading to abnormal bleeding and ischemic necrosis of tissues (especially the kidneys).

B. **Self-limiting febrile transfusion reaction.** This is not a hemolytic reaction. It typically occurs in a patient who has had numerous previous transfusions or in a multiparous woman. It is often secondary to sensitization to white blood cell or platelet antigens. This type of reaction is fairly frequent. It is estimated to cause 30% of all transfusion reactions.

C. **Transfusion of blood contaminated with microorganisms.** Fortunately, this is an infrequent transfusion reaction; however, as little as 50 mL of contaminated blood may contain sufficient microorganisms to produce fever, chills, or shock. Blood may be contaminated by cold-growing organisms such as **Pseudomonas.**

IV. Database

A. Physical examination key points

1. **Vital signs.** If a constellation of signs is present including fever, tachycardia, and hypotension, the diagnosis must be considered to be a severe hemolytic reaction.
2. **Skin and mucous membranes.** Generalized bleeding may be part of a severe hemolytic reaction.
3. **Chest.** Wheezing or rales are consistent with a life-threatening reaction.

B. Laboratory data

1. **Hemogram.** May point to contaminated blood or show evidence of hemolysis.
2. **Prothrombin time, partial thromboplastin time, thrombin time, fibrinogen, and fibrin split products.** Rule out DIC.
3. **Peripheral smear.** Should be reviewed. Look for schistocytes as evidence for DIC.
4. **Urine for hemoglobinuria.** Evidence of hemolysis.
5. **Serum for free hemoglobin.** Indicates hemolysis.
6. **Repeat type and cross-match.** To show blood group incompatibility (antibodies in the recipient reacting with blood group antigens on transfused cells).
7. **Gram stain of remaining untransfused blood.** Rule out bacterial contamination.

V. Plan. The treatment plan depends on the type of reaction.

A. Severe hemolytic reaction

1. If a serious transfusion reaction is suspected, the transfusion should be stopped immediately.
2. Supportive care is indicated in the presence of a severe hemolytic transfusion reaction.
   - **a.** Intravenous access should be maintained and intravenous fluids administered.
   - **b.** Prevention of renal complications depends on maintaining renal blood flow. Urine output should be closely monitored and systolic blood pressure should be maintained above 100 mm Hg. If urine output falls, diuretics or mannitol may be required to prevent the development of oliguria or anuria and subsequent renal failure.
   - **c.** In generalized bleeding related to DIC, heparin may be helpful. The use of heparin in DIC is controversial, however, and may be associated with increased risk.

B. Self-limiting febrile transfusion reaction

1. The transfusion can be continued if more serious symptoms are absent. A previous history of febrile reactions would sway you to continue the transfusion.
   - **a.** Antihistamines and antipyretics may control symptoms.
   - **b.** Steps to prevent this type of reaction will require further transfusions include washing PRBCs and/or pretreating the patient with antihistamines and acetaminopen (Tylenol) prior to transfusion.

C. Transfusion of blood contaminated with microorganisms

1. Broad-spectrum antibiotics should be instituted.

REFERENCE

Holland PV. Other adverse effects of transfusion. In Petz LD, Swansen SN, eds. *Clinical Practice of Blood Transfusion.* New York: Churchill Livingstone; 1981:783–804.

■ VAGINAL BLEEDING

I. Problem. You are called to see a 44-year-old white woman with vaginal bleeding who was admitted the day before with pyelonephritis.

II. Immediate Questions

A. When was the patient's last menstrual period? Inquire in detail about her menstrual history, specifically, the date of the last period, the frequency of periods, and the volume and character of the flow. Vaginal bleeding could represent a normal menstrual period. If the patient is postmenopausal (absence of menses for 1 year), vaginal bleeding could be a manifestation of endometrial carcinoma or some other pathologic process. If the patient has missed a period, bleeding could represent a complication of pregnancy.

B. Is the patient sexually active and if so, does she use birth control? Vaginal bleeding could be a complication of pregnancy, either a spontaneous abortion or an ectopic pregnancy.

C. Are there any associated symptoms? Lower abdominal pain with associated vaginal bleeding could arise from a ruptured tubal ectopic pregnancy, which usually occurs between weeks 8 and 16 after conception.

D. Is there any evidence of shock? Vaginal bleeding can be profuse. In some cases, the actual blood loss may represent only a fraction of the actual blood loss such as a ruptured ectopic pregnancy.

E. What is the quantity of blood loss? The rate of bleeding has both diagnostic and therapeutic implications. If a volume estimate of blood loss cannot be given, ask about number of pads/tampons used and degree of saturation.

F. Could the bleeding be from another source? Occasionally, hematuria (see Hematuria, p 124) or rectal bleeding (see Hematochezia, p 121) could be the actual source of bleeding.

III. Differential Diagnosis

A. Normal menstrual period. Most common cause of vaginal bleeding.

B. Dysfunctional bleeding (related to menstrual cycle)

1. **Perimenopausal bleeding.** Periods are often irregular.
2. **Luteal phase defect.** Often a problem with luteinizing hormone (LH) or follicle-stimulating hormone (FSH).
3. **Oral contraceptives.** Breakthrough bleeding may occur with birth control pills that contain low doses of estrogen.
4. **Physiologic causes.** At midcycle, there is a fall in estrogen. Light bleeding may occur either with every cycle or intermittently. Often there is associated sharp unilateral lower abdominal pain from ovulation (Mittelschmerz).

- **C. Anovulatory abnormal uterine bleeding**
  1. **Hypothalamic/pituitary disorders.** Pituitary tumors or failure resulting in inadequate LH or FSH. Often cause primary amenorrhea but may cause abnormal bleeding.
  2. **Stress**
  3. **Endocrine disorders.** Hypothyroidism or hyperthyroidism, and hypoadrenalism or hyperadrenalism can result in irregular periods.
  4. **Endometriosis.** Ectopic endometrial tissue. Cervical or vaginal lesions can cause abnormal bleeding.
- **D. Pregnancy-related causes**
  1. **Ectopic pregnancy.** Triad of lower abdominal pain, vaginal bleeding, and positive pregnancy test (previously missed period).
  2. **Threatened/spontaneous abortion**
  3. **Retained products of gestation.** Bleeding may occur after an abortion or delivery if there are retained products of gestation.
- **E. Neoplasia**
  1. **Uterine fibroids.** Periods are usually heavy and prolonged, and may be irregular.
  2. **Cervical polyps.** Most often asymptomatic but may cause excessive bleeding.
  3. **Carcinoma (cervical, uterine, ovarian, vaginal)**
     - **a. Endometrium.** Risk increases with age. Bleeding is most common symptom of endometrial cancer.
     - **b. Cervix.** Bleeding is an unusual presentation. Indicates advanced disease.
     - **c. Ovaries.** Abnormal vaginal bleeding may be presenting symptom.
     - **d. Vagina or vulva.** Rare cancer, bleeding, or spotting is common.
- **F. Infection**
  1. **Pelvic inflammatory disease (PID).** Lower abdominal pain and fever are often present. May be secondary to intrauterine device.
  2. **Vaginitis**
- **G. Trauma.** History of trauma should be present.
- **H. Bleeding diathesis.** Vaginal bleeding secondary to thrombocytopenia or a coagulopathy will usually not occur unless there is a defect in the mucosa. If vaginal bleeding occurs in the presence of a bleeding diathesis, you must rule out a mucosal lesion such as uterine fibroid. Bleeding may also be present at other sites.

IV. Database

- **A. Physical examination key points**
  1. **Vital signs.** Orthostatic changes indicate a significant loss of blood and emphasize urgency in diagnosis and treatment. Orthostatic changes are a decrease in systolic blood pressure

of 10 mm Hg and/or an increase in heart rate of 20 per minute 1 minute after movement from a supine to the standing position. A fever suggests an infectious etiology such as PID.

2. **Skin.** Pallor points to significant blood loss. Bruising and petechiae suggest bleeding diathesis.
3. **Abdomen.** Observe for peritoneal signs, tenderness, and distension. Peritoneal signs may be present from a ruptured ectopic pregnancy or PID. Distension may be from ascites secondary to ovarian carcinoma.
4. **Female genitalia.** Look for source and note rate of bleeding. On inspection, carcinoma of the cervix, cervical polyps, or tissue fragments may be present. Note if the cervical os is open or closed. Examine for vaginal, cervical, uterine, or adnexal mass. Pregnancy (uterine or ectopic), uterine fibroid, or ovarian carcinoma may present as a palpable mass. Tenderness with manipulation of the cervix (Chandler's sign) points to PID.

B. Laboratory data

1. **Hemogram.** Leukocytosis suggests PID. Microcytic anemia suggests a long history of blood losses.
2. **Platelet count.** Rule out thrombocytopenia.
3. **Prothrombin time, partial thromboplastin time.** To rule out coagulopathy. Check fibrinogen and fibrin split products if disseminated intravascular coagulation is suspected.
4. **Type and cross-match for blood.** Indicated with heavy bleeding and if patient is orthostatic.
5. **Serum/urine human chorionic gonadotropin.** A pregnancy test will be positive with an ectopic pregnancy or spontaneous abortion.
6. **Pap smear of cervix.** May reveal endometrial as well as cervical carcinoma.
7. **Cervical culture for *Neisseria gonorrhea* and *Chlamydia trachomatis*.** If PID is suspected.

C. Radiologic and other studies

1. **Culdocentesis.** If ectopic pregnancy is possible.
2. **Pelvic ultrasound.** To evaluate for intrauterine and intratubal lesions. Rules out ectopic pregnancy or any pelvic mass.
3. **CT scan of pelvis.** To further evaluate a mass. Usually not as easily obtained in emergencies as an ultrasound. Be sure there is not a salvagable intrauterine pregnancy **prior to** obtaining a CT scan.

V. Plan. Most vaginal bleeding does not require specific treatment as it represents normal menstrual bleeding. Virtually all the causes of significant vaginal bleeding require evaluation by gynecology.

A. Emergency management

1. Resuscitate the patient from acute blood loss as needed.
2. Establish large-bore intravenous access, administer crystal-

loid, type and cross-match for blood, monitor urine output, and follow serial hematocrits. The patient should also be NPO as urgent operative procedures may be indicated.

B. Ectopic pregnancy. If lower abdominal pain is a part of the symptom complex and the patient is of childbearing age, ectopic pregnancy must be ruled out even if the pregnancy tests are negative. The diagnostic procedure of choice is pelvic ultrasound or culdocentesis if ultrasound is not available. Emergency surgical exploration is usually indicated.

REFERENCES

Cope E. The treatment of unexplained menorrhagia. In *J Med Sci* 1983;152(suppl 2):29.

Riddick DH. Disorders of menstrual function. In: Scott JR, DiSaia PJ, Hammond CB, et al, eds. *Danforth's Obstetrics and Gynecology,* 6th ed. Philadelphia: JB Lippincott; 1990:747–771.

■ WHEEZING

I. Problem. You are cross-covering a patient recently admitted with chest pain who develops respiratory distress and wheezing.

II. Immediate Questions

A. What are the vital signs? A respiratory rate greater than 40/min may indicate the need for immediate treatment. Associated hypotension may suggest an anaphylactic reaction or an acute myocardial infarction (MI). Fever may point to an underlying infection or new pulmonary embolism.

B. Were any diagnostic tests recently performed or medicines administered? A beta blocker given to a stable asthmatic may precipitate an acute attack of bronchospasm. Wheezing after the administration of a drug such as penicillin or radiocontrast dye suggests an anaphylactic reaction.

C. What was the patient admitted for? A patient admitted to rule out MI may have developed acute pulmonary edema. A patient with a gastric ulcer may have gastric outlet obstruction and have aspirated.

D. Is there a history of asthma? Childhood asthma may reactivate at any age, given the right stimuli.

E. Does the patient have any allergies to medications or other substances such as shellfish? It is prudent to inquire about known allergies.

III. Differential Diagnosis

A. Diffuse wheezing

1. Acute bronchospasm. May be caused by asthma, exacerbation of chronic obstructive pulmonary disease (COPD), or an anaphylactic reaction.

2. **Aspiration.** May trigger bronchospasm from mucosal irritation or from impacted foreign bodies.
3. **Cardiogenic pulmonary edema.** The primary finding in "cardiac asthma" may be wheezing. Other findings of pulmonary edema should be present and the chest x-ray will be diagnostic.
4. **Pulmonary embolism (PE).** Mediators may be released that cause not only hypoxemia but also transient bronchospasm.

B. Stridor (upper airway wheezing)

1. **Laryngospasm.** This may be part of an anaphylactic reaction or secondary to aspiration.
2. **Laryngeal or tracheal tumor.** History of dysphagia, hoarseness, cough, or weight loss and anorexia may be present.
3. **Epiglottis.** The patient is often unable to speak or to swallow secretions.
4. **Foreign body aspiration**
5. **Vocal cord dysfunction.** Bilaterally paralyzed vocal cords may result in severe stridor and dyspnea. A subgroup of patients has recently been recognized to have "factitious asthma": they voluntarily adduct their vocal cords for psychogenic reasons.

C. Localized wheezing

1. **Tumors.** May obstruct one bronchus leading to localized wheezing.
2. **Mucous plugging**
3. **Aspirated foreign body**

IV. Database

A. Physical examination key points. Localization of wheezing allows categorization as outlined in the differential diagnosis.

1. **Vital signs.** A fever may indicate an infectious etiology. A pulsus paradoxus greater than 20 mm Hg indicates severe respiratory distress. Hypotension requires immediate assessment and action.
2. **HEENT.** Check the mouth carefully. Examine the neck for angioneurotic edema. Palpate the sternocleidomastoid muscles for accessory muscle use. Auscultate over the mouth and larynx in an effort to localize the wheezing.
3. **Chest.** Carefully auscultate for localized wheezing. Listen for bibasilar rales, which may be present in pulmonary edema. Rales, increased fremitus, and egophony suggest pneumonia.
4. **Heart.** Check carefully for evidence of an S_3 or S_4 gallop or jugular venous distension, which points to pulmonary edema.
5. **Extremities.** Clubbing may indicate underlyihng lung cancer. Cyanosis indicates underlying hypoxemia. Edema may signify chronic congestive heart failure.
6. **Skin.** Urticaria probably indicates an acute allergic reaction. A malar rash points toward acute systemic lupus erythematosus, which can present with acute pneumonitis.

B. Laboratory data

1. **Arterial blood gases.** An elevated $PaCO_2$ indicates significant ventilatory failure. Also check for hypoxemia.
2. **Complete blood count.** An increased white blood cell count may indicate an underlying infection; however, an increase in WBCs without a left shift can be seen with an acute MI and PE. Eosinophilia suggests an allergic or asthmatic etiology to the wheezing.

C. Radiologic and other studies

1. **Electrocardiogram.** An ECG may show an acute MI or ischemia. Occasionally it will be suggestive of a PE, showing an S wave in lead I, a Q wave in III, T wave inversion in lead III ($S_1Q_3T_3$), new right bundle branch block (RBBB), and right-axis shift. It may also show a change in rhythm.
2. **Chest radiograph.** A PE (with infarction) severe enough to cause wheezing may be evident on the chest film. Look for a pleural-based, wedge-shaped lesion. Kerley B lines, bilateral pleural effusions, vascular redistribution, and cardiomegaly may also suggest congestive heart failure or pulmonary edema. Look for localized infiltrates or masses suggesting other causes.

V. Plan. Treatment plans depend on the diagnosis. The preceding differential diagnoses and studies should enable you to form a tentative categorization on which to base initial therapy.

A. Bronchospasm (asthma, COPD, allergic reaction)

1. Methylprednisolone (Solumedrol) 200 mg IV stat dose.
2. Nebulized albuterol (Ventolin) 0.5 mL (2.5 mg) or metaproterenol (Alupent) 0.3 mL of 5% solution in 3.0 mL normal saline stat and then every 2–4 hours.
3. Aminophylline loading dose of 6 mg/kg (assuming the patient is not already on aminophylline) and then a maintenance IV of 0.2–0.6 mg/kg/h (15–30 mg/h). Aminophylline is now considered to be of only modest acute benefit and may cause worsening of arrhythmias. Therefore, initial dosing should be on the "low side" and blood levels need to be closely monitored.

B. Stridor

1. Methylprednisolone 200 mg IV stat dose.
2. Nebulized racemic epinephrine (Micronephrine) 0.5 mL in 3 mL normal saline.
3. Consider intubation or tracheostomy.

C. Pulmonary edema

1. Furosemide (Lasix) 20–80 mg IV.
2. Nitroglycerin 0.4 mg sublingually, or paste $\frac{1}{2}$ in. on skin, or nitroglycerin drip 10–20 μg/min and increase by 5–10 μg every 10 minutes.
3. Afterload reduction with agents such as intravenous Nipride or oral agents such as captopril (Captopen) or enalapril (Vasotec).

4. Intravenous morphine for venodilation and to relieve anxiety. (Be prepared to intubate the patient.)
5. Oxygen. Start with two liters by nasal cannula.

D. **Miscellaneous disorders.** Treatment varies with the disease. Obviously, PE should be treated with anticoagulants. Suspected tumors require additional tests such as bronchoscopy before reasonable treatment can be initiated.

REFERENCE

Hollingsworth HW. Wheezing and stridor. *Clin Chest Med* 1987;8:231–240.

2 Laboratory and Diagnosis

The ranges of normal values are given below the test, first in conventional units such as metric (e.g., milligrams per liter), and then in international units if there is a difference. Reference ranges for each laboratory may vary from the values given; therefore, interpret the results of a patient's laboratory value in light of an individual facility's range.

■ ACTH (Adrenocorticotropic Hormone)

8 A.M.: 20–100 pg/mL or 20–100 ng/L; midnight value: approximately 50% of AM value.

Increased. Addison's disease, ectopic ACTH production (oat cell carcinoma, pancreatic islet cell tumors, thymic tumors, renal cell carcinoma).

Decreased. Adrenal adenoma or carcinoma, nodular adrenal hyperplasia, pituitary insufficiency.

■ ACTH STIMULATION TEST

Used to help diagnose adrenal insufficiency. Cortrosyn (an ACTH analog) is given at a dose of 0.25 mg IM or IV. Collect blood at time 0 and 30 and 60 minutes for cortisol.

Normal Response. Basal level cortisol of at least 5 μg/dL, an increase of at least 7 μg/dL, and a final cortisol of 16 μg/dL at 30 minutes or 18 μg/dL at 60 minutes.

Addison's Disease (Primary Adrenal Insufficiency) and Secondary Adrenal Insufficiency. Secondary insufficiency is caused by pituitary insufficiency or suppression by exogeneous steroids. An ACTH level and pituitary stimulation tests can be used to differentiate primary from secondary adrenal insufficiency.

■ ACID FAST STAIN

Negative.

Positive. *Mycobacterium* species (tuberculosis and atypical mycobacteria such as *avium-intracellulare*), *Nocardia, Actinomyces.*

■ ACID PHOSPHATASE

<3.0 ng/mL or 0.11–0.60 U/L.
Radioimmunoassay determination usually specific for the prostate.

Increased. Carcinoma of the prostate (usually metastatic), prostatic surgery or trauma, excessive platelet destruction (idiopathic thrombocytopenic purpura), rarely in bone disease.

■ ALBUMIN

3.5–5.0 g/dL or 35–50 g/L.

Decreased. Malnutrition, nephrotic syndrome, cystic fibrosis, multiple myeloma, Hodgkin's disease, leukemia, protein-losing enteropathies, chronic glomerulonephritis, cirrhosis, inflammatory bowel disease, collagen-vascular diseases, hyperthyroidism.

■ ALDOSTERONE

Serum—supine: 3–10 ng/dL or 0.083–0.28 nmol/L early AM, normal sodium intake; upright: 5–30 ng/dL or 0.138–0.83 nmol/L. Urinary—2–16 μg/24 h or 5.4–44.3 nmol/d.

Increased. Hyperaldosteronism (primary or secondary). Should confirm after oral or intravenous salt loading.

Decreased. Adrenal insufficiency.

■ ALKALINE PHOSPHATASE

Adult 20–70 U/L.
A γ-glutamyltransferase (GGT) is often useful to differentiate whether an elevated alkaline phosphatase has its origin in bone or liver. A normal GGT suggests bone origin.

Increased. Increased calcium deposition in bone (hyperparathyroidism), Paget's disease, osteoblastic bone tumors (metastatic or osteogenic sarcoma), osteomalacia, rickets, pregnancy, childhood, liver disease such as biliary obstruction (masses, drug therapy), hyperthyroidism.

Decreased. Malnutrition, excess vitamin D ingestion.

■ ALPHA-FETOPROTEIN (AFP)

<30 ng/mL or <30 μg/L

Increased. Hepatoma, testicular tumor (embryonal carcinoma, malignant teratoma), spina bifida (in mother's serum).

■ ALT (Alanine Aminotransaminase) (SGPT: Serum Glutamic-Pyruvic Transaminase)

8–20 U/L.

Increased. Liver disease–liver metastasis, biliary obstruction, pancreatitis, liver congestion, hepatitis (ALT is more elevated than AST in viral hepatitis; AST is more elevated than ALT in alcoholic hepatitis).

■ AMMONIA

Arterial: 15–45 μg N/dL or 11–32 μmol N/L.

Increased. Hepatic encephalopathy, Reye's syndrome.

■ AMYLASE

25–125 U/L.

Increased. Acute pancreatitis, pancreatic duct obstruction (stones, stricture, tumor, sphincter spasm secondary to drugs), alcohol ingestion, mumps, parotiditis, renal disease, macroamylasemia, cholecystitis, peptic ulcers, intestinal obstruction, mesenteric thrombosis, after surgery (upper abdominal), ovarian cancer, ruptured ectopic pregnancy, and diabetic ketoacidosis.

Decreased. Pancreatic destruction (pancreatitis, cystic fibrosis), liver damage (hepatitis, cirrhosis).

■ ANION GAP

8–12 mmol/L.
Anion gap is a calculated estimate of unmeasured anions and is used to help differentiate the cause of metabolic acidosis.

Anion gap = $(Na^+) - (Cl^- + HCO_3)$

Increased (High). (> 12 mmol/L): Lactic acidosis, ketoacidosis (diabetic, alcoholic, starvation), uremia, toxins (salicylates, methanol, ethylene glycol, paraldehyde), hyperalimentation.

Decreased (Low). (< 8 mmol/L): Seen with bromide ingestion, hypernatremia, multiple myeloma, dilutional, and hypoalbuminemia.

■ ANTINUCLEAR ANTIBODIES (ANA)

Negative.
A useful screening test in patients with symptoms suggesting collagen-vascular disease, especially if titer is ≥1:160.

Positive. Systemic lupus erythematosus (SLE), drug-induced lupuslike syndromes (procainamide, hydralazine, isoniazid, etc.), scleroderma, mixed connective tissue disease (MCTD), rheumatoid arthritis, polymyositis, juvenile rheumatoid arthritis (5% to 20%). Low titers are also seen in non–collagen-vascular disease.

SPECIFIC IMMUNOFLUORESCENT ANA PATTERNS

ANA Patterns

Homogenous. Nonspecific, from antibodies to deoxyribonucleoproteins (DNP) and native double-stranded deoxyribonucleic acid (DNA). Seen in SLE and a variety of other diseases. Antihistone is consistent with drug-induced lupus.

Speckled. Pattern seen in many connective tissue disorders. From antibodies to extractable nuclear antigens (ENA) including antiribonucleoproteins (anti-RNP), anti-Sm, anti-PM-1, and anti-SS. Anti-RNP is positive in MCTD and SLE. Anti-Sm is found in SLE. Anti-SS-A and anti-SS-B are seen in Sjögren's syndrome and subacute cutaneous lupus. The speckled pattern is also seen with scleroderma.

Peripheral RIM Pattern. From antibodies to native double-stranded DNA and DNP. Seen in SLE.

Nucleolar Pattern. From antibodies to nucleolar ribonucleic acid (RNA). Positive in Sjögren's syndrome and scleroderma.

Other Autoantibodies

Antimitochondrial. Primary biliary cirrhosis.

Anti–Smooth Muscle. Low titers are seen in a variety of illnesses; high titers (>1:100) are suggestive of chronic active hepatitis.

Antimicrosomal. Hashimoto's thyroiditis.

■ AST (Aspartate Aminotransaminase) (SGOT: Serum Glutamic-Oxaloacetic Transaminase)

8–20 U/L.
Generally parallels changes in ALT in liver disease.

Increased. Liver disease, acute myocardial infarction, Reye's syndrome, muscle trauma and injection, pancreatitis, intestinal injury or surgery, factitious increase (erythromycin, opiates), burns, brain damage.

Decreased. Beri-beri, severe diabetes with ketoacidosis, liver disease.

■ B_{12} (Vitamin B_{12})

140–700 pg/mL or 189–516 pmol/L.

Increased. Leukemia, polycythemia vera.

Decreased. Pernicious anemia, bacterial overgrowth, dietary deficiency (rare—normally 2 to 3 years of stores), malabsorption, pregnancy.

■ BASE EXCESS/DEFICIT

See Table 2–1. A decrease in base (bicarbonate) is termed *base deficit;* an increase in base is termed *base excess.*

Excess. Metabolic alkalosis (see Chapter 1, Alkalosis, p 19), respiratory acidosis (see Chapter 1, Acidosis, p 11).

Deficit. Metabolic acidosis (see Chapter 1, Acidosis, p 11), respiratory alkalosis (see Chapter 1, Alkalosis, p 19).

■ BENCE-JONES PROTEINS—URINE

Negative.

Positive. Multiple myeloma, idiopathic Bence-Jones proteinuria.

■ BICARBONATE (Serum HCO_3^-)

22–29 mmol/L.
See Tables 2–1 and 2–2. Also see **Carbon Dioxide, Arterial,** for pCO_2 values.

TABLE 2–1. NORMAL BLOOD GAS VALUES

Measurement	Arterial	Mixed Venous	Venous
pH (range)	7.40 (7.38–7.44)	7.36 (7.31–7.41)	7.36 (7.31–7.41)
pO_2 (decreases with age)	80–100 mm Hg	35–40 mm Hg	30–50 mm Hg
pCO_2	35–45 mm Hg	41–51 mm Hg	40–52 mm Hg
O_2 saturation (decreases with age)	>95%	60%–80%	60%–85%
HCO_3^-	22–26 mmol/L	22–26 mmol/L	22–29 mmol/L
Base difference (deficit/ excess)	−2 to +2	−2 to+2	−2 to +2

[a]From right atrium.
From Gomella LG, ed. Clinician's Pocket Reference, *6th ed. East Norwalk, Conn: Appleton & Lange; 1989. Used with permission.*

TABLE 2–2. ACID-BASE DISORDERS WITH APPROPRIATE COMPENSATION

	Changes in Normal Values		
Disorder	***pH***	***HCO_3^-***	***pCO_2***
Metabolic acidosis	↓	↓↓	↓
Metabolic alkalosis	↑	↑↑	↑
Respiratory acidosis	↓	↑	↑↑
Respiratory alkalosis	↑	↓	↓↓

Increased. Metabolic alkalosis, compensation for respiratory acidosis. (See Chapter 1, Alkalosis, p 19, and Acidosis, p 11.)

Decreased. Metabolic acidosis, compensation for respiratory alkalosis. (See Chapter 1, Acidosis, p 11, and Alkalosis, p 19.)

■ BILIRUBIN

Total: <0.2–1.0 mg/dL or 3.4–17.1 μmol/L; direct: <0.2 mg/dL or <3.4 μmol/L; indirect: <0.8 mg/dL or <13.7 μmol/L.

Increased Total. Hepatic damage (hepatitis, toxins, cirrhosis), biliary obstruction (stone or tumor), hemolysis, fasting.

Increased Direct (Conjugated). Biliary obstruction (gallstone, tumor, stricture), drug-induced cholestasis, Dubin-Johnson syndrome, and Rotor's syndrome.

Increased Indirect (Unconjugated). Hemolytic anemia (transfusion reaction, sickle cell, collagen-vascular disease), Gilbert's disease, Crigler-Najjar syndrome.

■ BLEEDING TIME

Duke, Ivy: <6 min; Template: <10 min.

Increased. Thrombocytopenia, thrombocytopenic purpura, von Willebrand's disease, defective platelet function (aspirin, nonsteroidal anti-inflammatory drugs, uremia).

■ BLOOD GAS, ARTERIAL

See Tables 2–1 and 2–2. For acid-base disorders, see Chapter 1, Acidosis, p 9, and Alkalosis, p 17.

■ BLOOD GAS, VENOUS

See Table 2–1. There is little difference between arterial and venous pH and bicarbonate (except with congestive heart failure and shock); therefore, the venous blood gas may be occasionally used to assess acid-base status, but venous oxygen levels are significantly less than arterial levels.

■ BLOOD UREA NITROGEN (BUN)

7–18 mg/dL or 1.2–3.0 mmol urea/L.

Increased. Renal failure, prerenal azotemia (decreased renal perfusion secondary to congestive heart failure, shock, volume depletion), postrenal obstruction, gastrointestinal bleeding, hypercatabolic states.

Decreased. Starvation, liver failure (hepatitis, drugs), pregnancy, infancy, nephrotic syndrome, overhydration.

■ CBC (Complete Blood Count, Hemogram)

For normal values, see Table 2–3. For differential, see specific tests.

TABLE 2–3. NORMAL CBC VALUES—ADULTS[a]

WBC	4800–10,800 cells/μL
RBCs	M: 4.7–6.1 × 10^6 cells/μL
	F: 4.2–5.4 × 10^6 cells/μL
Hemoglobin	M: 14–18 g/dL
	F: 12–16 g/dL
Hematocrit	M: 40–54%
	F: 37–47%
MCV	M: 80–94 fL
	F: 81–99 fL
MCH	27–31 pg
MCHC (%)	33%–37%
RDW	11.5–14.5
Platelets	150–450,000/μL
■ **DIFFERENTIAL**	
Segmented neutrophils	41%–71%
Stab neutrophils	5%–10%
Lymphocytes	24%–44%
Monocytes	3%– 7%
Eosinophils	1%– 3%
Basophils	0%– 1%

[a]Refer to hospital reference values.
Modified from Gomella LG, ed. Clinician's Pocket Reference. *6th ed. East Norwalk, Conn: Appleton & Lange; 1989. Used with permission.*

■ C-PEPTIDE

Fasting: ≤4.0 ng/mL or ≤4.0 μg/L; male >60 years: 1.5–5.0 ng/mL or 1.5–5.0 μg/L; female: 1.4–5.5 ng/mL or 1.4–5.5 μg/L.

Decreased. Diabetes (insulin-dependent diabetes mellitus), insulin administration, hypoglycemia.

■ CALCITONIN

<100 pg/mL or <100 ng/L

Increased. Medullary carcinoma of the thyroid, pregnancy, chronic renal insufficiency, Zollinger-Ellison syndrome, pernicious anemia.

■ CALCIUM, SERUM

8.4–10.2 mg/dL (4.2–5.1 mEq/L) or 2.10–2.55 mmol/L; ionized: 4.5–4.9 mg/dL (2.2–2.5 mEq/L) or 1.1–1.2 mmol/L.

When interpreting a total calcium value, the albumin must be known. If the albumin is not within normal limits, a corrected calcium can be roughly calculated with the following formula. Values for ionized calcium need no special corrections.

$$\text{Corrected total Ca} = 0.8\,(\text{normal albumin} - \text{measured albumin}) + \text{reported Ca}$$

Increased. See Chapter 1, Hypercalcemia, p 133.

Decreased. See Chapter 1, Hypocalcemia, p 153.

■ CALCIUM, URINE

Calcium-free diet: <540 mg or 0.13–1.00 mmol per 24-hour urine; average calcium diet: 100–300 mg per 24-hour urine

Increased. Hyperparathyroidism, hyperthyroidism, hypervitaminosis D, distal renal tubular acidosis (type I), sarcoidosis, immobilization, osteolytic lesions (bony metastasis, multiple myeloma), Paget's disease, glucocorticoid excess (either endogenous or exogenous), furosemide.

Decreased. Thiazide diuretics, hypothyroidism, renal failure, steatorrhea, rickets, osteomalacia.

■ CARBON DIOXIDE, ARTERIAL (pCO_2)

35–45 mm Hg. See Tables 2–1 and 2–2, p 266.

Increased. Respiratory acidosis, compensation for metabolic alkalosis. (See Chapter 1, Acidosis, p 11,and Alkalosis, p 19.)

Decreased. Respiratory alkalosis, compensation for metabolic acidosis. (See Chapter 1, Acidosis, p 11, and Alkalosis, p 19.)

■ CARBOXYHEMOGLOBIN

Nonsmoker: <2%; smoker: <6%; toxic: >15%.

Increased. Smokers, smoke inhalation, automobile exhaust inhalation, inadequate ventilation with faulty heating units.

■ CARCINOEMBRYONIC ANTIGEN (CEA)

Nonsmoker: <3.0 ng/mL or <3.0 μg/L; smoker: <5.0 ng/mL or <5.0 μg/L.

Increased. Carcinoma (colon, pancreas, lung, stomach), smokers, nonneoplastic liver disease, Crohn's disease, and ulcerative colitis. Used predominantly in monitoring patients for recurrence of carcinoma, especially status post resection for colon carcinoma.

■ CATECHOLAMINES, FRACTIONATED

Values are variable and depend on the lab and method of assay used. Normal levels listed here are based on high-performance liquid chromatography technique.

	Plasma (Supine)	Urine
Norepinephrine	70–750 pg/mL	14–80 μg/24 h
	414–4435 pmol/L	82.7–473 nmol/d
Epinephrine	0–100 pg/mL	0.5–20 μg/24 h
	0–546 pmol/L	2.73–109 nmol/d
Dopamine	< 30 pg/mL	65–400 μg/24 h
	< 196 pmol/L	424–2612 nmol/d

Increased. Pheochromocytoma, neural crest tumors (neuroblastoma). With extra-adrenal pheochromocytoma norepinephrine may be markedly elevated compared with epinephrine.

■ CATECHOLAMINES, URINE, UNCONJUGATED

>15 years old: <100 μg/24 h.
Measures free (unconjugated) epinephrine, norepinephrine, and dopamine.

Increased. Pheochromocytoma, neural crest tumors (neuroblastoma).

■ CHLORIDE, SERUM

98–106 mEq/L

Increased. Diarrhea, renal tubular acidosis, mineralocorticoid deficiency, hyperalimentation, medications (acetazolamide, ammonium chloride).

Decreased. Vomiting, diabetes mellitus with ketoacidosis, mineralocorticoid excess, renal disease with sodium loss.

■ CHLORIDE, URINE

110–250 mmol per 24-hour urine
See **Urinary Electrolytes.**

■ CHOLESTEROL (Total)

140–240 mg/dL or 3.63–6.22 mmol/L; desired level: <200 mg/dL or 5.18 mmol/L.

Increased. Primary hypercholesterolemia (types IIA, IIB, III), elevated triglycerides (types I, IV, V), biliary obstruction, nephrosis, hypothyroidism, diabetes, pregnancy.

Decreased. Liver disease (eg, hepatitis), hyperthyroidism, malnutrition (cancer, starvation), chronic anemias, steroid therapy, lipoproteinemias.

High-Density Lipoprotein (HDL) Cholesterol

Fasting male: 30–70 mg/dL or 0.78–1.81 mmol/L; female: 30–80 mg/dL or 0.78–2.07 mmol/L.
HDL has the best correlation with the development of coronary artery disease; decreased HDL in males leads to an increased risk.

Increased. Estrogen (females), exercise, ethanol.

Decreased. Males, uremia, obesity, diabetes, liver disease, Tangier's disease.

Low-Density Lipoprotein (LDH) Cholesterol

Desired: <130–160 mg/dL or 3.36–4.14 mmol/L.

Increased. Excess dietary saturated fats, myocardial infarction, hyperlipoproteinemia, biliary cirrhosis, endocrine disease (diabetes, hypothyroidism).

Decreased. Malabsorption, severe liver disease, abetalipoproteinemia.

Triglycerides

See **Triglycerides.**

■ COLD AGGLUTININS

< 1:32.

Increased. Mycoplasma pneumonia, viral infections (especially mononucleosis, measles, mumps), cirrhosis, some parasitic infections.

■ COMPLEMENT C3

80–155 mg/dL or 800–1550 ng/L; >60 years: 80–170 mg/dL or 80–1700 ng/L. Normal values may vary greatly depending on the assay used.

Increased. Rheumatic fever, various neoplasms (gastrointestinal, prostate, others).

Decreased. Systemic lupus erytheratosus, glomerulonephritis (poststreptococcal and membranoproliferative), vasculitis, severe hepatic failure.

Variable. Rheumatoid arthritis.

■ COMPLEMENT C4

20–50 mg/dL or 200–500 ng/L.

Increased. Neoplasma (gastrointestinal, lung, others).

Decreased. Systemic lupus erythematosus, chronic active hepatitis, cirrhosis, glomerulonephritis, hereditary angioedema.

Variable. Rheumatoid arthritis.

■ COMPLEMENT CH50 (TOTAL)

33–61 mg/mL or 330–610 ng/L. Tests for complement deficiency in the classical pathway.

Increased. Acute-phase reactants (eg, tissue injury, infections).

Decreased. Hereditary complement deficiencies, any cause of deficiency of individual complement components.

■ COOMBS' TEST, DIRECT

Negative.
Uses patient's erythrocytes; tests for the presence of antibody or complement on the patient's red blood cells.

Positive. Autoimmune hemolytic anemia (leukemia, lymphoma, collagen-vascular diseases, systemic lupus erythematosus), hemolytic transfusion reaction, sensitization to some drugs (methyldopa, levodopa, penicillins, cephalosporins).

■ COOMBS' TEST, INDIRECT

Negative.
More useful for red cell typing. Uses serum that contains antibody from the patient.

Positive. Isoimmunization from previous transfusion, incompatible blood as a result of improper cross-matching.

■ CORTISOL

Serum—8 AM: 5.0–23.0 μg/dL or 138–635 nmol/L; 4 PM: 3.0–15.0 μg/dL or 83–414 nmol/L. Urine (24 hour)—10–100 μg/d or 27.6–276 nmol/d.

Increased. Adrenal adenoma, adrenal carcinoma, Cushing's disease, nonpituitary ACTH-producing tumor, steroid therapy, oral contraceptives.

Decreased. Primary adrenal insufficiency (Addison's disease), Waterhouse-Friderichsen syndrome, ACTH deficiency.

■ CORTROSYN STIMULATION TEST

See **ACTH Stimulation Test.**

■ COUNTERIMMUNOELECTROPHORESIS (CIE)

Negative.
An immunologic technique that allows rapid identification of infecting organisms from fluids including serum, urine, cerebrospinal fluid, and other body fluids. Organisms that can be identified include *Neisseria meningitidis, Streptococcus pneumoniae, Hemophilus influenzae,* and group B streptococcus.

■ CREATINE PHOSPHOKINASE (CPK)

25–145 mU/mL or 25–145 U/L.

Increased. Cardiac muscle (acute myocardial infarction, myocarditis, defibrillation), skeletal muscle (intramuscular injection, hypothyroidism, rhabdomyolysis, polymyositis, muscular dystrophy), brain infarction.

CPK Isoenzymes MM, MB, BB. MB (normal $< 6\%$) increased in acute myocardial infarction (begins in 4–8 hours, peaks at 24 hours), cardiac surgery; BB not frequently seen or useful.

■ CREATININE CLEARANCE

Male: 100–135 mL/min or 0.963–1.300 mL/s/m^2; female: 85–125 mL/min or 0.819–1.204 mL/s/m^2. A concurrent serum creatinine and a

24-hour urine creatinine are needed. A shorter time interval can be used and corrected for in the formula. A quick formula for estimation is also found on p 499, Table 7–13, on Aminoglycoside Dosing.

$$\text{Creatinine clearance} = \frac{\text{urine creatinine} \times \text{total urine volume}}{\text{plasma creatinine} \times \text{time in minutes}}$$

To verify if the urine sample is a complete 24-hour collection, determine if the sample contains at least 18–25 mg/kg/24 h or 125–220 μmol/kg/d creatinine for adult males or 12–20 mg/kg/24 h or 106–177 μmol/kg/d for adult females. This test is not a requirement.

Decreased. A decreased creatinine clearance results in an increase in serum creatinine usually secondary to renal insufficiency. Clearance normally decreases with age. See **Creatinine, Serum, Increased.**

Increased. Pregnancy.

■ CREATININE, SERUM

Male: 0.7–1.3 mg/dL; female: 0.6–1.1 mg/dL.

Increased. Renal failure (prerenal, renal, or postrenal), acromegaly, ingestion of roasted meat, large body mass. Falsely elevated with ketones and certain cephalosporins depending on assay.

■ CREATININE, URINE

Male total creatinine: 14–26 mg/kg/24 h or 124–230 μmol/kg/d; female: 11–20 mg/kg/24 h or 97–177 μmol/kg/d. See **Creatinine Clearance.**

■ CRYOCRIT

$\leq$ **0.4%.** (Negative if qualitative.) Cryocrit, a quantitative measure, is preferred over the qualitative method. Should be collected in nonanticoagulated tubes and transported at body temperature. Positive samples can be analyzed for immunoglobulin class, and light chain type on request.

$>$ **0.4%** (Positive if qualitative.) *Monoclonal*—Multiple myeloma, Waldenström's macroglobulinemia, lymphoma, chronic lymphocytic leukemia.

Mixed polyclonal or mixed monoclonal—Infectious diseases (viral, bacterial, parasitic) such as subacute bacterial endocarditis or malaria, systemic lupus erythematosus, rheumatoid arthritis, essential cryoglobulinemia, lymphoproliferative diseases, sarcoidosis, chronic liver disease (cirrhosis).

■ DEXAMETHASONE SUPPRESSION TEST

Used in the differential diagnosis of Cushing's syndrome.

Overnight Dexamethasone Suppression Test

In the rapid version, a patient takes 1 mg of dexamethasone PO at 11 PM and a fasting 8 AM plasma cortisol is obtained. Normally, the cortisol level should be <5 μg/dL or <138 nmol/L. A value >5 μg/dL or >138 nmol/L suggests the diagnosis of Cushing's syndrome; however, suppression may not occur with obesity, alcoholism, or depression. In these patients, the best screening test is a 24-hour urine for free cortisol.

Low-Dose Dexamethasone Suppression Test

After collection of baseline serum cortisol and 24-hour urine free cortisol levels, dexamethasone 0.5 mg PO is administered every 6 hours for eight doses. Serum cortisol and 24-hour urine for free cortisol are repeated on the second day. Failure to suppress to a serum cortisol of <5 μg/dL (138 nmol/L) and a urine free cortisol <30 μg/dL (82 nmol/L) confirms Cushing's syndrome.

High-Dose Test

After the low-dose test, dexamethasone 2 mg PO every 6 hours for eight doses is administered. A fall in urinary free cortisol to 50% of the baseline value occurs in patients with Cushing's disease, but not in patients with adrenal tumors or ectopic ACTH production.

■ ETHANOL LEVEL

See Drug Levels, Table 7–11, p 498.

■ FERRITIN

Male: 15–200 ng/mL or 15–220 μg/L; female: 12–150 ng/mL or 12–150 μg/L.

Decreased. Iron deficiency, severe liver disease.

Increased. Hemochromatosis, hemosiderosis, sideroblastic anemia.

■ FIBRIN DEGRADATION PRODUCTS (FDP)

< 10 μg/mL.

Increased. Any thromboembolic condition (deep venous thrombosis, myocardial infarction, pulmonary embolus), disseminated intravascular coagulation, hepatic dysfunction.

■ FIBRINOGEN

150–450 mg/dL or 150–450 g/L.

Decreased. Congenital, disseminated intravascular coagulation (sepsis, amniotic fluid embolism, abruptio placentae, prostatic or cardiac surgery), burns, neoplastic and hematologic malignancies, acute severe bleeding, snake bite.

Increased. Inflammatory processes (acute-phase reactant).

■ FOLATE RED BLOOD CELL

160–640 ng or 360–1450 nmol/mL RBC.
More sensitive for detecting folate deficiency from malnourishment if the patient has started proper nutrition before the serum folate is measured.

Increased. See **Folic Acid.**

Decreased. See **Folic Acid.**

■ FOLIC ACID (Serum Folate)

2–14 ng/mL or 4.5–31.7 nmol/L.

Increased. Folic acid administration.

Decreased. Malnutrition, malabsorption, massive cellular growth (cancer), hemolytic anemia, pregnancy.

■ FTA-ABS (Fluorescent Treponemal Antibody Absorbed)

Nonreactive.

Positive. Syphilis (test of choice to confirm diagnosis). May be negative in early primary syphilis and can remain positive after adequate treatment.

■ FUNGAL SEROLOGIES

Negative (< 1:8). This is a complement-fixation fungal antibody screen that usually detects antibodies to *Histoplasma, Blastomyces, Aspergillus,* and *Coccidiodes.*

■ GASTRIN

Male: <100 pg/mL or <100 ng/L; Female: < 75 pg/mL.

Increased. Zollinger-Ellison syndrome, pyloric stenosis, pernicious anemia, atrophic gastritis, ulcerative colitis, renal insufficiency, steroid and calcium administration.

■ GLUCOSE

Fasting: 70–105 mg/dL or 3.89–5.83 nmol/L: 2 hours postprandial: 70–120 mg/dL or 3.89–6.67 mmol/L.

Increased. (See Chapter 1, Hyperglycemia, p 137.)

Decreased. (See Chapter 1, Hypoglycemia, p 157.)

■ GAMMA-GLUTAMYLTRANSFERASE (SGGT)

Male: 9–50 U/L; female: 8–40 U/L. Generally parallels changes in serum alkaline phosphatase and 5′-nucleotidase in liver disease.

Increased. Liver disease (hepatitis, cirrhosis, obstructive jaundice), pancreatitis.

■ GLYCOHEMOGLOBIN (Hemoglobin A_{1c})

4.6%–7.1%.

Increased. Diabetes mellitus.

■ GRAM STAIN

Rapid Technique

Spread thin layer of specimen onto glass slide and allow to dry. Fix with heat. Apply Gentian violet (15–20 seconds); follow with iodine (15–20 seconds), then alcohol (just a few seconds until effluent is barely decolorized). Rinse with water and counterstain with safranin (15–20 seconds). Examine under oil immersion lens: gram positives are dark blue and gram negatives are red.

Gram-Positive Cocci. *Staphylococcus, Streptococcus, Micrococcus, Peptococcus* (anaerobic), and *Peptostreptococcus* (anaerobic) species.

Gram-Positive Rods. *Clostridium* (anaerobic), *Corynebacterium, Listeria, Bacillus,* and *Bacteroides* (anaerobic) species.

Gram-Negative Cocci. *Neisseria* species.

Gram-Negative Coccoid Rods. *Hemophilus, Pasteurella, Brucella, Francisella, Yersinia,* and *Bordetella* species.

Gram-Negative Straight Rods. *Acinetobacter* (Mima, Herellea), *Aeromonas, Bacteroides* (anaerobic), *Campylobacter* (comma-shaped) species, *Eikenella, Enterobacter, Escherichia, Fusobacterium* (anaerobic), *Klebsiella, Legionella, Proteus, Providencia, Pseudomonas, Salmonella, Serratia, Shigella, Vibrio, Yersenia.*

■ HAPTOGLOBIN

26–185 mg/mL.

Increased. Obstructive liver disease, any inflammatory process.

Decreased. Hemolysis (eg, transfusion reaction), severe liver disease.

■ HEMATOCRIT

See Table 2–3, p 268, for normal values.

Increased. See Chapter 1, Polycythemia, p 223.

Decreased. See Chapter 1, Anemia, p 25.

■ HEMOGLOBIN

See Table 2–3, p 268, for normal values. Also see Chapter 1, Anemia, p 25.

Increased. See **Hematocrit, Increased.**

Decreased. See **Hematocrit, Decreased.**

■ HEPATITIS TESTS

See Table 2–4, p 280.

HBsAg Hepatitis B surface antigen (formerly Australia antigen). Indicates either chronic or acute infection with hepatitis B. Used by blood banks to screen donors.

Total Anti-HB_c IgG and IgM antibody to hepatitis B core antigen. Confirms either previous exposure to hepatitis B virus (HBV) or ongoing infection. Used by blood banks to screen donors.

Anti-HB_c IgM IgM antibody to hepatitis B core antigen. Early and best indicator of acute infection with hepatitis B.

HB_eAg Hepatitis B_e antigen. When present, indicates high degree of infectivity. Order **only** when evaluating a patient with chronic HBV infection.

Anti-HB_e Antibody to hepatitis B_e antigen. Presence is associated with resolution of active inflammation but often means virus is integrated into host DNA, especially if host remains HB_sAg positive.

Anti-HB_s Antibody to hepatitis B surface antigen. Typically indicates immunity associated with clinical recovery from an HBV infection or previous immunization with hepatitis B vaccine. Order **only** to assess effectiveness of vaccine and ask for titer.

Anti-HAV Total antibody to hepatitis A virus. Confirms previous exposure to hepatitis A virus.

Anti-HAV IgM IgM antibody to hepatitis A virus. Indicates recent, acute infection with hepatitis A virus.

Anti-HDV Total antibody to delta hepatitis. Confirms previous exposure. Order **only** in patients with known acute or chronic HBV infection.

Anti-HDV IgM IgM antibody to delta hepatitis. Indicates recent infection. Order **only** in patients with known acute or chronic HBV infection.

Anti-HCV Antibody against hepatitis C, formerly known as non-A non-B virus and the major cause of posttransfusion hepatitis. Test is now commercially available. Is being used by blood banks to screen donors and in patients with chronic hepatitis.

■ HUMAN CHORIONIC GONADOTROPIN, SERUM (HCG Beta Subunit)

<3.0 mIU/mL; 7–10 days postconception: >3 mIU/mL; 30 days: 100–5000 mIU/mL; 10 weeks: 50,000–140,000 mIU/mL; >16 weeks: 10,000–50,000 mIU/mL; thereafter: levels slowly decline.

Increased. Pregnancy, testicular tumors, trophoblastic disease (hydatidiform mole, choriocarcinoma levels usually > 100,000 mIU/mL).

TABLE 2–4. HEPATITIS PANEL TESTING

Profile Name	Markers	Purpose
SCREENING TESTS		
Admission: High-risk patients (homosexuals, dialysis patients)	HB_sAg	To screen for chronic or active infection
Percutaneous inoculation	HB_sAg Anti-HB_c IgM	Test serum of patient for possible infectivity with HBV when a health care worker is exposed.
	HB_sAg Anti-HB_c	Test exposed person for immunity or chronic infection; in particular, dialysis patients and health care workers
Pre-HBV vaccine in high-risk patients	HB_sAg Anti-HB_c	To determine if an individual is infected or has antibodies
DIAGNOSTIC TESTS		
Differential diagnosis	HB_sAg Anti-HB_c IgM Anti-HAV IgM	To differentiate between hepatitis A, hepatitis B, and non-A/non-B in acute infection (up to 12 weeks after the onset of symptoms)
Acute hepatitis B	HB_sAg Anti-HB_c IgM	To diagnose acute hepatitis B infection (2–12 weeks after onset of hepatitis symptoms)
	Anti-HDV IgM	To diagnose delta virus in patients with acute or chronic hepatitis B
Acute hepatitis A	Anti-HAV IgM	To diagnose recent infection with hepatitis A
MONITOR		
Chronic	HB_sAg HB_eAg/Anti-HB_e Anti-HB_c IgM	To test for late seroconversion and/or disease resolution in known hepatitis B carrier
Postvaccination screening	Anti-HB_s	To ensure immunity has been achieved after vaccination
Sexual contact	Hb_sAg Anti-HB_c	To monitor sexual partners with acute or chronic hepatitis B

Courtesy Abbott Laboratories, North Chicago, Illinois. Modified by Steven Shedlofsky, MD.

■ 5-HIAA (5-Hydroxyindoleacetic Acid)

2–8 mg or 10.4–41.6 μmol/24-h urine collection. 5-HIAA is a serotonin metabolite.

Increased. Carcinoid tumors, certain foods (banana, pineapple, tomato).

■ HUMAN IMMUNODEFICIENCY VIRUS (HIV) ANTIBODY TEST

Negative. Used in the diagnosis of acquired immunodeficiency syndrome (AIDS) and HIV infection and to screen blood for use in transfusion.

ELISA

Enzyme-linked immunoabsorbent assay to detect HIV antibody. A positive test is usually confirmed by Western blot.

Positive. AIDS, asymptomatic HIV infection, false-positive test.

Western Blot

The technique used as the reference procedure for confirming the presence or absence of HIV antibody, usually after a positive HIV antibody by ELISA determination.

Positive. AIDS, asymptomatic HIV infection.
Note: In the future, polymerase chain reaction may become a viable tool for detection of the HIV virus. At this point, it is used on a research basis only. It will be useful especially in very early infection, when antibody may not be present.

■ IRON

Males: 65–175 μg/dL or 11.64–31.33 μmol/L; females: 50–170 μg/dL or 8.95–30.43 μmol/L.

Increased. Hemochromatosis, hemosiderosis caused by excessive iron intake, excess destruction or decreased production of erythrocytes, liver necrosis.

Decreased. Iron deficiency anemia, nephrosis (loss of iron-binding proteins), anemia of chronic disease.

■ IRON BINDING CAPACITY, TOTAL (TIBC)

250–450 μg/dL or 44.75–80.55 μmol/L.
The normal iron/TIBC ratio is 20% to 50%; $<$15% is characteristic of iron deficiency anemia. An increased ratio is seen with hemochromatosis.

Increased. Acute and chronic blood loss, iron deficiency anemia, hepatitis, oral contraceptives.

Decreased. Anemia of chronic disease, cirrhosis, nephrosis, hemochromatosis.

■ 17-KETOGENIC STEROIDS (17-KGS)

Males: 5–23 mg or 17–80 μmol/24-h urine; females: 3–15 mg or 10–52 μmol/24-h urine.

Increased. Adrenal hyperplasia.

Decreased. Panhypopituarism, Addison's disease, acute steroid withdrawal.

■ 17-KETOSTEROIDS (17-KS)

Males: 9–22 mg or 31–76 μmol/24-h urine; females: 6–15 mg or 21–52 μmol/24-h urine.

Increased. Cushing's syndrome, 11- and 21-hydroxylase deficiency, severe stress, exogenous steroids, excess ACTH or androgens.

Decreased. Addison's disease, anorexia nervosa, panhypopituitarism.

■ KOH PREP

Negative.

Positive. Superficial mycoses (*Candida, Trichophyton, Microsporum, Epidermophyton, Keratinomyces*).

■ LACTATE DEHYDROGENASE (LDH)

45–100 U/L.

Increased. Acute myocardial infarction, cardiac surgery, hepatitis, pernicious anemia, malignant tumors, pulmonary embolus, hemolysis, renal infarction.

LDH Isoenzymes (LDH 1 to LDH 5). Normally, the ratio LDH 1/LDH 2 is < 0.6–0.7. If the ratio becomes larger than 1 or approaches 1, suspect a recent myocardial infarction. With an acute myocardial infarction, the LDH begins to rise at 10 to 12 hours, peaks at 48 to 72 hours, and remains elevated for 7–10 days. LDH 5 is increased in hepatitis.

■ LACTIC ACID (Lactate)

4.5–19.8 mg/dL or 0.5–2.2 mmol/L.

Increased. Lactic acidosis resulting from hypoxia, hemorrhage, circulatory collapse, sepsis, cirrhosis, exercise.

■ LE (Lupus Erythematosus) PREPARATION

"No cells seen" is normal.

Positive. Systemic lupus erythematosus, scleroderma, rheumatoid arthritis, drug-induced lupus (procainamide, others). ANA is more sensitive.

■ LEUKOCYTE ALKALINE PHOSPHATASE SCORE (LAP Score)

70–140.

Increased. Leukemoid reaction, Hodgkin's disease, polycythemia vera, myeloproliferative disorders, pregnancy, liver disease, acute inflammation.

Decreased. Chronic myelogenous leukemia, pernicious anemia, paroxysmal nocturnal hemoglobinuria, nephrotic syndrome.

■ LIPASE

Variable depending on the method; 10–150 U/L by turbidimetric method.

Increased. Acute pancreatitis, pancreatic duct obstruction (stone, stricture, tumor, drug-induced spasm), fat emboli. Usually normal in mumps.

■ LYMPHOCYTES, TOTAL

1800–3000/mL.
Often used to assess nutritional status. Calculated by multiplying the white cell count by the percentage of lymphocytes: <900, severe; 900–1400, moderate; 1400–1800, minimal nutritional deficit. Lymphopenia is also seen with certain viral infections including human immunodeficiency virus.

■ MAGNESIUM

1.6–2.4 mg/dL or 0.80–1.20 mmol/L.

Increased. Renal failure, hypothyroidism, magnesium-containing antacids, Addison's disease, severe dehydration.

Decreased. See Chapter 1, Hypomagnesemia, p 164.

■ MAGNESIUM, URINE

6.0–10.0 mEq/d or 3.00–5.00 mmol/d.

Increased. Hypermagnesemia, diuretics, hypercalcemia, metabolic acidosis, hypophosphatemia.

Decreased. Hypomagnesemia, hypocalcemia, hypoparathyroidism, metabolic alkalosis.

■ METANEPHRINES, URINE

Total: <1.0 mg or 0.574 mmol/24-h urine; fractionated metanephrines-normetanephrines: <0.9 mg or 0.517 mmol/24-h urine; fractionated metanephrines: <0.4 mg or 0.230 mg/24-h urine.

Increased. Pheochromocytoma, neural crest tumors (neuroblastoma), false positives with drugs (phenobarbital, hydrocortisone, others).

■ MONOSPOT

Negative.

Positive. Mononucleosis.

■ MYOGLOBIN, URINE

Qualitative negative.

Positive. Disorders affecting skeletal muscle (crush injury, rhabdomyolysis, electrical burns, delirium tremens, surgical procedures), acute myocardial infarction.

■ NITROGEN BALANCE

+4 to +20 g/d or +275 to +1400 mmol/d; urinary nitrogen: 12–24 g/24-h urine or 850–1700 mmol/24-h urine.
Most often used in the assessment of patients on hyperalimentation. A positive nitrogen balance is usually the goal.

$$\text{Nitrogen balance} = \frac{\text{24-hour protein intake (g)}}{6.25} - (\text{24 hr urine nitrogen} + 4)$$

■ 5′-NUCLEOTIDASE

2–15 U/L.

Increased. Obstructive liver disease.

■ OSMOLALITY, SERUM

275–295 mOsm/kg.
A rough estimation of osmolality is [2(sodium) + BUN/2.8 + glucose/18]). Will not be accurate if foreign substances that increase the osmolality are present, such as mannitol.

Increased. Hyperglycemia, alcohol ingestion, increased sodium resulting from water loss (diabetes, hypercalcemia, diuresis), ethylene glycol ingestion, mannitol.

Decreased. Low serum sodium, diuretics, Addison's disease, hypothyroidism, syndrome of inappropriate antidiuretic hormone (SIADH), iatrogenic causes (poor fluid balance).

■ OSMOLALITY, URINE

Spot 50–1400 mOsm/kg; > 850 mOsm/kg after 12 hours of fluid restriction.
The loss of the ability to concentrate urine, especially during fluid restriction, is an early indicator of impaired renal function.

■ OXYGEN, ARTERIAL (pO_2)

See Table 2–1, p 266. Also see Chapter 6.

Decreased. *Ventilation-Perfusion (V/Q) Abnormalities*—COPD, asthma, atelectasis, pneumonia, pulmonary embolus, respiratory distress syndrome, pneumothorax, cystic fibrosis, obstructed airway.

Alveolar Hypoventilation—Skeletal abnormalities, neuromuscular disorders, Pickwickian syndrome.

Decreased pulmonary diffusing capacity—Pneumoconiosis, pulmonary edema, pulmonary fibrosis.

Right-to-left shunt—Congenital heart disease (tetralogy of Fallot, transposition, others).

■ pH, ARTERIAL

See Table 2–1 and Table 2–2, p 266.

Increased. Metabolic and respiratory alkalosis. See Chapter 1, Alkalosis, p 19.

Decreased. Metabolic and respiratory acidosis. See Chapter 1, Acidosis, p 11.

■ PARATHYROID HORMONE (PTH)

Normal based on relationship to serum calcium, usually provided on the lab report. Also, reference values will vary depending on the laboratory and whether N-terminal, C-terminal, or midmolecule is measured. PTH midmolecule: 0.29–0.85 ng/mL or 29–85 pmol/L with calcium 8.4–10.2 mg/dL or 2.1–2.55 mmol/L.

Increased. Primary hyperparathyroidism, secondary hyperparathyroidism (hypocalcemic states such as chronic renal failure, others).

Decreased. Hypoparathyroidism and hypercalcemia not resulting from hyperparathyroidism, hypoparathyroidism.

■ PARTIAL THROMBOPLASTIN TIME (PTT)

27–38 seconds.

Prolonged. Heparin and any defect in the intrinsic clotting mechanism such as severe liver disease or disseminated intravascular coagulation (includes factors I, II, V, VIII, IX, X, XI, and XII), prolonged use of a tourniquet before drawing a blood sample, hemophilia A and B, lupus coagulant, liver disease. See Chapter 1, Coagulopathy, p 61.

■ PHOSPHORUS

2.7–4.5 mg/dL or 0.87–1.45 mmol/L.

Increased. Hypoparathyroidism, pseudohypoparathyroidism, excess vitamin D, secondary hypoparathyroidism, acute and chronic renal failure, acromegaly, tumor lysis (lymphoma or leukemia treated with chemotherapy), alkalosis, glucose, factitious increase (hemolysis of specimen).

Decreased. See Chapter 1, Hypophosphatemia, p 172.

■ PLATELETS

See Table 2–3, p 268.
Platelet counts may be normal in number, but abnormal in function as with aspirin therapy; platelet function with a normal platelet count can be assessed by using bleeding time.

Increased. Primary thrombocytosis (idiopathic myelofibrosis, agnogenic myeloid metaplasis, polycythemia vera, primary thrombocythemia, chronic myelogenous leulsemia). Secondary thrombocytosis (collagen-vascular diseases, chronic infection [ostemyelitis, tuberculosis], hepatic cirrhosis, sarcoidosis, hemolytic anemia, iron deficiency anemia, recovery from B_{12} deficiency or iron deficiency, solid tumors and lymphomas; after surgery, especially postsplenectomy; response to drugs such as epinephrine or withdrawal of myelosuppressive drugs).

Decreased. See Chapter 1, Thrombocytopenia, p 247.

■ POTASSIUM, SERUM

3.5–5.1 mmol/L.

Increased. See Chapter 1, Hyperkalemia, p 142.

Decreased. See Chapter 1, Hypokalemia, p 160.

■ POTASSIUM, URINE

25–125 mmol/24-h urine; varies with diet. See **Urine Electrolytes**.

■ PROLACTIN

Females: 1–25 ng/mL; males: 1–20 ng/mL.

Increased. Pregnancy, nursing after pregnancy, prolactinoma, hypothalamic tumors, sacroidosis or granulomatous disease of the hypothalamus, hypothyroidism, renal failure, Addison's disease, phenothiazines, butyrophenones—haloperidol (Haldol).

Decreased. Sheehan's syndrome.

■ PROSTATIC-SPECIFIC ANTIGEN (PSA)

< 4 ng/dL.
Most useful as a measure of response to therapy for prostate cancer.

Values greater than 8.0 ng/dL are associated with carcinoma at the 90% confidence level.

Increased. Prostate cancer, some cases of benign prostatic hypertrophy, prostatic infarction.

Decreased. Total prostatectomy, response to therapy for prostatic carcinoma.

■ PROTEIN ELECTROPHORESIS, SERUM AND URINE (Serum Protein Electrophoresis [SPEP]; Urine Protein Electrophoresis [UPEP])

Quantitative analysis of the serum proteins is often used in the workup of hypoglobulinemia, macroglobulinemia, α_1-antitrypsin deficiency, collagen disease, liver disease, myeloma, and occasionally in nutritional assessment. Serum electrophoresis yields five different bands (see Figure 2–1, p 289, and Table 2–5, p 290). If a monoclonal gammopathy or a low globulin fraction is detected, quantitative immunoglobulins should be checked.

Urine protein electrophoresis can be used to evaluate proteinuria and can detect Bence-Jones (light-chain) protein that is associated with myeloma, Waldenström's macroglobulinemia, and Fanconi's syndrome.

■ PROTEIN, SERUM

6.0–7.8 g/dL or 60–78 g/L.

Increased. Multiple myeloma, Waldenström's macroglobulinemia, benign monoclonal gammopathy, lymphoma, sarcoidosis, chronic inflammatory disease.

Decreased. Any cause of decreased albumin or any cause of hypogammaglobulinemia such as common variable hypogammaglobulinemia.

■ PROTEIN, URINE

<100 mg/24-h urine; spot: < 10 mg/dL (< 20 mg/dL if early-morning collection); dipstick: negative.

Increased. Nephrotic syndrome, glomerulonephritis, lupus nephritis, amyloidosis, venous congestion of kidney (renal vein thrombosis, severe congestive heart failure), multiple myeloma, pre-eclampsia, postural proteinuria, polycystic kidney disease, diabetic nephropathy, radiation nephritis, malignant hypertension.

False positive. Gross hematuria, very concentrated urine, pyridium, very alkaline urine.

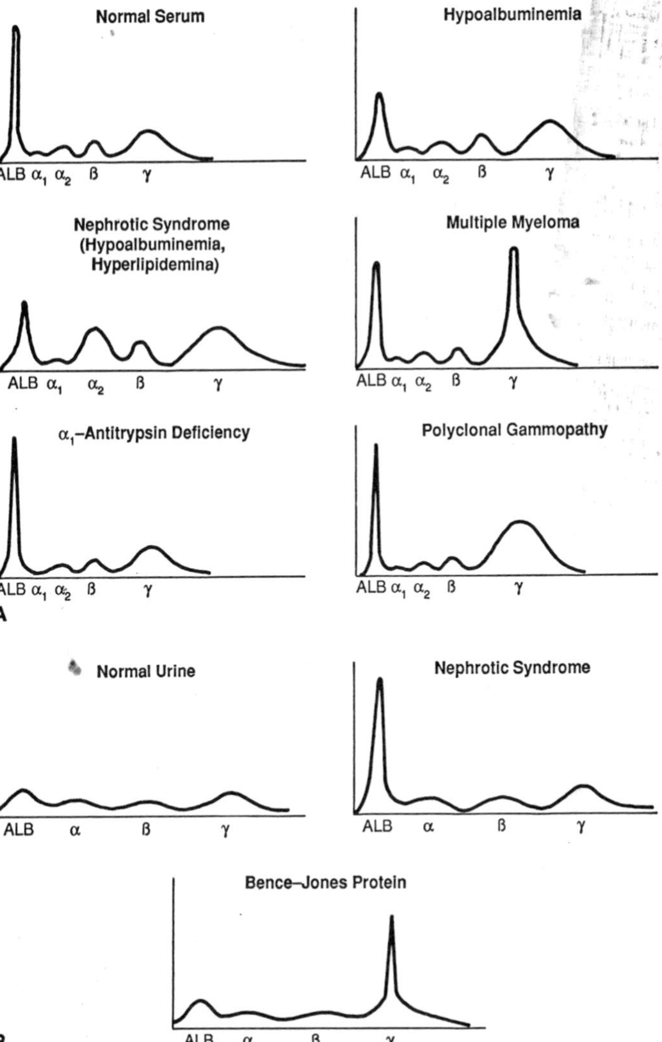

Figure 2–1. Protein electrophoresis patterns. Examples of (**A**) serum and (**B**) urine protein electrophoresis patterns.

TABLE 2–5. NORMAL SERUM PROTEIN COMPONENTS AND FRACTIONS AS DETERMINED BY ELECTROPHORESIS ALONG WITH ASSOCIATED CONDITIONS

Protein Fraction	Percentage of Total Protein	Constituents	Increased	Decreased
Albumin	52–68	Albumin	Dehydration (only known cause)	Nephrosis, malnutrition, chronic liver disease
α_1-Globulin	2.4–4.4	Thyroxine-binding globulin, antitrypsin, lipoproteins, glycoprotein, transcortin	Inflammation, neoplasia	Nephrosis, α_1-antitrypsin deficiency (emphysema related)
α_2-Globulin	6.1–10.1	Haptoglobin, glycoprotein, macroglobulin, ceruloplasmin	Inflammation, infection, neoplasia, cirrhosis	Severe liver disease, acute hemolytic anemia
β-Globulin	8.5–14.5	Transferrin, glycoprotein, lipoprotein	Cirrhosis, obstructive jaundice	Nephrosis
γ-Globulins (immunoglobulins)	10–21	IgA, IgG, IgM, IgD, IgE	Infections, collagen-vascular diseases, leukemia, myeloma	Agammaglobulinemia, hypogammaglobulinemia, nephrosis

From Gomella LG, ed. Clinician's Pocket Reference. *6th ed. East Norwalk, Conn: Appleton & Lange; 1989. Used with permission.*

■ PROTHROMBIN TIME (PT)

11.5–13.5 seconds.
Evaluates the extrinsic clotting mechanism that includes factors I, II, V, VII, and X.

Prolonged. Drugs such as sodium warfarin (Coumadin), decreased vitamin K, fat malabsorption, liver disease, prolonged use of a tourniquet before drawing a blood sample, disseminated intravascular coagulation, lupus anticoagulant (usually selectively increased PTT). See Chapter 1, Coagulopathy, p 61.

■ QUANTITATIVE IMMUNOGLOBULINS

IgG: 650–1500 mg/dL or 6.5–15 g/L; **IgM:** 40–345 mg/dL or 0.4–3.45 mg/L; **IgA:** 76–390 mg/dL or 0.76–3.90 g/L; **IgE:** 0–380 IU/mL or KIU/L; **IgD:** 0–8 mg/dL or 0–80 mg/L.

Increased. Multiple myeloma (myeloma immunoglobulin increased, other immunoglobulins decreased), Waldenström's macroglobulinemia (IgM increased, others decreased), lymphoma, carcinoma, bacterial infection, liver disease, sarcoidosis, amyloidosis, myeloproliferative disorders.

Decreased. Hereditaryimmunodeficiency, leukemia, lymphoma, nephrotic syndrome, protein-losing enteropathy, malnutrition.

■ RED BLOOD CELL COUNT

See Table 2–3, p 268. Also see **Hematocrit.**

■ RED BLOOD CELL INDICES

See Table 2–3, p 268.

MCV (Mean Cell Volume)

Increased. Megaloblastic anemia (B_{12}, folate deficiency), reticulocytosis, chronic liver disease, alcoholism, hypothyroidism, aplastic anemia.

Decreased. Iron deficiency, sideroblastic anemia, thalassemia, some cases of lead poisoning, hereditary spherocytosis.

MCH (Mean Cellular Hemoglobin)

Increased. Macrocytosis (megaloblastic anemias, high reticulocyte counts).

Decreased. Microcytosis (iron deficiency).

MCHC (Mean Cellular Hemoglobin Concentration)

Increased. Very severe, prolonged dehydration; spherocytosis.

Decreased. Iron deficiency anemia, overhydration, thalassemia, sideroblastic anemia.

RDW (Red Cell Distribution Width)

Measure of the degree of anisocytosis.

Increased. Combination of a macrocytic and microcytic anemia or recovery from iron deficiency anemia.

■ RED BLOOD CELL MORPHOLOGY

Poikilocytosis. Irregular RBC shape (sickle, Burr).

Anisocytosis. Irregular RBC size (microcytes, macrocytes).

Basophilic Stippling. Lead, heavy metal poisoning, thalassemia.

Howell-Jolly Bodies. After a splenectomy, some severe anemias.

Sickling. Sickle cell disease and trait.

Nucleated RBCs. Severe bone marrow stress (hemorrhage, hemolysis), marrow replacement by tumor, extramedullary hematopoiesis.

Target Cells. Thalassemia, hemoglobinopathies (sickle cell disease), obstructive jaundice, any hypochromic anemia, after splenectomy.

Spherocytes. Hereditary spherocytosis, immune or microangiopathic hemolysis.

Helmet Cells (Schistocytes). Microangiopathic hemolysis, hemolytic transfusion reaction, other hemolytic anemias.

Burr Cells (Acanthocytes). Severe liver disease; high levels of bile, fatty acids, or toxins.

Polychromasia. Appearance of a bluish-gray red cell on routine Wright's stain suggests reticulocytes.

■ RETICULOCYTE COUNT

0.5%–1.5%.
If the patient's hematocrit is abnormal, a corrected reticulocyte count should be calculated as follows:

$$\text{Corrected reticulocyte count} = \text{\% reticulocyte} \times \frac{\text{patient's hematocrit}}{45\%}$$

Increased. Hemolysis, acute hemorrhage, therapeutic response to treatment for iron, vitamin B_{12}, or folate deficiency.

Decreased. Infiltration of bone marrow by carcinoma, lymphoma or leukemia, marrow aplasia, chronic infections such as osteomyelitis, toxins, drugs (> 100 reported), many anemias.

■ RETINOL BINDING PROTEIN (RBP)

3–6 mg/dL.

Increased. Chronic renal disease.

Decreased. Malnutrition states, vitamin A deficiency, intestinal malabsorption of fats, chronic liver disease.

■ RHEUMATOID FACTOR (RA Latex Test)

<15 IU by microscan kit or <1:40.

Increased. Rheumatoid arthritis, systemic lupus erythematosus, Sjogren's syndrome, scleroderma, dermatomyositis, polymyositis, syphilis, chronic inflammation, subacute bacterial endocarditis, hepatitis, sarcoidosis, interstitial pulmonary fibrosis.

■ SCHLICTER TEST

Bactericidal ≥ 1:8 dilution.
Used most frequently to ensure adequate antimicrobial levels in patients with osteomyelitis or bacterial endocarditis.

■ SEDIMENTATION RATE (ESR)

Wintrobe Scale. Males: 0–9 mm/h; females: 0–20 mm/h.

ZETA Scale. 40%–54%, normal; 55%–59%, mildly elevated; 60–64%, moderately elevated; >65%, markedly elevated.

Westergren Scale. Males < 50 years: 15 mm/h; males > 50 years: 20 mm/h; females < 50 years, 25 mm/h; females > 50 years: 30 mm/h.

This is a very nonspecific test. ZETA method is not affected by anemia. The Westergren scale remains the preferred method.

Increased. Any type of infection, inflammation, rheumatic fever, endocarditis, neoplasm, acute myocardial infarction.

■ SGGT (Serum Gamma-Glutamyltransferase)

See **Gamma-Glutamytransferase (GGT).**

■ SGOT (Serum Glutamic-Oxaloacetic Transaminase) OR AST (Serum Aspartate Aminotransaminase)

See **AST.**

■ SGPT (Serum Glutamic-Pyruvic Transaminase) OR ALT (Serum Alanine Aminotransaminase)

See **ALT.**

■ SODIUM, SERUM

136–145 mmol/L.

Increased. See Chapter 1, Hypernatremia, p 146.

Decreased. See Chapter 1, Hyponatremia, p 168.

■ SODIUM, URINE

40–210 mmol/24-h urine. See **Urinary Electrolytes.**

■ STOOL FOR OCCULT BLOOD (Hemoccult Test)

Negative.

Positive. See Chapter 1, Hematochezia, p 121, and Hematemesis, Melena, p 118. Swallowed blood, ingestion of red meat, any gastrointestinal tract lesion (ulcer, carcinoma, polyp), large doses of vitamin C (> 500 mg/d).

■ STOOL FOR WBC

Occasional WBC.

Increased. (Usually polyps). *Shigella, Salmonella,* enteropathogenic *Escherichia coli,* ulcerative colitis, pseudomembranous colitis.

■ T3 (Triiodothyronine) RADIOIMMUNOASSAY

120–195 ng/dL or 1.85–3.00 nmol/L.

Increased. Hyperthyroidism, T3 thyrotoxicosis, oral estrogen, pregnancy, hepatitis, exogenous T4, any cause of increased thyroid-binding globulin.

Decreased. Hypothyroidism, euthyroid sick state, any cause of decreased thyroid-binding globulin.

■ T3 RU (Resin Uptake)

24%–34%.

Increased. Hyperthyroidism, medications (phenytoin [Dilantin], steroids, heparin, aspirin, others), nephrotic syndrome.

Decreased. Hypothyroidism, pregnancy, medications (estrogens, iodine, propylthiouracil, others).

■ T4 TOTAL (Thyroxine)

5–12 μg/dL or 65–155 nmol/L; males > 60 years: 5–10 μg/dL or 65–129 nmol; females: 5.5–10.5 μg/dL or 71–135 nmol/L.

Increased. Hyperthyroidism, exogenous thyroid hormone, estrogens, pregnancy, severe illness, any cause of increased thryroid-binding globulin.

Decreased. Hypothyroidism, euthyroid sick state, any cause of decreased thyroid-binding globulin.

■ THROMBIN TIME

10–14 seconds.

Increased. Systemic heparin, disseminated intravascular coagulation, elevated fibrin degradation products, fibrinogen deficiency, congenitally abnormal fibrinogen molecules. See Coagulopathy, p 61.

■ THYROGLOBULIN

0–60 ng/mL or <60 μg/L.
Used primarily to detect recurrence in patients who undergo surgical resection for nonmedullary thyroid carcinoma.

Increased. Differentiated thyroid carcinomas (papillary, follicular), thyroid adenoma, Grave's disease, toxic goiter, nontoxic goiter, thyroiditis.

Decreased. Hypothyroidism, testosterone, steroids, phenytoin.

■ THYROID-BINDING GLOBULIN (TBG)

1.5–3.4 mg/dL or 15–34 mg/L.

Increased. Hypothyroidism, pregnancy, oral contraceptives, estrogens, hepatitis, acute porphyria, familial.

Decreased. Hyperthyroidism, androgens, anabolic steroids, corticosteroids, nephrotic syndrome, severe illness, phenytoin, liver failure, malnutrition.

■ THYROID-STIMULATING HORMONE (TSH)

0.7–5.3 mU/mL.
Newer sensitive assay is an excellent screening test for hyperthyroidism as well as hypothyroidism. Allows you to distinguish between a low normal and a decreased TSH.

Increased. Hypothyroidism.

Decreased. Hyperthyroidism. Less than 1% of hypothyroidism is from pituitary or hypothalamic disease resulting in a decreased TSH.

■ TRANSFERRIN

220–400 mg/dL or 2.20–4.00 g/L.

Increased. Acute and chronic blood loss, iron deficiency anemia, hepatitis, oral contraceptives.

Decreased. Anemia of chronic disease, cirrhosis, nephrosis, hemochromatosis.

■ TRIGLYCERIDES

Males: 40–160 mg/dL or 0.45–1.81 mmol/L; females: 35–135 mg/dL or 0.40–1.53 mmol/L. Can vary with age.

Increased. Hyperlipoproteinemias (types I, IIb, III, IV, V), hypothyroidism, liver diseases, alcoholism, pancreatitis, acute myocardial infarction, nephrotic syndrome.

Decreased. Malnutrition, congenital abetalipoproteinemia.

■ URIC ACID

Males: 4.5–8.2 mg/dL or 0.27–0.48 mmol/L; females: 3.0–6.5 mg/dL or 0.18–0.38 mmol/L.

Increased. Gout, renal failure, destruction of massive amounts of nucleoproteins (tumor lysis after chemotherapy, leukemia or lymphoma), toxemia of pregnancy, drugs (especially diuretics), hypothyroidism, polycystic kidney disease, parathyroid diseases.

Decreased. Uricosuric drugs (salicylates, probenecid, allopurinol), Wilson's disease, Fanconi's syndrome, pregnancy.

■ URINALYSIS, ROUTINE

Appearance

Normal	Yellow, clear, straw-colored
Pink/red	Blood, hemoglobin, myoglobin, food coloring, beets
Orange	Pyridium, bile pigments
Brown/black	Myoglobin, bile pigments, melanin, cascara bark, iron, Macrodantin, Flagyl, sickle cell crisis
Blue	Methylene blue, *Pseudomonas* urinary tract infection (rare), hereditary tryptophan metabolic disorders
Cloudy	Urinary tract infection (pyuria), blood, myoglobin, chyluria, mucus (normal in ileal loop specimens), phosphate salts (normal in alkaline urine), urates (normal in acidic urine), hyperoxaluria
Foamy	Proteinuria, bile salts

pH

(4.6–8.0)

Acidic High-protein diet, Mandelamine, acidosis, ketoacidosis (starvation, diabetic), diarrhea, dehydration.

Basic Urinary tract infection, renal tubular acidosis, diet (high vegetable, milk, immediately after meals), sodium bicarbonate or Diamox therapy, vomiting, metabolic alkalosis, chronic renal failure.

Specific Gravity

1.001–1.035.

Increased. Volume depletion, congestive heart failure, adrenal insufficiency, diabetes mellitus, syndrome of inappropriate antidiuretic hormone, increased proteins (nephrosis). If markedly increased (1.040–1.050), suspect artifact or excretion of radiographic contrast medium or some other osmotic agent.

Decreased. Diabetes insipidus, pyelonephritis, glomerulonephritis, water load with normal renal function.

Bilirubin

Negative dipstick.

Positive. Obstructive jaundice, hepatitis, cirrhosis, congestive heart failure with hepatic congestion, congenital hyperbilirubinemia (Dubin-Johnson syndrome).

Blood (Hemoglobin)

Negative dipstick.

Positive. Hematuria (See Chapter 1, Hematuria, p 125), free hemoglobin (from trauma, transfusion reaction, or lysis of red cells) or myoglobin (crush injury, burn, or tissue ischemia).

Glucose

Negative dipstick.

Positive. Diabetes mellitus, other endocrine disorders (pheochromocytoma, hyperthyroidism, Cushing's syndrome, hyperadrenalism), stress states (sepsis, burns), pancreatitis, renal tubular disease, iatrogenic causes (steroids, thiazides, birth control pills), false positive with vitamin C ingestion.

Ketones

Negative dipstick.

Positive. Starvation, high-fat diet, alcoholic and diabetic ketoacidosis, vomiting, diarrhea, hyperthyroidism, pregnancy, febrile states.

Nitrite

Negative dipstick.

Positive. Infection (a negative test does not rule out infection).

Protein

Negative dipstick.

Positive. See **Protein, Urine.**

Leukocyte Esterase

Negative dipstick.

Positive. Infection (test detects 5 or more WBC/HPF or lysed WBCs).

Reducing Substance

Negative dipstick.

Positive. Glucose, fructose, galactose.

False Positives. Vitamin C, antibiotics.

Urobilinogen

Negative dipstick.

Positive. Bile duct obstruction, suppression of gut flora with antibiotics.

Microscopy

Note: If the dipstick is negative and the gross appearance is normal, many laboratories are no longer performing urine microscopy on a routine basis.

RBCs. (Normal 0–3/HPF.) Trauma, urinary tract infection, prostatic hypertrophy, genitourinary tuberculosis, stones, malignant and benign tumors, glomerulonephritis and any cause of blood on dipstick (see earlier).

WBCs. (Normal 0–4/HPF.) Infection anywhere in the urinary tract, genitourinary tuberculosis, renal tumors, acute glomerulonephritis, radiation damage, interstitial nephritis (analgesic abuse). (Glitter cells represent WBCs lysed in hypotonic solution.)

Epithelial Cells. (Normal occasional.) Acute tubular necrosis, necrotizing papillitis.

Parasites. (Normal none.) *Trichomonas vaginalis, Schistosoma hematobium.*

Yeast. (Normal none.) *Candida albicans* (especially in diabetics and immunosuppressed patients or if a vaginal infection is present).

Spermatozoa. (normal if after intercourse or nocturnal emission)

Crystals. Normal in acid urine—Calcium oxalate (small square crystals with a central cross), uric acid.

Normal in alkaline urine—Calcium carbonate, triple phosphate (resemble coffin lids).

Abnormal—Cystine, sulfonamide, leucine, tyrosine, cholesterol, or excessive amounts of the crystals noted earlier.

Contaminants. Cotton threads, hair, wood fibers, amorphous substances (all usually unimportant).

Mucus. (Small amounts normal.) Large amounts suggest urethral disease. Ileal loop urine normally has large amounts.

Hyaline Cast. (Normal occasional.) Benign hypertension, nephrotic syndrome.

RBC Cast. (Normal none.) Acute glomerulonephritis, lupus nephritis, subacute bacterial endocarditis, Goodpasture's disease, vasculitis, malignant hypertension.

WBC Cast. (Normal none.) Pyelonephritis.

Epithelial Cast. (Normal occasional.) Tubular damage, nephrotoxin, viral infections.

Granular Cast. (Normal none.) Breakdown of cellular casts, leads to waxy casts.

Waxy Cast. (Normal none.) End stage of a granular cast, severe chronic renal disease, amyloidosis.

Fatty Cast. (Normal none.) Nephrotic syndrome, diabetes mellitus, damaged renal tubular epithelial cells.

Broad Cast. (Normal none.) Chronic renal disease.

■ URINARY ELECTROLYTES

These "spot urines" are of limited value because of large variations in daily fluid and salt intake. Results are usually indeterminate if a diuretic has been given. Sodium is most useful in the differentiation of volume depletion, oliguria, or hyponatremia. Chloride is useful in the diagnosis and treatment of metabolic alkalosis. Urinary potassium levels are often used in the evaluation of hypokalemia.

Chloride < 10 mmol/L. Chloride-sensitive metabolic alkalosis (see Chapter 1, Alkalosis, p 19).

Chloride* $>$ *20 mmol/L. Chloride-resistant metabolic alkalosis (see Chapter 1, Alkalosis, p 19).

Potassium* $<$ *10 mmol/L. Hypokalemia, potassium depletion, extrarenal loss.

Potassium* $>$ *10 mmol/L. Renal potassium wasting (diuretics, brisk urinary output).

Sodium* $<$ *20 mmol/L. Volume depletion, hyponatremic states, prerenal azotemia (congestive heart failure, shock, others), hepatorenal syndrome, edematous states

Sodium* $>$ *40 mmol/L. Acute tubular necrosis, adrenal insufficiency, renal salt wasting, syndrome of inappropriate antidiuretic hormone.

Sodium* $>$ *20–40 mmol/L. Indeterminate.

■ URINARY INDICES

See Table 2—6. These are used in determining the etiology of oliguria. (See Chapter 1, Oliguria/Anuria, p 213.)

TABLE 2–6. URINARY INDICES IN ACUTE RENAL FAILURE ACCOMPANIED BY OLIGURIA: DIFFERENTIAL DIAGNOSIS OF OLIGURIA

Index	Prerenal	Renal (ATN)
Urine osmolality	> 500	< 350
Urinary sodium	$< 10–20$	$> 30–40$
Urine/serum creatinine	> 40	< 20
Urine/serum osmolality	> 1.2	< 1.2
Fractional excreted sodium[a]	< 1	> 1
Renal failure index[b]	< 1	> 1

[a]Fractional excreted sodium $= \dfrac{\text{(urine/serum sodium)}}{\text{(urine/serum creatinine)}} \times 100.$

[b]Renal failure index $= \dfrac{\text{(urine sodium} \times \text{serum creatinine)}}{\text{urine creatinine}}.$

Modified from Gomella LG, ed. Clinician's Pocket Reference. *6th ed. East Norwalk, Conn: Appleton & Lange; 1989. Used with permission.*

■ VANILLYMANDELIC ACID (VMA), URINE

2–7 mg/dL or 10.1–35.4 μmol/d.
VMA is urinary metabolite of both epinephrine and norepinephrine.

Increased. Pheochromocytoma, neural crest tumors (neuroblastoma, ganglioneuroma). False positive with methyldopa, chocolate, vanilla, others.

■ VDRL TEST (Venereal Disease Research Laboratory) OR RAPID PLASMA REAGIN (RPR)

Nonreactive.
Good for screening syphilis. Almost always positive in secondary syphilis, but frequently becomes negative in late syphilis. Also, in some patients with HIV infection, the VDRL can be negative in primary and secondary syphilis.

Positive (Reactive). Syphilis, systemic lupus erythematosus, pregnancy and drug addicts. If reactive, confirm with FTA-ABS (false positives with bacterial or viral illnesses).

■ WHITE BLOOD CELL COUNT

See Table 2–3.

Increased. See Chapter 1, Leukocytosis, p 199.

Decreased. See Chapter 1, Leukopenia, p 204.

■ WHITE BLOOD CELL DIFFERENTIAL

See Table 2–3. Many hospitals are now performing the "3 Cell Differential Count" on automated machines. *Small cells* correlate to lymphocytes; *middle size cells* are monocytes, eosinophils, and basophils; and *large cells* are related to neutrophils (both segmented and banded).

Neutrophils

40%–70% segmented neutrophils, 5%–10% banded neutrophils.

Increased. Exercise, pain, stress, infection, burns, drugs, thyrotoxicosis, steroids, malignancy, chronic inflammatory disease (vasculitis, collagen-vascular disease, colitis), lithium, epinephrine, asplenia, idiopathic.

Decreased. Congenital, immune-mediated, drug-induced, infectious (viral, rickettsial, parasitic).

Lymphocytes

24%–44%.

Increased. Measles, German measles, mumps, whooping cough, smallpox, chicken pox, influenza, hepatitis, infectious mononucleosis, virtually any viral infection, acute and chronic lymphocytic leukemias.

Decreased. After stress, burns, trauma, normal finding in 22% of population, uremia, some viral infections.

Lymphocytes, Atypical

0%–3%.

$>$ ***20%.*** Infectious mononucleosis, cytomegalovirus infection, infectious hepatitis, toxoplasmosis.

$<$ ***20%.*** Viral infections (mumps, rubeola, varicella), rickettsial infections, tuberculosis.

Monocytes

3%–7%.

Increased. Subacute bacterial endocarditis, brucellosis, typhoid fever, kala-azar (visceral leishmaniasis), trypanosomiasis, rickettsial infection, ulcerative colitis, sarcoidosis, Hodgkin's disease, monocytic leukemias, collagen-vascular diseases.

Decreased. Myelodysplasia, aplastic anemia, hairy cell leukemia, cyclic neutropenia, thermal injuries, collagen-vascular diseases.

Eosinophils

0%–3%.

Increased. Allergy, parasites, skin diseases, malignancy, drugs, asthma, Addison's disease, collagen-vascular diseases. (A handy mnemonic is **NAACP: N**eoplasm, **A**llergy, **A**ddison's disease, **C**ollagen-vascular diseases, **P**arasites).

Decreased. After steroids, ACTH, after stress (infection, trauma, burns), Cushing's syndrome.

Basophils

0%–1%.

Increased. Chronic myeloid leukemia, rarely in recovery from infection and from hypothyroidism.

Decreased. Acute rheumatic fever, lobar pneumonia, after steroid therapy, thyrotoxicosis, stress.

■ WHITE BLOOD CELL MORPHOLOGY

Auer Rod. Acute myelogenous leukemias.

Döhle Bodies. Severe infection, burns, malignancy, pregnancy.

Hypersegmentation. Megaloblastic anemias, iron deficiency, myeloproliferative disorders, drug induced.

Toxic Granulation. Severe illness (sepsis, burns, high temperature).

■ ZINC

60–130 μg/dL or 9–20 μmol/L.

Increased. Atherosclerosis, coronary artery disease.

Decreased. Inadequate dietary intake (parenteral nutrition, alcoholism), malabsorption, increased needs such as pregnancy or wound healing, acrodermatitis enteropathica.

Reference

Tietz NW, ed. *Textbook of Clinical Chemistry,* 1st ed. Philadelphia: WB Saunders; 1986.

3 Procedures

■ ARTERIAL LINE PLACEMENT

(See also Chapter 1, Arterial Line Problems, p 30.)
Indications. Frequent sampling of arterial blood; hemodynamic monitoring when continuous blood pressure readings are needed, such as a patient being treated for malignant hypertension on nitroprusside or a patient in shock, where indirect cuff pressures may be inaccurate.

Contraindications. Poor collateral circulation. Avoid the femoral artery if severe aortoiliac atherosclerosis is present. Coagulopathy is a relative contraindication. (See Chapter 1, Coagulopathy, p 60.)

Materials. Twenty-gauge (or smaller) 1.5- to 2-in. catheter-over-needle assembly (Angiocath TM), arterial line setup per ICU routine (transducer, tubing, and pressure bag with heparinized saline), armboard, sterile dressing, lidocaine.

Procedure

1. The radial artery is most frequently used and this approach is described here. Other sites, in decreasing order of preference, are the dorsalis pedis, femoral, brachial, and axillary arteries. Axillary arteries are infrequently used and catheters in these arteries should be placed by an intensivist or anesthesiologist.
2. Verify the patency of the collateral circulation between the radial and ulnar arteries using the Allen test (see Chapter 3, Arterial Puncture, p 306).
3. Place the extremity on an armboard with a roll of gauze behind the wrist to hyperextend the joint. Prep with povidone-iodine and drape with sterile towels. The operator should wear gloves and a mask.
4. Raise a very small skin wheal at the puncture site with 1% lidocaine using a 25-gauge needle. Carefully palpate the artery and choose the puncture site where it appears most superficial.
5. While palpating the path of the artery with the nondominant hand, advance the 20-gauge catheter-over-needle assembly into the artery at a 30° angle to the skin with the needle bevel up. Once a "flash" of blood is seen in the hub, hold the needle steady and advance the entire unit 1–2 mm so that the needle and catheter are in the artery. Advance the catheter over the needle into the artery.

Briefly occlude the artery with manual pressure while the pressure tubing is being connected.

6. Suture in place with 3-O silk and apply a sterile dressing.
7. Splint the dorsum of the wrist to limit mobility and provide catheter stability.
8. Kits are available with a needle and guide wire that allow the Seldinger technique to be used, especially for femoral artery cannulation.
9. Arterial lines should be replaced using a different site every 4 days to decrease risk of infection.

Complications. Thrombosis, hematoma, arterial embolism, arterial spasm, infection, hemorrhage, pseudoaneurysm formation.

■ ARTERIAL PUNCTURE

Indications. Blood gas determination and when arterial blood is needed for chemistry determinations such as ammonia levels.

Contraindications. Thrombolytic therapy is a relative contraindication to arterial puncture.

Materials. Blood gas sampling kit *or* 3- to 5-mL syringe, 23- to 25-gauge needle (20–22 gauge for femoral artery), 1 mL heparin (1000 U/mL), alcohol or povidone/iodine swabs, and a cup of ice.

Procedure

1. Use a heparinized syringe for blood gas and a nonheparinized syringe for chemistry determinations. Obtain a blood gas kit (contains a preheparinized syringe) or a small syringe (3–5 mL) with a small-gauge needle (23–25 gauge for radial artery, 20–22 gauge acceptable for femoral artery). Heparinize the syringe by drawing up about 0.5–1 mL of heparin, pulling the plunger all the way back, and discarding the heparin.
2. Arteries, in the order of preference, are radial, femoral, and brachial. If using the radial artery, perform the **Allen test** to verify collateral flow from the ulnar artery. Have the patient make a tight fist. Occlude both the radial and ulnar arteries at the wrist and have the patient open her or his hand. While maintaining pressure on the radial artery, release the ulnar artery. If the ulnar artery is patent, the hand should flush red within 10 seconds. If the Allen test is positive (the radial distribution will remain white beyond 10 seconds), the artery should not be used. Hyperextension of the wrist joint or elbow will often bring the radial and brachial arteries closer to the surface.
3. If using the femoral artery, the mnemonic NAVEL will aid in locating the important structures in the groin. Palpate the femoral artery just two fingerbreadths below the inguinal ligament. From lateral to medi-

al, the structures are nerve, artery, vein, empty space, lymphatic. You may wish to inject 1% lidocaine subcutaneously for anesthesia. Palpate the artery proximally and distally with two fingers or trap the artery between two fingers placed on either side of the vessel.

4. Prep the area with either a povidone-iodine solution or an alcohol swab. Hold the syringe like a pencil with the needle bevel up and enter the skin at a 60° to 90° angle. Maintain slight negative pressure on the syringe.
5. Obtain blood on the downstroke or on slow withdrawal. Aspirate very slowly. A good arterial sample should require only minimal back pressure. If a glass or special blood-gas syringe is used, the barrel will usually rise spontaneously. You should obtain 2–3 mL.
6. If the vessel cannot be located, redirect the needle without coming out of the skin.
7. Withdraw the needle quickly and apply FIRM pressure at the site for at least 5–10 minutes, even if the sample was not obtained to avoid a hematoma.
8. If the sample is for a blood gas, expel any air from the syringe, mix the contents thoroughly by twirling the syringe between your fingers, and make the syringe airtight with a cap. Place the syringe in an ice bath before the sample is processed.

Complications. Localized bleeding; thrombosis of the artery, which may lead to arterial insufficiency; infection.

■ ARTHROCENTESIS (Diagnostic and Therapeutic)

Indications. Diagnostic. Arthrocentesis is helpful in the diagnosis of new-onset arthritis; to rule out infection in acute or chronic, unremitting joint effusion. Therapeutic. To instill steroids and maintain drainage of septic arthritis.

Contraindications. None. Care must be taken not to induce excessive trauma if coagulopathy or thrombocytopenia is present or if the patient is anticoagulated.

Materials. Betadine, alcohol swabs, sterile gloves, lidocaine or ethyl chloride spray, an 18- or 20-gauge needle (a smaller-gauge needle if aspirating a joint of the finger or toe), a large syringe (size is dependent on the amount of fluid present), a 3-mL syringe with a 25-gauge needle, and two heparinized tubes for cell count and crystal examination.

Discuss with your microbiology lab their preference for transporting fluid for bacterial, fungal, acid-fast bacillus (AFB) culture, and gram stain. A Thayer-Martin plate is needed if *Neisseria gonorrhoeae* (GC) is suspected. A small syringe containing a long-acting corticosteroid such as depomedrol or triamcinolone is optional for therapeutic arthrocentesis.

Procedure

General

1. Obtain a consent form describing the procedure and complications.
2. Determine the optimal site for aspiration and mark with indelible ink.
3. Wear gloves (universal precautions) to protect yourself against AIDS. When aspiration is to be followed by corticosteroid injection, maintaining a sterile field with sterile implements minimizes the risk of infection to the patient.
4. Clean the area with betadine, and dry and wipe over the aspiration site with alcohol. Betadine can render cultures negative. Let the alcohol dry before beginning the procedure.
5. Anesthetize the area with lidocaine using a 25-gauge needle, taking care not to inject into the joint space. Lidocaine is bactericidal. Avoid preparations containing epinephrine, especially in a small digit. Alternatively, spray the area with ethyl chloride just prior to needle aspiration.
6. Insert the aspirating needle applying a small amount of vacuum to the syringe. Remove as much fluid as possible, repositioning the syringe if necessary.
7. If corticosteroid is to be injected, remove the aspirating syringe from the needle, which is still in the joint space. It is helpful to ensure that the syringe can easily be removed from the needle before step 6. Attach the syringe containing corticosteroid, pull back on the plunger to ensure you are not in a vein, and inject contents. Never inject steroids when there is a possibility of an infected joint. Remove the needle and apply pressure to the area. Generally, the equivalent of 40 mg of methylprednisolone is injected into large joints such as the knee and 20 mg into medium-sized joints such as the ankle or wrist.
8. Joint fluid is sent for cell count and differential, crystal exam, gram stain, and cultures for bacteria, fungi, and AFB as indicated. (See Chapter 1, Joint Swelling, p 193.)

Arthrocentesis of the Knee

1. The knee should be fully extended with the patient supine. Wait until the patient has a relaxed quadriceps muscle, as its contraction plants the patella against the femur, making aspiration painful.
2. The needle is inserted posterior to the **medial** portion of the patella into the patellar-femoral groove. The advancing needle is directed slightly posteriorly and inferiorly. (See Figure 3–1.)

Arthrocentesis of the Wrist. The easiest site for aspiration is between the navicular bone and radius on the dorsal wrist.

1. Locate the distal radius between the tendons of the extensor pollicus

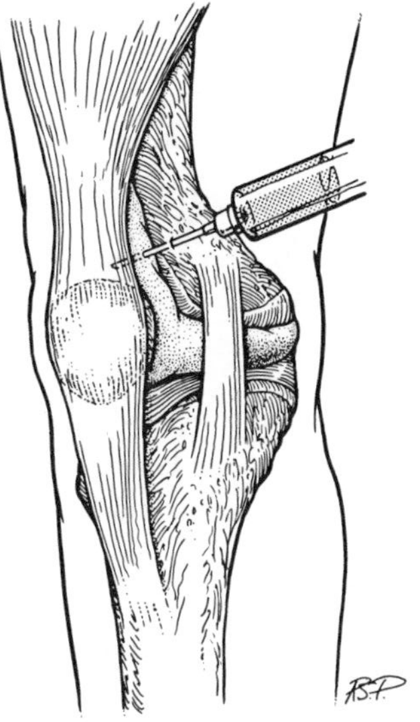

Figure 3–1. Arthrocentesis of the knee.

longus and the extensor carpi radialis longus to the second finger. This site is just ulnar to the anatomic snuff box.

2. The needle is directed perpendicular to the mark. (See Figure 3–2.)

Arthrocentesis of the Ankle

1. The most accessible site is between the tibia and the talus. The angle of the foot to leg is positioned at 90°. A mark is made lateral and anterior to the medial malleolus and medial and posterior to the tibialis anterior tendon. The advancing needle is directed posteriorly toward the heel.
2. The subtalar ankle joint does not communicate with the ankle joint and is difficult to aspirate even by an expert. One should be aware that "ankle pain" may originate in the subtalar joint rather than in the ankle. (See Figure 3–3.)

Complications. Infection, bleeding, pain. Postinjection flare of joint pain and swelling can occur after steroid injection and can persist up to 24 hours. This complication is felt to be a crystal-induced synovitis resulting from the crystalline suspension used in long-acting steroids.

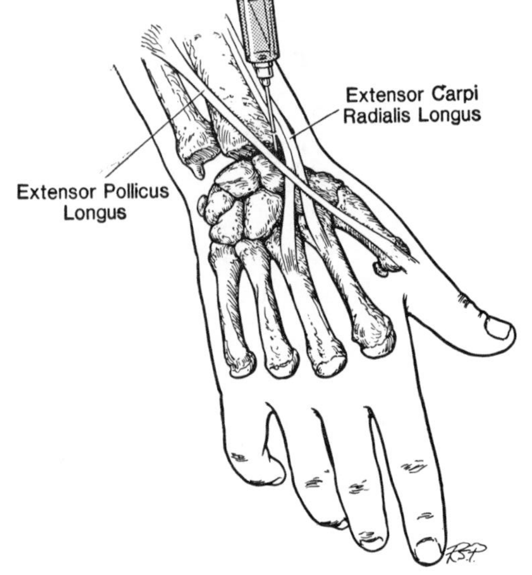

Figure 3–2. Arthrocentesis of the wrist.

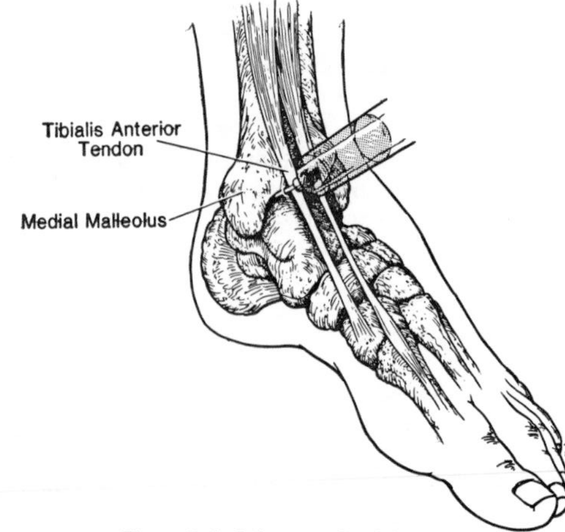

Figure 3–3. Arthrocentesis of the ankle.

■ BLADDER CATHETERIZATION

(See also Chapter 1, Foley Catheter Problems, p 104.)
Indications. Relieve urinary retention; collect an uncontaminated urine sample; monitor urinary output in critically ill patients; perform bladder tests (cystogram, cystometrogram, determine amount of postvoid residual urine).

Contraindications. Urethral disruption associated with pelvic fracture, acute prostatitis (relative).

Materials. Prepackaged Foley catheter tray (may need to add a catheter), catheter of choice (16- to 20-French Foley in adults).

Procedure

1. Have the patient in a well-lighted area in a supine position. With females, knees are flexed wide and heels placed together to get adequate exposure of the meatus.
2. Open the kit and put on the gloves. Get all the materials ready before you attempt to insert the catheter. Open the prep solution and soak the cotton balls. Apply the sterile drapes.
3. Inflate and deflate the balloon of the Foley catheter with 5–10 mL of sterile water to ensure its proper function. Coat the end of the catheter with lubricant jelly.
4. In females, use one gloved hand to prep the urethral meatus in a pubis-toward-anus direction; hold the labia apart with the other gloved hand. With uncircumsized males, retract the foreskin to prep the glands; use a gloved hand to hold the penis still.
5. The hand used to hold the penis or labia should not touch the catheter while it is being inserted. A disposable forceps in the kit can be used to insert it, or the forceps can be used to prep and then the gloved hand can insert the catheter.
6. In the male, stretch the penis upward perpendicular to the body to eliminate any folds in the urethra that might lead to a false passage. GENTLE pressure should be used to slowly advance the catheter. Any significant resistance that is encountered may represent a stricture and requires urologic consultation. In males with benign prostatic hypertrophy (BPH), a Coude-tip catheter may facilitate passage. Other means to facilitate catheter passage are to ensure that the penis is well-stretched and to instill 30–50 mL of sterile surgical lubricant into the urethra with a catheter-tipped syringe.
7. In both males and females, insert the catheter to the hilt of the drainage end. Compress the penis toward the pubis. These maneuvers ensure that the balloon will be inflated in the bladder and not in the urethra. The balloon is inflated with 5–10 mL of sterile water. After inflation, pull the catheter back so that the balloon will come to rest on the bladder neck. There should be good urine return when

the catheter is in place. ANY MALE WHO IS UNCIRCUMSIZED SHOULD HAVE THE FORESKIN REPOSITIONED TO PREVENT MASSIVE EDEMA OF THE GLANS AFTER THE CATHETER IS INSERTED.

8. If no urine returns, attempt to irrigate with 25–50 mL of sterile saline and a catheter-tipped syringe. A CATHETER THAT WILL NOT IRRIGATE IS IN THE URETHRA, NOT THE BLADDER.
9. Catheters in females can be taped to the leg. In males, the catheter should be taped to the abdominal wall to decrease urethral stricture formation (avoids catheter damage to urethra at penoscrotal junction).

Complications. Infection, bleeding, false passage.

■ BONE MARROW ASPIRATION AND BIOPSY

Indications. Evaluation of anemia, thrombocytopenia, leukopenia; evaluation of leukocytosis, thrombocytosis, malignancy primary to the marrow (leukemia, myeloma) or metastatic to the marrow (lung cancer, breast cancer); evaluation of iron stores; evaluation of possible disseminated infection (tuberculosis, fungal disease).

Contraindications. Infection near the puncture site. Relative contraindications include severe coagulopathy or thrombocytopenia uncorrected by platelet transfusion.

Materials. Commercial kits are available that contain all the materials necessary. If such a kit is not available, the following items will be needed: bone marrow biopsy needle (Jamshidi, Westerman, or similar type), sterile gloves and surgical drapes, iodine prep solution, alcohol, 22- and 26-gauge needles, at least two 10-mL syringes, 1% lidocaine solution, No. 11 scalpel blade, 4 × 4 gauze pads, and several microscope slides for staining.

Procedure

1. The procedure must be explained in detail to the patient and/or legally responsible individual and informed consent obtained.
2. Usually local anesthesia is all that is required; however, in extremely anxious patients, premedication with an anxiolytic or sedative such as diazepam (Valium) or midazolam (Versed) and/or an analgesic is reasonable.
3. Bone marrow can be obtained from numerous sites, the most common being the sternum, the anterior iliac crest, and the posterior iliac crest. The posterior iliac crest is the safest and is the method described here. The patient may be positioned on either the abdomen or on the side opposite the side to be biopsied.
4. The posterior iliac crest is identified with palpation and the desired biopsy site is marked with indelible ink.

5. Sterile gloves are used and strict aseptic technique is followed for the remainder of the procedure.
6. The biopsy site is prepped with sterile iodine solution and the skin is allowed to dry. Then the site is wiped free of the iodine with sterile alcohol. Surgical drapes are then used to cover the surrounding areas.
7. With a 26-gauge needle, 1% lidocaine solution is administered subcutaneously to raise a skin wheal. Then, with the 22-gauge needle, the deeper tissues are infiltrated with lidocaine until the periosteum is reached. At this point, the needle should be advanced just through the periosteum and lidocaine infiltrated subperiosteally. An area approximately 2 cm in diameter should be infiltrated, using repeated periosteal punctures.
8. Once local anesthesia has been obtained, a No. 11 scalpel blade is used to make 2- to 3-mm skin incision over the biopsy site.
9. The bone marrow biopsy needle is inserted through the skin incision and then advanced with a rotating motion and gentle pressure until the periosteum is reached. Once it is firmly seated on the periosteum, the needle is advanced through the outer table of bone into the marrow cavity with the same rotating motion and gentle pressure. Generally, a slight change in the resistance to needle advancement signals entry into the marrow cavity. At this point, the needle should be advanced 2–3 mm.
10. The stylet is removed from the biopsy needle and a 10-mL syringe is attached to the hub of the biopsy needle. The plunger on the syringe is then withdrawn briskly and 1–2 mL of marrow aspirated into the syringe. This may cause severe, instantaneous pain. Slow withdrawal of the plunger or collection of more than 1–2 mL of marrow with each aspiration will result in excessive contamination of the specimen with peripheral blood.
11. The marrow aspiration specimen can be used to prepare coverslips for viewing under the microscope, sent for special studies such as cytogenetics and cell markers or for culture. Repeat aspirations may be required to obtain enough marrow to perform all of the preceding studies. Also note that certain studies may require heparin or EDTA for collection. The appropriate laboratory should be contacted prior to the procedure to be sure that specimens are collected in the appropriate solution.
12. If a biopsy is to be obtained, the stylet is replaced and the needle withdrawn. The needle is then reinserted at a slightly different angle and location, still within the area of periosteum previously anesthetized. Once the marrow cavity has been reentered, the stylet is again removed and the needle is advanced 5–10 mm using the same rotating motion with gentle pressure. The needle is withdrawn several millimeters (but not outside of the marrow cavity) and is redirected at a slightly different angle and then advanced again. This is repeated several times. This should result in 2–3 cm

of core material entering the needle. The needle is rotated rapidly on its long axis in a clockwise and then a counterclockwise manner. This will sever the biopsy specimen from the marrow cavity. The needle is withdrawn completely without replacing the stylet. Some operators prefer to hold their thumb over the open end of the needle to create a negative pressure in the needle as it is withdrawn. This may help prevent loss of the core biopsy.

13. The core biopsy is removed from the needle by inserting a probe (provided with the biopsy needle) into the distal end of the needle and then gently pushing the specimen the full length of the needle and finally out of the hub end of the needle. This is important as an attempt to push the specimen out the distal end may damage the biopsy as most biopsy needles are tapered at this end, presumably allowing the specimen to expand once in the needle and preventing specimen loss when the needle is withdrawn from the patient.
14. The core biopsy is usually collected in formalin solution. Again, plans for special studies should be made prior to the procedure so that any special handling of the biopsy can be done.
15. The biopsy site is observed for excess bleeding and local pressure is applied for several minutes. The area is cleaned thoroughly with alcohol and a band-aid or gauze patch applied. The patient is instructed to assume a supine position and a pressure pack is placed between the bed or table and the biopsy site to apply pressure for 10–15 minutes. This is not an absolute requirement in patients without an underlying coagulopathy or thrombocytopenia, but still serves to decrease local hematoma formation. Patients with an underlying bleeding tendency should maintain pressure 20–25 minutes. A patient who is stable at this point may resume normal activities.

Complications. Local bleeding and hematoma, pain, possible infection.

■ CENTRAL VENOUS CATHETERIZATION

(See also Chapter 1, Central Venous Line Problems, p 47.)
Indications. Administration of fluids and medications when peripheral administration is impossible, inappropriate, or unreliable; hemodynamic monitoring; transvenous pacemaker placement.

Contraindications. A coagulopathy dictates the use of the femoral or median basilic vein approach to avoid bleeding complications.

Materials. Generally, two approaches are used to place central venous lines. One of these involves puncturing the vein with a relatively small needle through which a thin guide wire is placed in the vein. After the needle has been withdrawn, the intravascular appliance or a sheath through which a smaller catheter will be placed is introduced into the vein over the guide wire. The other technique involves puncturing the vein with a larger-bore needle through which the intravascular catheter will fit. There are commercially available disposable trays that provide all necessary needles, wires, sheaths, dilators, suture materials, and topical anesthetics. Some hospitals insist that these materials be assembled when central line placement becomes necessary. If needles, guide wires, and sheaths are collected from different places, it is very important to make sure that the needle will accept the guide wire, that the sheath and dilator will pass over the guide wire, and that the appliance to be passed through the sheath will indeed fit the inside lumen of the sheath. Supplies should include the following items:

1. Small needle (16–18 gauge)
2. Guide wire
3. 5- to 10-mL syringe
4. Scalpel
5. Intravascular appliance (triple-lumen catheter or a sheath through which a Swan-Ganz pulmonary artery catheter could be placed).
6. Heparinized flush solution 1 mL of 1:100 U heparin in 10 mL of normal saline (to be used to fill all lumens prior to placement to prevent clotting of the catheter during placement)
7. Lidocaine 1% with or without epinephrine
8. Povidone-iodine (Betadine) prep solution
9. Alcohol pads
10. Sterile towels
11. 4 × 4 gauze sponges
12. 21-gauge needle to draw up the lidocaine.

Also, sterile procedure is highly recommended (mask, sterile gown, and gloves).

Note: If the catheter is introduced through a large-bore needle, an appropriately sized large-bore needle is required (12–14 gauge) and a smaller needle and guide wire are not required.

There seems to be little rationale for placement of a single-lumen catheter when multiple lumens can be installed for potential use at virtually the same risk. For these reasons, the ensuing discussion focuses on the over-the-guide wire technique and placement of either a triple-lumen catheter or a sheath through which a smaller catheter will eventually be placed.

Right Internal Jugular Vein Approach

Actually, three different sites are described and used in accessing the right internal jugular vein: anterior (medial to the sternocleidomastoid muscle belly), middle (between the two heads of the sternocleidomastoid muscle belly), and posterior (lateral to the sternocleidomastoid muscle belly). The middle approach is most commonly used and has the advantage of well-defined landmarks.

Procedure

1. Sterilize the site with povidone-iodine and drape with sterile towels.
2. Administer local anesthesia with lidocaine in the area to be explored.
3. Place the patient in Trendelenburg (head down) position.
4. Use a small-bore thin-walled needle with syringe attached to locate the internal jugular vein. It may be helpful to have a small amount of anesthetic in the syringe to inject during exploration for the vein if the patient notes some discomfort.
5. The internal diameter of the needle used to locate the internal jugular vein should be large enough to accommodate the passage of the guide wire.
6. Percutaneous entry should be made at the apex of the triangle formed by the two heads of the sternocleidomastoid muscle and the clavicle.
7. The needle should be directed slightly lateral toward the ipsilateral breast and kept as superficially as possible.
8. Often a notch can be palpated on the posterior surface of the clavicle. This actually can help locate the vein in the lateral/medial plane, as the vein lies deep to this shallow notch.
9. Successful puncture of the vein is accomplished at an unnerving depth of needle insertion, and is heralded by sudden aspiration of nonpulsatile venous blood.
10. After the needle is detached from the syringe, the guide wire should pass with ease all the way to the right atrium. Once the wire is passed, remove the needle.
11. Leave enough wire outside the patient to accommodate the length of the intravascular catheter, sheath, etc., with an adequate amount to allow control over the distal end of the guide wire at all times.
12. Nick the skin with a No. 11 scalpel blade.
13. The catheter or sheath should be introduced over the guide wire while the depth of the guide wire is kept relatively constant to avoid irritation of the right atrium or ventricle and possible ventricular ectopy.
14. When the sheath or catheter is placed over the guide wire, the proximal end of the guide wire should be held until the catheter or sheath completely passes over the distal end of the guide wire.
15. Then the distal end of the guide wire is controlled while the catheter or sheath is advanced through the incised skin and into the vein.
16. Once the catheter or sheath is in place the guide wire is removed.
17. An occlusive sterile dressing should be applied.
18. A chest x-ray should be obtained to verify position of the line as well as to identify complications such as a pneumothorax.

Complications

1. Remarkably safe, with the literature describing literally thousands of attempts uncomplicated by pneumothorax.
2. It is likely that errant attempts at internal jugular puncture will end up in the mediastinum. It is possible to perforate endotracheal tube cuffs by this approach. This usually is not a subtle event and generally requires prompt replacement of the now faulty endotracheal tube before safe deep line placement can proceed.
3. The other procedural miscue is inadvertent puncture of the carotid artery. Common if the needle is inserted medial to where it should be on the middle approach and common with the anterior approach. With arterial puncture, the syringe fills without negative pressure because of arterial pressure, and bright red blood pulsates from the needle after the syringe is removed. The needle should be removed and manual pressure applied for 10–15 minutes to ensure adequate hemostasis.
4. A chest x-ray should always be obtained after the procedure to check for positioning of the catheter and to rule out pneumothorax.

Advantages. Central venous access from this site allows virtually every potential use of the deep line, including hemodynamic assessment (both central venous pressure and pulmonary artery measurements are easily done), temporary pacemaker placement, endomyocardial biopsy, as well as administration of fluids, drugs, and parenteral nutrition.

Disadvantages

1. The major disadvantage of this site is patient discomfort. The site is difficult to dress and is uncomfortable for patients who have the capacity to turn their heads.
2. The risk of infectious contamination for this line is intermediate between that for femoral lines and that for subclavian lines and is probably related to the difficulty in keeping the site occlusively dressed.

Left Internal Jugular Vein Approach

The left internal jugular vein is not commonly used for central line placement. Better options exist and should be exhausted before resorting to this approach.

Procedure. Similar to right internal jugular vein approach.

Complications. In addition to the usual procedural complications common to central lines, this approach has some unique complications.

1. There are case reports of inadvertent left brachiocephalic vein and superior vena cava puncture with intravascular wires, catheters, and sheaths.
2. Laceration of the thoracic duct.

Advantages. None over right internal jugular vein approach.

Disadvantages. See complications for right internal jugular vein approach. Laceration of the thoracic duct and puncture of the left brachiocephalic vein and superior vena cava are also possible.

Subclavian Approach (Left or Right)

Procedure

1. A small, rolled-up towel placed between the shoulder blades facilitates this approach.
2. Place the patient in the Trendelenburg position.
3. Use sterile preparation and appropriate draping.
4. Anesthetize the skin with local anesthetic.
5. Percutaneous entry is then made at the distal third of the clavicle.
6. A small amount of topical anesthetic in the syringe can be used to anesthetize periosteal surfaces while the vein is located, but hopefully only one puncture will be needed.
7. The guide wire should fit inside the lumen of the needle used to find the vein.
8. Direct the needle under the clavicle, above the first rib and toward the jugular notch. (See Figure 3–4.)
9. Apply constant negative pressure while the needle is advanced.
10. Successful entry is marked by free flow of nonpulsatile venous blood.
11. The patient's head should be directed to face the operator while the guide wire is inserted. This facilitates guide wire placement down the superior vena cava as opposed to up the internal jugular vein.
12. Remove the syringe.
13. Advance the guide wire through the needle.
14. The guide wire should slide easily through the needle, essentially to the hub of the needle.
15. If there is resistance to passage of the guide wire it is important to reattach the syringe and reposition the needle so that the blood flows freely.
16. If the resistance is more distal than the tip of the needle the guide wire is likely coursing cephalad at the internal jugular vein (an awake patient may remark that the ipsilateral ear hurts). Another pass of the guide wire with the entry needle pulled back slightly is appropriate. Placing the guide wire in the internal jugular vein from the subclavian approach accomplishes nothing. The catheter placed over the guide wire will also end up in the internal jugular vein.
17. Once the guide wire is passed remove the needle.
18. Follow steps 11 through 18 for placement via the right internal jugular vein.

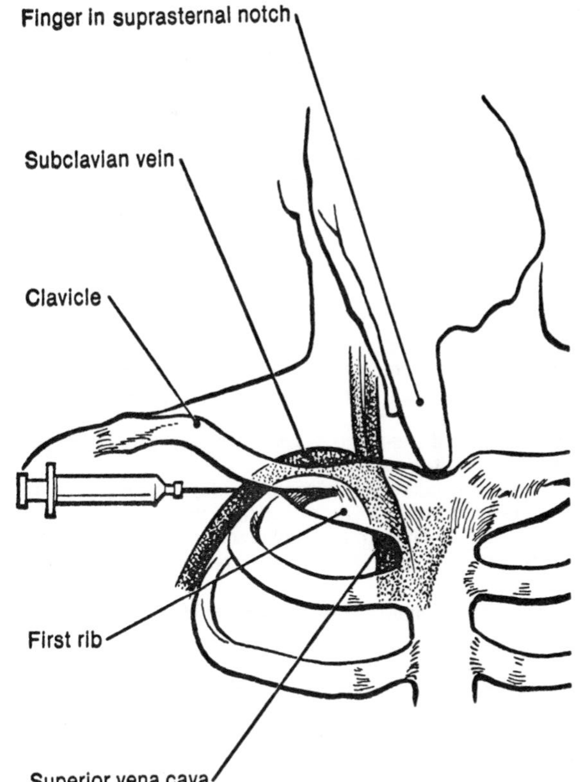

Figure 3–4. Catheterization of the right subclavian vein. (*From Gomella LG, ed.* Clinician's Pocket Reference. *6th ed. East Norwalk, Conn: Appleton & Lange; 1989. Used with permission.*)

Complications

1. Arterial puncture is usually obvious, as bright red blood spurts from the needle when the syringe is detached or the syringe spontaneously fills without negative pressure. The needle is then withdrawn and manual pressure applied to stop arterial bleeding. A significant bleed deep to the clavicle may occur and is heavily dependent on the patient's coagulation system and the size of the puncture. This underscores the importance of knowing the coagula-

tion profile before making the decision of where to place a central line.

2. Pneumothorax can be detected when a sudden gush of air is aspirated instead of blood. A postprocedure chest x-ray should always be done to rule out pneumothorax and check for line placement. A pneumothorax requires chest tube placement in virtually all cases, especially when the patient is being supported on a ventilator. The left-sided approach is associated with higher risk for pneumothorax because of the higher dome of the left pleura compared with the right.
3. Hemothorax.
4. Air embolus.

Advantages

1. The left subclavian approach affords a gentle, sweeping curve to the apex of the right ventricle and is the preferred entry site for placement of a temporary transvenous pacemaker without fluoroscopic assistance.
2. Hemodynamic measurements are often easier to record from the left subclavian approach.
3. From the left subclavian vein approach, the catheters do not have to negotiate an acute angle as is commonly the case at the junction of the right subclavian with the right brachiocephalic vein en route to the superior vena cava. This is also a common site for kinking of the deep line.
4. Lowest risk of infection of various central line sites.

Disadvantages. Risk of pneumothorax.

Femoral Vein Approach

The femoral line is an option probably underutilized in critical care settings.

Procedure

1. Place the patient in the supine position.
2. Use sterile preparation and appropriate draping. Administer local anesthesia in the area to be explored.
3. Palpate the femoral artery.
4. Guard the artery with the fingers of one hand.
5. Explore for the vein just medial to the operator's fingers with a needle and syringe.
6. It may be helpful to have a small amount of anesthetic in the syringe to inject with exploration.
7. The needle is directed cephalad at about a 30° angle and should be inserted below the femoral crease.
8. Puncture is heralded by the return of venous, nonpulsatile blood on application of negative pressure to the syringe.

9. Advance the guide wire through the needle.
10. The guide wire should pass with ease into the vein to a depth at which the distal tip of the guide wire is always under the operator's control even when the sheath/dilator or catheter is placed over the guide wire.
11. Remove the needle once the guide wire has advanced into the femoral vein.
12. If the catheter is 6 French or larger, a skin incision with a scalpel blade is generally needed. The catheter can then be advanced along with the guide wire in unison into the femoral vein. Be sure always to control the distal end of the guide wire.
13. Follow steps 14 through 17 for the right internal jugular vein approach.

Complications

1. The femoral deep line has the highest incidence of contamination and sepsis. If an occlusive dressing can remain in place and remain free from contamination, this is a safe option.
2. Deep vein thrombosis (DVT) has occurred from femoral vein catherization. The risk for DVT increases if the catheter remains in place for prolonged periods.

Advantages

1. The procedure is safe, in that arterial and venous sites are compressible.
2. It is impossible to cause pneumothorax from this site.
3. Placement can be accomplished without interrupting cardiopulmonary resuscitation.
4. This site can be used to place a variety of intravascular appliances, including temporary pacemakers, pulmonary artery catheters (expertise with fluoroscopy is needed), and triple-lumen catheters.

Disadvantages

1. Highest rate of infection.
2. Fluroscopy is required for placement of pulmonary artery catheters or transvenous pacemakers.

Median Basilic Vein Approach

It is possible in some patients, particularly men with well-developed upper extremities, to place an 8-French-sized introducer into the median basilic vein. The median basilic vein is directed medially at the antecubital fossa. The cephalic vein should be avoided. It runs laterally at the antecubital fossa and should not be relied on to pass a deep line because the line will commonly hang up at the origin of the axillary vein. Passage to the central circulation may occur via the cephalic vein but should be tested using a long, thin guide wire and fluoroscopy before this approach is counted on for central access.

Procedure

1. Use sterile preparation with appropriate draping.
2. Administer local anesthesia with lidocaine.
3. Place an intracath needle into the vein through which the guide wire will pass.
4. Advance the guide wire through the intracath.
5. Once the guide wire has passed into the median vein remove the intracath.
6. Incise the skin with a No. 11 scalpel. Advance the sheath/dilator system or triple-lumen catheter over the wire and into the vein while controlling either the proximal or distal end of the guide wire at all times.
7. Follow steps 14 through 17 for the right internal jugular vein approach.

Complications. Thrombophlebitis (should be removed in 48–72 hours).

Advantages

1. Noncompressible bleeding is avoided. This route or femoral route is preferred in the presence of coagulopathy or severe lung disease.
2. No risk of pneumothorax.

Disadvantages

1. Cannot be used in all patients.
2. Fluoroscopy is required for placement of pulmonary artery catheters or temporary pacemakers.
3. Uncomfortable and immobilizing.

■ CHEST TUBE INSERTION

Indications. Pneumothorax (simple or tension); hemothorax; hydrothorax; empyema.

Materials. Chest tube (28–36 French for adults), water-sealing drainage system (eg, Pleurevac) with connecting tubing, minor procedure and instrument tray, silk suture (0 or 2-0), Vaseline gauze.

Procedure

1. For a pneumothorax, choose a high anterior site, such as the second or third intercostal site, midclavicular line, or subaxillary position (more cosmetic). For fluid drainage, place a low lateral chest tube in the fifth or sixth intercostal space in the midaxillary line, directed posteriorly. For a traumatic pneumothorax, use a low lateral tube as this condition is usually associated with bleeding. Use a 24- to 38-French tube for pneumothorax and a 36-French tube for fluid removal.
2. If the procedure is elective, sedation may be helpful. Prep the area

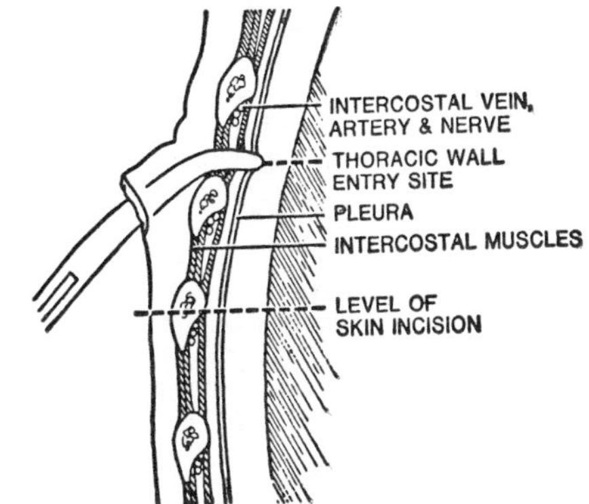

Figure 3–5. Chest tube technique demonstrating the procedure for creating a subcutaneous tunnel. (*From Gomella TL, ed.* Neonatology: Basic Management, On Call Problems, Diseases, Drugs. *San Mateo, Calif: Appleton & Lange; 1988. Used with permission.*)

with antiseptic and drape with towels. Use 1% lidocaine (with or without epinephrine) to anesthetize the skin and periosteum of the rib; start at the center of the rib and gently work over the top. Remember, the neurovascular bundle runs under the rib. (See Figure 3–5.)

3. Make a 2- to 3-cm transverse incision over the center of the rib. Use a hemostat to bluntly dissect over the top of the rib and create a subcutaneous tunnel. Injection of additional lidocaine into the muscle helps ease the pain.
4. Puncture the parietal pleura with the hemostat and spread the opening. Insert a gloved finger into the pleural cavity to gently clear any clots or adhesions and to help ensure that the lung is not accidentally punctured by the tube.
5. Carefully insert the tube superiorly into the desired position with a hemostat or gloved finger. Make sure all the holes in the tube are in the chest cavity. Attach the end of the tube to a water-sealed Pleurevac suction system.
6. Suture the tube in place. Place a heavy silk (0 or 2-0) suture through the incision next to the tube. Tie the incision together; then tie the ends around the chest tube. Alternatively, a pursestring suture can be placed. Make sure all of the suction holes are beneath the skin before the tube is secured.
7. Wrap the tube with Vaseline gauze and cover with plain gauze. Make the dressing as airtight as possible with tape.
8. Start suction (usually −20 cm in adults) and take a chest x-ray

immediately to check the placement of the tube and to evaluate for residual pneumothorax or fluid.

9. **To remove a chest tube,** make sure the pneumothorax or hemothorax is cleared. Check for an air leak by having the patient cough; observe the water-seal system for bubbling that indicates either a system (tubing) leak or a persistent pleural air leak.
10. Take the tube off suction BUT NOT OFF WATER-SEAL and cut the retention suture. (Some advocate clamping the tube before pulling it.) Have the patient perform the Valsalva maneuver while you apply pressure with Vaseline gauze and 4 × 4 gauze squares. Pull the tube rapidly and make an airtight seal with the Vaseline gauze as the tube is removed. Tape over the gauze to maintain an airtight seal. Check an upright chest x-ray for pneumothorax.

Complications. Infection, bleeding, lung damage, subcutaneous emphysema, persistent pneumothorax or fluid collection, poor tube placement.

■ ENDOTRACHEAL INTUBATION

(See also Chapter 6, Ventilator Management, p 355.)

Indications. Airway management during cardiopulmonary resuscitation; any indication for using mechanical ventilation such as coma, respiratory failure, or surgery.

Contraindications. (Relative) massive maxillofacial trauma; fractured larynx; suspected cervical spinal cord injury. Nasotracheal intubation is contraindicated in suspected basilar skull fractures.

Materials. Endotracheal tube (ETT), usually 7.0–9.0 mm in internal diameter for most adults; laryngoscope handle and blade (No. 3 straight or curved); 10-mL syringe; adhesive tape; suction equipment; malleable stylet (optional).

Procedure

1. Orotracheal intubation is most commonly used and is described here. The use of orotracheal intubation should be strongly discouraged in the case of suspected cervical spine injuries; nasotracheal intubation is preferred.
2. Any patient who is hypoxic or apneic must be ventilated with 100% oxygen using a bag and mask prior to attempting endotracheal intubation. Remember to avoid prolonged periods without ventilation if the intubation is difficult.
3. Extend the laryngoscope blade to 90° to verify that the light is working and check the balloon on the tube for leaks.
4. Place the patient's head in the so-called "sniffing position" (neck extended anteriorly and head extended posteriorly). Use suction to clear the upper airway if needed.
5. Hold the laryngoscope in the nondominant hand, hold the mouth

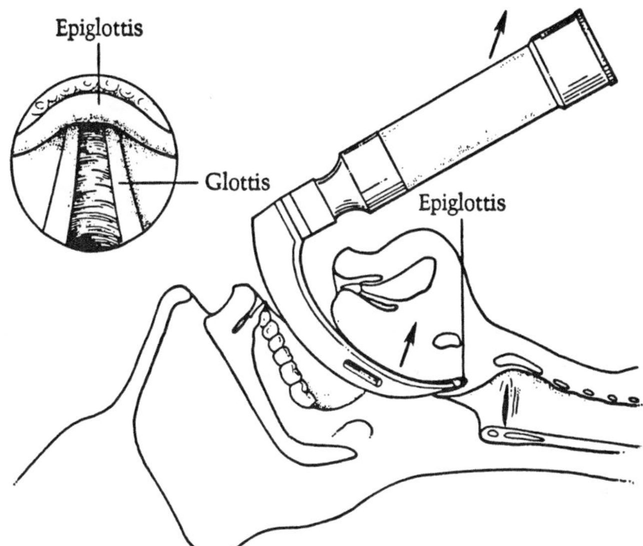

Figure 3–6. Endotracheal intubation. Advance blade to groove between base of tongue and epiglottis. (*From Vander Salm TJ, ed.* Atlas of Bedside Procedures, *2nd ed. Boston, Mass: Little, Brown; 1988: chap 21. Used with permission.*)

open with the dominant hand, and use the blade to push the tongue to the patient's left and make certain the tongue remains anterior to the blade. Advance carefully toward the midline until the epiglottis is seen.

6. With the STRAIGHT LARYNGOSCOPE BLADE pass the blade under the epiglottis, and lift the blade upward and the vocal cords should be visualized. If they are not, have an assistant push down on the thyroid cartilage. When using a CURVED blade, place it anterior to the epiglottis and gently lift anteriorly. The handle should not be used to pry the epiglottis open, but rather should be gently lifted in both cases. (See Figure 3–6.)
7. While maintaining visualization of the cords, grasp the ETT in the dominant hand and pass it through the cords. With more difficult intubations, a malleable stylet can be used to direct the tube.
8. Gently inflate the balloon with air from a 10-mL syringe until there is an adequate seal (about 5 mL). Ventilate the patient while auscultating laterally and visualizing both sides of the chest to verify positioning. If the left side does not seem to be ventilating, it may signify that

the tube has been advanced down the right mainstem bronchus. Withdraw the tube 1–2 cm and recheck the breath sounds. Confirm positioning with a stat chest x-ray.

9. Tape the tube in position and insert an oropharyngeal airway to prevent the patient from biting the ETT.

Complications. Bleeding; oral or pharyngeal trauma; improper tube positioning (esophageal or right mainstream bronchus intubation); aspiration; obstruction of the ETT or kinking.

■ GASTROINTESTINAL TUBES

Indications. Gastrointestinal (GI) decompression (paralytic ileus, obstruction, postoperatively); lavage of the stomach with GI bleeding or drug overdose; prevention of aspiration in obtunded patient (should protect the airway by endotracheal intubation first); feeding a patient who is unable to swallow.

Contraindications. Nasal fractures, basilar skull fracture.

Materials. Gastrointestinal tube of choice, lubricant jelly, catheter tip syringe, glass of water with a straw, stethoscope.

1. **Nasogastric tubes**
   a. **Levine:** Single-lumen tube that must be placed on intermittent suction to evacuate gastric contents.
   b. **Salem sump:** The best tube for continuous suction. A double-lumen tube, with the smaller tube acting as an air intake vent. Use 14- to 18-French size in adults.
   c. **Ewald:** Large (18–36 French) double-lumen tube, especially suited for gastric lavage of drug overdose, more often inserted by the orogastric route.
2. **Feeding tubes.** Although any small-bore nasogastric tube can be used as a feeding tube, certain weighted tubes are designed to pass into the duodenum and decrease the risk of aspiration of gastric contents.
   a. **Dobhoff, Entriflex, Keogh:** Weighted mercury tip with stylet.
   b. **Vivonex:** Tungsten-tipped.
3. **Sengsten-Blakemore tube:** A triple-lumen tube used exclusively for tamponade to control bleeding from esophageal varices. One lumen is for aspiration, one is for the gastric balloon, and the third is for the esophageal balloon.

Procedure

1. Inform the patient of the nature of the procedure and encourage cooperation by the patient. Choose the nasal passage that appears most patent by occluding one nostril and having the patient sniff.
2. Lubricate the distal 3–4 in. of the tube with a water-soluble jelly (K-Y

Jelly or viscous 2% lidocaine) and insert the tube gently along the floor of the nasal passageway. Maintain gentle pressure that will allow the tube to pass into the nasopharynx. Running the tube under warm water prior to lubrication makes it more pliable and may help facilitate the placement of the tube.

3. When the patient can feel the tube in the back of the throat, ask him or her to swallow small amounts of water through a straw as you advance the tube 2–3 in. at a time.
4. To be sure that the tube is in the stomach, aspirate gastric contents or blow air into the tube and listen over the stomach with your stethoscope for a "pop" or "gurgle."
5. Attach sump tubes (Salem sump) to continuous low wall suction and the single-lumen tube (Levin) to intermittent suction.
6. Feeding tubes are more difficult to insert because they are more flexible. A stylet or guide wire can be used or the smaller tube can be attached to a larger, stiffer tube by wedging both into a gelatin capsule. Pass the tube in the usual fashion and allow it to remain in the stomach for 10–15 minutes. After this time, the capsule dissolves and the larger tube can be removed.
7. Always verify the position of feeding tubes by chest x-ray before beginning the feedings.
8. Tape the tube securely in place but do not allow it to apply pressure to the ala of the nose. Patients have been disfigured because of ischemic necrosis of the nose caused by a poorly positioned tube.

Complications. Inadvertent passage into the trachea; coiling of the tube in the mouth or pharynx; bleeding from the nose, pharynx, or stomach.

■ INTRAVENOUS TECHNIQUES

Indications. To establish intravenous access for the administration of fluids, blood, or medications.

Materials. Intravenous fluid, connecting tubing, tourniquet, alcohol swab, intravenous cannulas (a catheter over a needle, such as Intracath, Angiocath, and Jelco or a butterfly needle), antiseptic ointment, dressing, and tape (it helps to rip the tape into strips and to flush the air out of the tubing with the intravenous fluid before you begin).

Procedure

1. An upper, nondominant extremity is the site of choice for an IV. Choose a distal vein so that if the vein is damaged, you can reposition the IV more proximally. Avoid veins that cross a joint space. Also avoid the leg, as there is a high incidence of thrombophlebitis. If no extremity vein can be found, try the external jugular vein. If all these fail, the only alternative is a central line or a cutdown.
2. Apply a tourniquet above the proposed IV site. Techniques to help

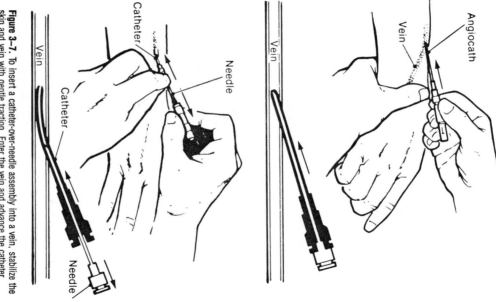

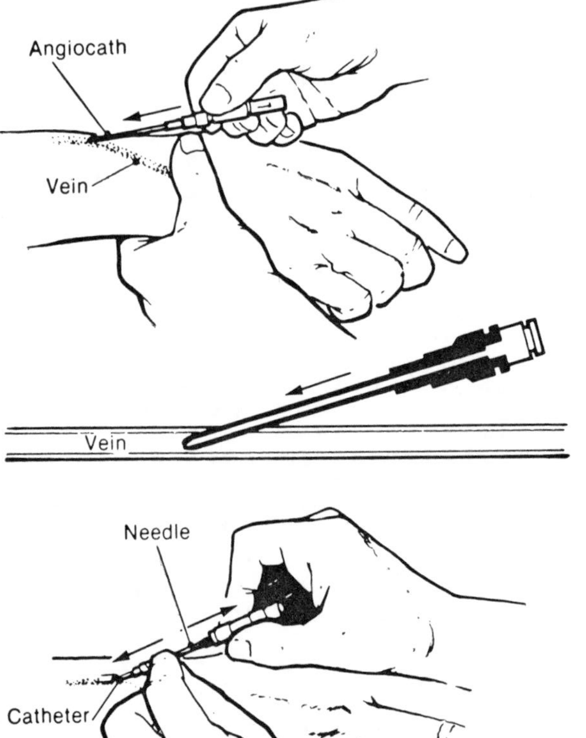

Figure 3–7. To insert a catheter-over-needle assembly into a vein, stabilize the skin and vein with gentle traction. Enter the vein and advance the catheter while holding the needle steady; then remove the needle. (*From Gomella LG, ed.* Clinician's Pocket Reference. *6th ed. East Norwalk, Conn: Appleton & Lange; 1989. Used with permission.*)

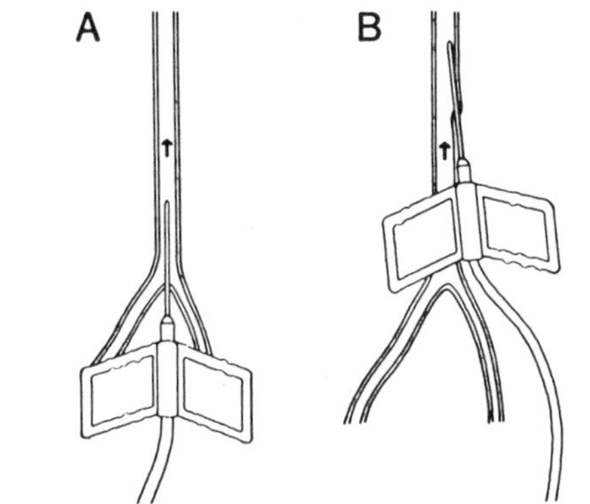

Figure 3–8. Example of a "butterfly" assembly and the two different techniques of entering a vein for intravenous access. (**A**) direct puncture and (**B**) side entry. (*From Gomella TL, ed.* Neonatology: Basic Management, On Call Problems, Diseases, Drugs. *San Mateo, Calif: Appleton & Lange, 1988. Used with permission.)*

expose difficult-to-locate veins include wrapping the extremity in a warm towel, leaving the arm in a dependent position for a few minutes after the tourniquet is applied, or using a blood pressure cuff as a tourniquet, inflated so that the arterial flow is still maintained. Carefully clean the site with an alcohol or povidone-iodine swab. If a large-bore IV is to be used (16 or 14 French), local anesthesia with 1% lidocaine may be helpful.

3. Stabilize the vein distally with the thumb of your free hand. Using the catheter-over-needle assembly (Intracath or Angiocath), enter the skin alongside the vein first, and then stick the vein along the side at about a 20° angle. Once the vein is punctured, blood should appear in the "flash" chamber. Advance a few more millimeters to be sure that BOTH the needle AND the tip of the catheter have entered the vein. Carefully withdraw the needle as you advance the catheter into the vein. (See Figure 3–7.) *NEVER WITHDRAW THE CATHETER OVER THE NEEDLE AS THIS PROCEDURE CAN SHEAR OFF THE PLASTIC TIP AND CAUSE A CATHETER EMBOLUS.* Apply pressure with your thumb over the vein just proximal to the site to prevent significant blood loss while you connect the IV line to the catheter.
4. Observe the site with the IV fluid running for signs of induration or swelling that indicate improper placement or damage to the vein.
5. Tape the IV securely in place; apply a drop of povidone-iodine or antibiotic ointment and a sterile dressing at the puncture site over

the needle. Ideally, the dressing should be changed every 24–48 hours to help reduce infections. Armboards are also useful to help maintain an IV site.

6. If the veins are deep and difficult to locate, a small 3- to 5-mL syringe can be mounted on the catheter assembly. Proper position inside the vein is determined by aspiration of blood.
7. If venous access is limited, a "butterfly" needle can be used (see Figure 3–8) or the external jugular vein may be considered as an alternative site.
8. All intravenous lines should be changed every 72 hours to decrease the risk of infection.

Complications. Thrombophlebitis; localized infection or sepsis.

■ LUMBAR PUNCTURE

Indications. Diagnostic purposes; measurement of cerebrospinal fluid pressure; injection of various agents (contrast medium, chemotherapy).

Contraindications. Increased intracranial pressure (papilledema, mass lesion); infection near the puncture site; planned myelography or pneumoencephalography; coagulopathy (see Chapter 1, Coagulopathy, p 60).

Materials. A sterile, disposable LP kit or minor procedure tray, spinal needles (21 gauge), sterile specimen tubes.

Procedure

1. Examine the optic disc for evidence of papilledema and review the CT scan of the head if available. Remember, a CT scan must be done prior to a lumbar puncture if there is papilledema or focal neurologic findings. Discuss the procedure with the patient and obtain informed consent from the patient or the legal representative.
2. Place the patient in the lateral decubitus position close to the edge of the bed or table. The patient (held by an assistant, if possible) should be positioned with knees pulled up toward the stomach and head flexed on the chest. This enhances flexion of the vertebral spine and widens the interspaces between the spinous processes. Try to position the patient so that the hips and spinal column are perpendicular to the bed. Place a pillow beneath the patient's side to prevent sagging and ensure alignment of the spinal column. In an obese patient or a patient with arthritis or scoliosis, the sitting position, leaning forward, may be preferred.
3. Draw an imaginary line between the iliac crests. This should cross the spine at the L4 vertebral body and assist in locating the L4–L5 interspace. You may want to make a mark in the skin with your

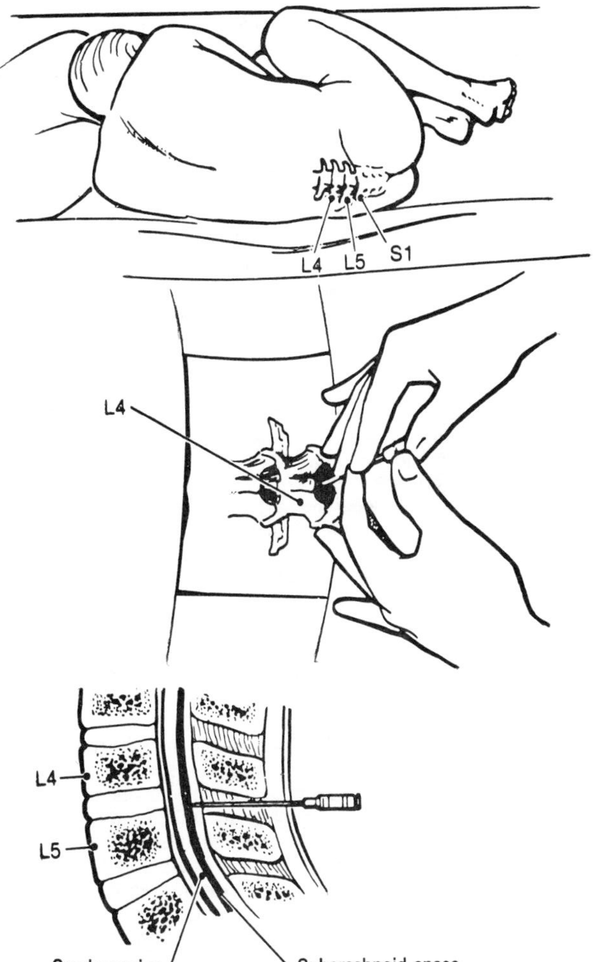

Figure 3–9. When performing a lumbar puncture, place the patient in the lateral decubitus position and locate the L4–L5 interspace. Control the spinal needle with two hands and enter the subarachnoid space. (*From Gomella LG, ed.* Clinician's Pocket Reference. *6th ed. East Norwalk, Conn: Appleton & Lange; 1989. Used with permission.)*

fingernail in the middle of the L4–L5 interspace prior to sterilizing the area for easier identification later.

4. Open the kit, put on sterile gloves, and prep the area with povidone-iodine solution in a circular fashion starting at the center and covering several interspaces. This step will need to be repeated twice. Next, drape the patient.
5. With a 25-gauge needle and 1% lidocaine, raise a skin wheal over the L4–L5 interspace. Anesthetize the deeper structures with a 22-gauge needle.
6. Examine the spinal needle and stylet for defects and then insert the needle with stylet into the skin wheal and into the spinous ligament. Hold the needle between the index fingers of both hands, with your thumbs holding the hub of the needle and stylet and guiding the needle. Direct the needle perpendicular to the long axis of the spine and parallel to the bed. Aim the needle toward the umbilicus. (See Figure 3–9.)
7. Advance through the major structures and "pop" into the subarachnoid space through the dura. An experienced operator can feel these layers, but an inexperienced one may need to remove the stylet periodically every 2–3 mm to look for return of fluid. Direct the bevel of the needle parallel to the long axis of the body so that the dural fibers are separated rather than sheared. This method helps cut down on "spinal headaches."
8. If no fluid returns, it is sometimes helpful to rotate the needle slightly. If there is still no fluid and you think that you are in the subarachnoid space, 1 mL of air can be injected as it is not uncommon for a piece of tissue to clog the needle. NEVER inject saline or distilled water. If no air returns and if spinal fluid cannot be aspirated, the bevel of the needle probably lies in the epidural space; advance it with the stylet in place.
9. If unsuccessful in the L4–L5 interspace, attempt the procedure one interspace above or below the current location.
10. When fluid returns, attach a manometer and stopcock and measure the pressure. Normal opening pressure is 70–180 mm water. Increased pressure may result from congestive heart failure (CHF), ascites, subarachnoid hemorrhage, infection, or a space-occupying lesion. Decreased pressure may result from needle position, obstructed flow, or severe volume depletion.
11. Collect 0.5- to 2.0-mL samples in serial, labeled containers. Send them to the lab in this order:
    - Tube 1 for cell count and differential
    - Tube 2 for glucose and protein
    - Tube 3 for bacterial culture and gram stain
    - Tube 4 for cell count and differential and special studies: VDRL, AFB, and fungal smear and culture, cryptococcal antigen, and counterimmune electrophoresis (CIE) or latex agglutination

TABLE 3–1. DIFFERENTIAL DIAGNOSIS OF CEREBROSPINAL FLUID

Condition	Color	Opening Pressure (mm H_2O)	Protein (mg/100 mL)	Glucose (mg/100 mL)	Cells (per mm^3)
Adult (normal)	Clear	70–180	45–80	45–80	0–5 lymphs
Viral infection	Clear or opalescent	Normal or slightly increased	Normal or slightly increased	Normal	10–500 lymphs (polys early)
Bacterial infection	Opalescent or yellow, may clot	Increased	50–1500	Decreased, usually < 20	25–10,000 polys
Granulomatous (TB, fungal)	Clear or opalescent	Often increased	Increased but usually < 500	Usually 20–40	10–500 lymphs
Subarachnoid hemorrhage	Bloody or usually xanthochromic after 2–8 hours	Usually increased	Increased	Normal	WBC/RBC ratio same as blood

WBC = white blood cell, RBC = white blood cell, lymphs = lymphocytes, polys = polymorphonuclear leukocytes, TB = tuberculosis.
Modified from Gomella LG, ed. Clinician's Pocket Reference. *6th ed. East Norwalk, Conn: Appleton and Lange; 1989. Used with permission.*

for *Streptococcus pneumoniae, Hemophilus influenzae, Neisseria meningitides,* as well as two less commonly found organisms, beta-hemolytic *streptococci* and *Stapholococcus aureus.*

Obtaining cell counts from tubes 1 and 4 permits better differentiation between a subarachnoid hemorrhage and a traumatic tap. In a traumatic tap, the number of red blood cells in the first tube should be much higher than that in the last tube. In a subarachnoid hemorrhage, the cell counts should be similar. Xanthochromia indicates the presence of old blood and suggests subarachnoid hemorrhage rather than a traumatic tap.

12. Withdraw the needle and place a sterile dressing over the site.
13. Instruct the patient to remain recumbent for 12–24 hours and encourage an increased fluid intake to help prevent "spinal headaches." Interpret the results based on Table 3–1.

Complications. Spinal headache (the most common complication seen about 20% of the time) typically is improved by recumbency and aggravated by upright posture. Its onset usually occurs within 24–48 hours of the procedure but may occur up to 1 week after the procedure. To help prevent spinal headaches, keep the patient recumbent for 12–24 hours, encourage the intake of fluids, use the smallest needle possible, and keep the bevel of the needle parallel to the long axis of the body to help prevent a persistent cerebrospinal fluid leak. If the headache is persistent and resistant to usual measures, refer to an anesthesiologist as a "blood patch" should be considered. Other complications include trauma to nerve roots, herniation of either the cerebellum or the medulla, and meningitis.

■ PARACENTESIS (Peritoneal)

Indications. To determine the cause of ascites; to rule out bacterial peritonitis; therapeutic removal of fluid as for respiratory distress.

Contraindications. Abnormal coagulation factors; multiple prior abdominal operations; uncooperative patient.

Materials. Minor procedure tray, Angiocath or Jelco (18- to 20-gauge with a $1\frac{1}{2}$-in. needle), 20- to 60-mL syringe, sterile specimen containers.

Procedure

1. Obtain informed consent. The patient's bladder needs to be empty.
2. If there is any doubt about whether or not ascites is present, confirmation should be made by ultrasound of the abdomen. If the amount of ascites is small, the ultrasound can be used to help locate the fluid during the procedure.
3. The entry site is usually the midline 3–4 cm below the umbilicus.

Avoid old surgical scars as the bowel may be clinging to the abdominal wall. Alternatively, the entry site can be in the left or right lower quadrant midway between the umbilicus and the anterior superior iliac spine or in the patient's flank, depending on percussion of the fluid wave.

4. Prep with povidone-iodine solution and drape the patient. Raise a skin wheal with 1% lidocaine over the proposed entry site.
5. With the Angiocath mounted on the syringe, go through the anesthetized area carefully while gently aspirating. You will meet some resistance as you enter the fascia. When you get free return of fluid, leave the catheter in place, remove the needle, reattach the syringe, and aspirate. Sometimes it is necessary to reposition the catheter because of abutting bowel.
6. Aspirate the amount of fluid needed for tests (20–30 mL). For a therapeutic tap, do not remove more than 500 mL in 10 minutes. A liter is the maximum that should be removed at one time. Otherwise, hypotension may result.
7. Quickly remove the needle, apply a sterile 4 × 4 gauze square, and apply pressure with tape.

TABLE 3–2. DIFFERENTIAL DIAGNOSIS OF ASCITIC FLUID

Transudative ascites: cirrhosis, nephrosis, congestive heart failure, hypoalbuminemia.

Exudative ascites: malignncy, peritonitis, tuberculosis, spontaneous perforated viscus, myxedema.

Lab Value	Transudate	Exudate
Specific gravity	< 1.016	> 1.016
Protein (ascitic fluid)	< 3 g/100 mL	> 3 g/100 mL
Protein (ascitic-to-serum ratio)	< 0.5	> 0.5
Lactic dehydrogenase (LDH) (ascitic-to-serum ratio)	< 0.6	> 0.6
Ascitic fluid LDH	< 200 IU	> 200 IU
Glucose (serum-to-ascitic ratio)	< 1	> 1
Fibrinogen (clot)	No	Yes
White blood cell count	< 500/mm³	> 1000/mm³
Red blood cell count		> 100 RBC/mm³

Food fibers: Found in most causes of a perforated viscus.

Cytology: Bizarre cells with large nuclei may represent reactive mesothelial cells and NOT a malignancy.

Malignant cells suggest a tumor.

Modified from Gomella LG, Lefor AT, eds. Surgery On Call Reference. *East Norwalk, Conn: Appleton & Lange; 1990. Used with permission.*

8. Depending on the clinical picture of the patient, send samples for total protein, specific gravity, lactate dehydrogenase, amylase, cytology, culture, stains, cell count, and differential. See Table 3–2 for the differential diagnosis of the fluid obtained.

Complications. Peritonitis; perforated bowel; intra-abdominal hemorrhage; perforated bladder.

■ PULMONARY ARTERY CATHETERIZATION

(See also Pulmonary Artery Catheter Problems, p 228.)

Indications. Pulmonary artery catheterization is generally undertaken in an acutely ill patient when a question exists regarding the patient's volume status or cardiac output. Some specific examples are (1) differentiating the etiology of pulmonary infiltrates between congestive heart failure and acute respiratory distress syndrome or pneumonia; (2) determining whether poor urine output is due to volume depletion, acute renal failure, or poor forward cardiac output; and (3) determining whether a patient with acute myocardial infarction and tachycardia has volume depletion, stress, or early left ventricular failure.

Contraindications. If a pulmonary artery catheter is needed to manage a patient in a critical care setting, there are no absolute contraindications. As with all indwelling catheters that are frequently manipulated, pulmonary artery catheters should be changed every 3 days to avoid the increased likelihood of an infection.

Materials. In most institutions, a single brand of a flow-directed balloon-tipped pulmonary artery catheter (often called Swan-Ganz catheter) is available. An insertion kit should be used that provides the catheter as well as a sheath and the various syringes, needles, preparation material, local anesthetic, and other items that will be used to insert the catheter.

The pulmonary artery catheter has four or five ports: air inflation port, thermistor, distal port, right atrial port, and (in some) a port for fluid or medication administration. (See Figure 3–10.) The air inflation port is used to inflate the balloon to facilitate passage of the catheter from the right cardiac chambers to the pulmonary artery. The thermistor can be used to measure cardiac outputs by thermal dilution when connected to a cardiac output computer. The distal port is used to measure pulmonary artery pressure and pulmonary capillary wedge pressure (PCWP) with the catheter in the pulmonary artery. The right atrial port is used to administer fluids, to measure right atrial pressure, or to inject fluid to measure cardiac output in conjunction with the thermistor and the cardiac output computer. (See Figure 3–10.) The catheter is often marked so it can be determined how far the distal tip is from the entry site. This may help in catheter placement without fluoroscopy.

Procedure

1. Informed consent is usually required.
2. A site is chosen and the area is prepped and draped. The choice of

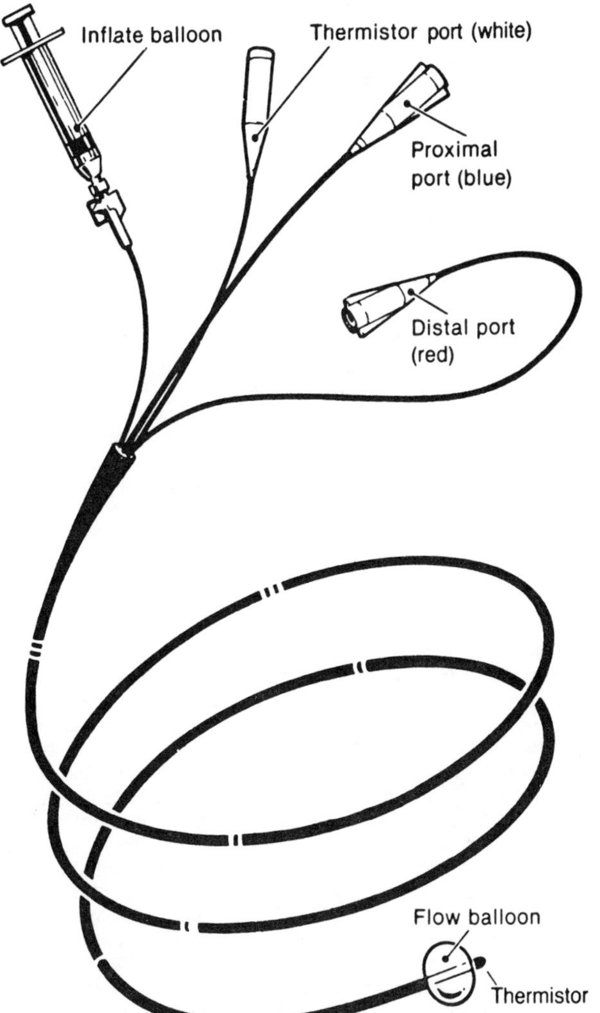

Figure 3–10. Pulmonary artery catheter (see text for complete description). (*From Gomella LG, ed.* Clinician's Pocket Reference. *6th ed. East Norwalk, Conn: Appleton & Lange; 1989. Used with permission.*)

site is dictated by patient variables and operator experience. The easiest sites to place a pulmonary artery catheter without fluoroscopic guidance are the right internal jugular vein and the left subclavian vein. In a patient who may receive thrombolytic therapy, femoral and median basilic veins are better routes.

3. A strict sterile approach with gown, gloves, and mask is generally used.
4. The pulmonary artery catheter is prepared by flushing the lumens with heparinized saline solution (1 mL of 1:100 U heparin in 10 mL of normal saline). Balloon function is checked, and the catheter is tapped to be sure that an appropriate waveform is present. The pressure transducer should be set level to the middle of the patient's chest.
5. The central vein is cannulated. (See Central Venous Catheterization, p 314, for details.) In general, never push a guide wire where it does not want to go and **always** keep one hand on the guide wire.
6. Once the sheath is in place, the prepared catheter can be advanced into the sheath. Once it has been advanced approximately 15 cm, the balloon will have cleared the tip of the sheath and can be gently inflated with 1.0–1.5 cm^3 of air. The maximum amount of air to be used with smaller catheters (5 French) is 1.0 cm^3. If there is resistance to full inflation, consider that the balloon may not have yet cleared the sheath or that it may be in an extravascular location.
7. Once the balloon is inflated, advance the catheter to the level of the right atrium under the guidance of the pressure waveform and the electrocardiogram. Monitor the waveform and electrocardiogram at all times while advancing the balloon catheter. Advance the catheter with the balloon inflated and withdraw it with the balloon deflated. Pulmonary artery catheters usually come with a preformed curve on the tip. The catheter should be inserted pointing the catheter tip anteriorly and to the left. Positioning in the right atrium is probably best determined by watching for the characteristic waveform. The right atrium is generally located approximately 20 cm from the right internal jugular or subclavian vein insertion site and approximately 25–30 cm from the left subclavian vein insertion site. The catheter should be advanced steadily. An abrupt change in the pressure tracing will occur as the catheter enters the right ventricle. There is generally little ectopy on entry into the right ventricle; however, as the catheter is advanced into the right ventricular outflow tract, premature ventricular contractions (PVCs) may occur. Keep advancing the catheter until the ectopy disappears and the pulmonary artery tracing is obtained. If this does not occur, the balloon should be deflated and the catheter withdrawn and another attempt made with the balloon inflated after slightly rotating the catheter. The PCWP will then be obtained after advancing the catheter another 10–15 cm. The catheter's final

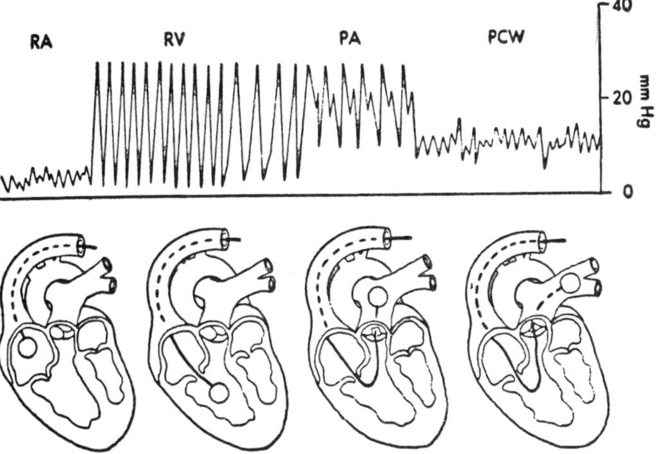

Figure 3–11. Pulmonary artery catheter pressure waveforms as the catheter is advanced from the right atrium to the pulmonary artery in the wedge position. RA = right atrial pressure, RV = right ventricular pressure, PA = pulmonary artery pressure, and PCW = pulmonary capillary wedge pressure. (*From Rosen P, ed.* Emergency Medicine Concepts and Clinical Practice. *St. Louis, Mo: C.V. Mosby; 1983. Used with permission.*)

position should be such that the PCWP is obtained with full balloon inflation and the pulmonary artery pressure (PAP) tracing is present with the balloon deflated. In the "ideal position," transition from PAP to PCWP (and vice versa) will occur within three or fewer heartbeats. NEVER withdraw the catheter with the balloon inflated. See Figure 3–11 for normal waveforms. See Table 3–3 for normal pulmonary artery catheter measurements.

8. The catheter is sutured in place and dressed according to each institution's practice. A chest x-ray should be obtained to document the catheter's present position as well as to rule out a pneumothorax or other complication from central venous catheterization.
9. Common problems. Catheter placement is much more difficult if severe pulmonary artery hypertension is present. If there is significant cardiac enlargement, particularly dilation of the right heart structures, the catheter may have a propensity to coil and get lost in its path to the right ventricular outflow tract. Fluoroscopy may be required to get the catheter into the correct position and it will hold this position poorly. Placement of the catheter in the pulmonary artery may also be difficult in the setting of a low cardiac output as

TABLE 3–3. NORMAL PULMONARY ARTERY CATHETER MEASUREMENTS

Parameter	Range
Right atrial pressure	1–7 mm Hg
Right ventricular systolic pressure	15–25 mm Hg
Right ventricular diastolic pressure	0–8 Hg
Pulmonary artery systolic pressure	15–25 mm Hg
Pulmonary artery diastolic pressure	8–15 mm Hg
Pulmonary artery mean pressure	10–20 mm Hg
Pulmonary capillary wedge pressure	6–12 mm Hg
Cardiac output	3.5–5.5 L/min
Cardiac index	2.8–3.2 L/min

From Gomella LG, ed. Clinician's Pocket Reference. *6th ed. East Norwalk, Conn: Appleton & Lange; 1989. Used with permission.*

the balloon-tipped catheter is dependent on blood flow to carry it through the right heart chambers.

10. Cardiac output can be measured by thermal dilution. First, connect the thermistor to the cardiac output computer. Then rapidly inject fluid (usually 10 mL of ice-cooled normal saline) through the right atrial port. Have someone set the computer as you inject. The computer will display the cardiac output. Repeat two more times. If all these values are approximately the same, then average the readings and record. For normal cardiac output and index, see Table 3–3.
11. Various clinical entities can often be differentiated by measuring the blood pressure, PCWP, and cardiac output while calculating the systemic vascular resistance. (See Table 3–4.) Abnormalities in various pressures obtained from pulmonary artery catheterization can often help diagnose various disease states. (See Table 3–5.)

Complications

1. Most complications that occur in the course of pulmonary artery catheterization are related to central vein cannulation and include arterial puncture and pneumothorax.
2. Arrhythmias are another common complication. The most common of these are transient PVCs that occur when the catheter is advanced into the right ventricular outflow tract. If a patient with a pulmonary artery catheter suddenly develops frequent premature ventricular complexes, displacement of the catheter should be suspected.
3. Ventricular tachycardia (VT) and ventricular fibrillation (VF) are rare occurrences.
4. Transient right bundle branch block (RBBB) occurs occasionally as the catheter passes through the right ventricular outflow tract. In a patient with preexisting left bundle branch block, this can result in

TABLE 3–4. COMMONLY ENCOUNTERED HEMODYNAMIC SUBSETS

	BP	PCWP	CO	SVR
Volume depletion	Decreased	Decreased	Decreased or normal	Increased
Volume overload (Normal left ventricular function)	Normal or increased	Increased	Increased	Normal or decreased
Sepsis, early	Normal or decreased	Normal or decreased	Increased	Decreased
Sepsis, late	Decreased	Decreased	Decreased	Decreased
Cardiogenic shock	Decreased	Increased	Decreased	Increased

$$SVR = \frac{80\ (\text{aortic mean pressure—right atrial mean pressure})}{\text{cardiac output}}$$

BP = Blood pressure, PCWP = pulmonary capillary wedge pressure, CO = cardiac output, SVR = systemic vascular resistance.
Modified from Gomella LG, Lefor AT, eds. Surgery On Call Reference, *East Norwalk, Conn: Appleton & Lange; 1990. Used with permission.*

TABLE 3–5. DIFFERENTIAL DIAGNOSIS OF COMMON PULMONARY ARTERY CATHETER READINGS

Low right atrial pressure	Volume depletion
High right atrial pressure	Volume overload, congestive heart failure, cardiogenic shock, increased pulmonary vascular resistance (hypoxia, ventilator effect of PEEP, pulmonary disease, primary pulmonary hypertension)
Low right ventricular pressure	Volume depletion
High right ventricular pressure	Volume overload, congestive heart failure, cardiogenic shock, increased pulmonary vascular resistance (hypoxia, ventilator effect of PEEP, pulmonary disease, primary pulmonary hypertension)
High pulmonary artery pressure	Congestive heart failure, increased pulmonary vascular resistance (hypoxia, ventilator effect of PEEP, pulmonary disease, primary pulmonary hypertension), cardiac tamponade
Low wedge pressure	Volume depletion
High wedge pressure	Cardiogenic shock, left ventricular failure, ventricular septal defect, mitral regurgitation and stenosis, volume overload, cardiac tamponade

PEEP = positive end expiratory pressure.
Modified from Gomella LG, Lefor AT, eds. Surgery On Call Reference. *East Norwalk, Conn: Appleton & Lange; 1990. Used with permission.*

complete heart block. In this setting, some form of backup pacing should be readily available. Complete heart block has been reported but occurs rarely.

5. Significant pulmonary infarcts and pulmonary artery rupture are serious but infrequent complications of pulmonary artery catheters secondary to permanent wedge or peripheral placement of the catheter.
6. Most complications and problems tend to increase with the time the catheter is in place. There is a significant risk of bacteremia and subacute bacterial endocarditis in chronically instrumented, severely ill patients. In the setting of unexplained fever, the catheter and sheath should always be removed and cultured. The catheter and sheath should be replaced at a different site if a pulmonary catheter is still indicated.

■ SKIN BIOPSY

Indications. Any skin lesion or eruption for which the diagnosis is unclear; any skin condition that has been unresponsive to therapy.

Contraindications. Any skin lesion that is suspected to be a malignancy should be referred to a dermatologist or plastic surgeon for excisional biopsy rather than a punch biopsy.

Materials. A 2-, 3-, 4-, or 5-mm skin punch; 3 mL lidocaine 1% solution; 3-mL syringe; 26-gauge needle; sterile gloves; 4 × 4 gauze pads; 70% alcohol solution; pair of curved iris scissors and fine-tooth forceps (ordinary forceps may distort a small biopsy specimen and should not be used); specimen bottle containing 10% formalin; suturing materials for 3- to 5-mm skin punch biopsies.

Procedure

1. If more than one lesion is present, choose one that is well developed and representative of the dermatosis. For patients with vesiculobullous disease, an early edematous lesion should be chosen rather than a vesicle. Avoid lesions that are excoriated or infected.
2. Mark the area to be biopsied with a skin marking pen. Inject the lidocaine to form a skin wheal over the site of the biopsy.
3. After putting on sterile gloves and preparing a sterile field, perform the punch biopsy. First, immobilize the skin with the fingers of one hand, applying pressure perpendicular to the skin wrinkle lines with the skin punch. Core out a cylinder of skin by twirling the punch between the fingers of the other hand. As the punch enters into the subcutaneous fat, resistance will lessen. At this point, the punch should be removed. The core of tissue usually pops up slightly and can be cut at the level of the subcutaneous fat with curved iris scissors without using forceps. If tissue core does not pop up, it may

be elevated by use of a hypodermic needle or fine-tooth forceps. Be sure to include a portion of the subcutaneous fat in the specimen.
4. Place the specimen in the specimen container.
5. Hemostasis can be achieved by pressure with the gauze pad.
6. Defects from 1.5- and 2-mm punches usually do not require suturing and will heal with very minimal scarring. Punch defects that are 2–4 mm can generally be closed with a single suture.
7. A dry dressing should be applied and removed the following day.
8. Sutures can be removed as early as 3 days from the face and 7 to 10 days from other areas.

Complications. Infection (unusual); hemorrhage (usually controlled by simple application of pressure); keloid formation, especially in a patient with a prior history of keloid formation.

■ THORACENTESIS

Indications. Diagnosis of pleural effusion; therapeutic removal of pleural fluid; instillation of sclerosing compounds such as tetracycline to obliterate the pleural space.

Contraindications. Pneumothorax, hemothorax, or respiratory impairment on the contralateral side; coagulopathy (relative); a patient receiving positive pressure ventilation (relative).

Materials. Prepackaged thoracentesis kit or minor procedure tray plus 20- to 60-mL syringe, 20- or 22-gauge $1\frac{1}{2}$-in. needle, three-way stopcock, specimen containers.

Procedure

1. It takes at least 300 mL of fluid to visualize a pleural effusion on a standard posteroanterior chest x-ray.
2. Discuss the procedure with the patient and obtain informed consent. Teach the patient the Valsalva maneuver or make sure the patient can hum.
3. The usual site for a thoracentesis is the posterolateral back above the diaphragm but under the fluid level. Percuss out the fluid level or use the chest x-ray and count ribs. The site will be above the rib to avoid the neurovascular bundle that travels below the rib.
4. Prep the area with povidone-iodine and drape. The patient should be sitting up comfortably; leaning too far forward causes the effusion to move anteriorly away from the thoracentesis site. The bed stand is helpful to keep the patient upright and leaning slightly forward.
5. Make a skin wheal over the proposed site with a 25-gauge needle and lidocaine. Change to a 22-gauge $1\frac{1}{2}$-needle and infiltrate up and over the rib; try to anesthetize the deeper structures and the pleura. During this time, you should be aspirating. (See Figure 3–12.) Once fluid returns, note the depth of the needle and mark it with a hemo-

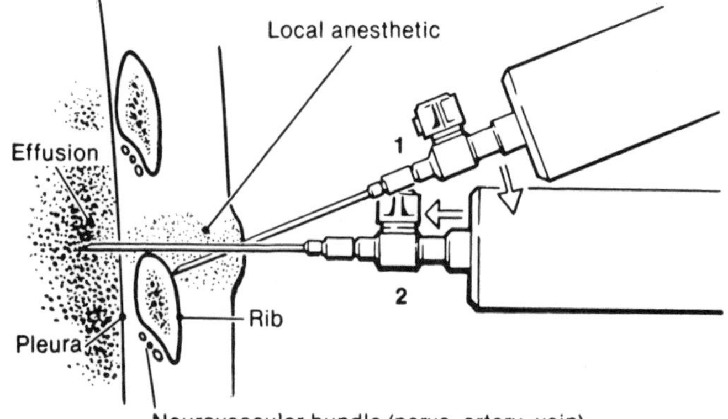

Figure 3–12. In a thoracentesis, the needle is passed over the top of the rib to avoid the neurovascular bundle. (*From Gomella, LG, ed.* Clinician's Pocket Reference. *6th ed. East Norwalk, Conn: Appleton & Lange; 1989. Used with permission.*)

stat. This gives you the approximate depth before entering the pleural space. Remove the needle.

6. Measure the 16- to 18-gauge thoracentesis needle to the same depth as the first needle with a hemostat. Penetrate through the anesthetized area with the thoracentesis needle. You may also use a catheter-over-needle assembly (Angiocath) and leave the plastic catheter in position to remove the fluid. Always go over the top of the rib to avoid the neuromuscular bundle that runs below the rib. (See Figure 3–12.) Never pull the catheter back over the needle or shearing of the catheter can occur. Attach the three-way stopcock and tubing and aspirate the amount needed. Turn the stopcock and evacuate the fluid through the tubing. NEVER REMOVE MORE THAN 1000 mL PER TAP!
7. Have the patient hum or do the Valsalva maneuver as you withdraw the needle. This maneuver increases intrathoracic pressure and decreases the chance of a pneumothorax. Bandage the site.
8. Obtain a chest x-ray to evaluate the fluid level and to rule out a pneumothorax. An expiratory film is best because a small pneumothorax is more likely to be visualized.
9. Distribute specimens in containers, label slips, and send to the lab. Always order pH, specific gravity, protein, LDH, cell count and differential, glucose, gram stain and cultures, and fungal and acid-fast cultures and smears. Optional lab studies are cytology if you suspect a malignancy, amylase if you suspect an effusion secondary to pan-

TABLE 3–6. DIFFERENTIAL DIAGNOSIS OF PLEURAL FLUID

Transudate: Nephrosis, congestive heart failure, cirrhosis.

Exudate: Infection (pneumonia, tuberculosis, malignancy, empyema, peritoneal dialysis, pancreatitis, chylothorax).

Lab value	Transudate	Exudate
Specific gravity	< 1.016	> 1.016
Protein (pleural fluid)	< 2.5 g/100 mL	> 3 g/100 mL
Protein ratio (pleural fluid-to-serum ratio)	< 0.5	> 0.6
LDH ratio (pleural fluid-to-serum ratio)	< 0.5	> 0.6
Pleural fluid LDH	< 200 IU	> 200 IU
Fibrinogen (clot)	No	Yes
Cell count and differential	Low WBC count	WBC count > 2500/mm^3; suspect an inflammatory exudate (early polys, later monos)

Grossly bloody tap: trauma, pulmonary infarction, tumor, and iatrogenic causes.

pH: The pH of pleural fluid is usually > 7.3. If between 7.2 and 7.3, suspect tuberculosis or malignancy or both. If < 7.2, suspect an empyema.

Glucose: Normal pleural fluid glucose is two-thirds serum glucose. If the pleural fluid glucose is MUCH, MUCH lower than the serum glucose,then consider empyema or rheumatoid arthritis (0–16 mg/100 mL) as the cause of the effusion.

Triglycerides and positive Sudan stain: Chylothorax.

LDH = lactic dehydrogenase, WBC = white blood cells, polys = polymorphonuclear leukocytes, monos = monocytes.

Modified from Gomella LG, Lefor AT, eds. Surgery On Call Reference. *East Norwalk, Conn: Appleton & Lange; 1990. Used with permission.*

creatitis (usually on the left), and a Sudan stain and triglycerides if a chylothorax is suspected. See Table 3–6 for the differential diagnosis.

Complications. Pneumothorax, hemothorax, infection, pulmonary laceration, hypoxemia, vasovagal attack.

4 Fluids and Electrolytes

Daily maintenance requirements for the average 70-kg man are as follows:

Fluid	2000–2500	mL
Dextrose	100–200	g
Sodium	60–100	mEq
Potassium	40–60	mEq

These requirements can be met with an infusion of $D_5 \frac{1}{4}$ NS with 20–30 mEq of potassium chloride per liter infused at 100 mL/h. The preceding combination of fluid and electrolytes may differ depending on other clinical parameters such as congestive heart failure, cirrhosis, hyponatremia, hypernatremia, hyperkalemia, and renal insufficiency. Maintenance fluids should be used for only 48–72 hours at which time more effective measures of nutritional support (enteral tube feedings) should be instituted. For patients with severe volume depletion, normal saline can be administered as rapidly as 500–1000 mL/h until the patient is stabilized. For patients undergoing nasogastric suction, measured losses can be replaced every 4 hours with an equal volume of normal saline. Additional potassium may have to be added to the maintenance fluids to replace that lost with gastric suction. (See Tables 4–1 and 4–2.)

TABLE 4–1. COMPOSITIONS OF COMMONLY USED CRYSTALLOID SOLUTIONS

Fluid	Glucose (g/L)	Na	Cl	K (mEq/L)	Ca	HCO_3	kcal/L
D5W (dextrose in 5% water)	50	—	—	—	—	—	170
D10W (dextrose in 10% water)	100	—	—	—	—	—	340
D20W (dextrose in 20% water)	200	—	—	—	—	—	680
D50W (dextrose in 50% water)	500	—	—	—	—	—	1700
½ NS (0.45% NaCl)	—	77	77	—	—	—	—
NS (0.9% NaCl)	—	154	154	—	—	—	—
3% NS	—	513	513	—	—	—	—
D 5% ¼ NS	50	34	34	—	—	—	170
D 5% ½ NS (0.45% NaCl)	50	77	77	—	—	—	170
D 5% NS (0.9% NaCl)	50	154	154	—	—	—	170
D 5% lactated ringer's (D5LR)	50	130	110	4	3	27	180
Lactated ringer's	—	130	110	4	3	27	<10

NS = normal saline.
Modified from Gomella LG, ed. Clinician's Pocket Reference. *6th ed. Norwalk, Conn: Appleton and Lange; 1989. Used with permission.*

TABLE 4–2. COMPOSITION AND DAILY PRODUCTION OF BODY FLUIDS

	Electrolytes (mEq/L)				Average Daily Production (mL)
Fluid	***Na***	***Cl***	***K***	***HCO_3***	
Sweat	50	40	5	0	Varies
Saliva	100	15	26	50	1500
Gastric juice	60–100	100	10	0	1500–2000
Duodenum	130	90	5	0–10	300–2000
Bile	145	100	5	15–35	100–800
Pancreatic juice	140	75	5	70–115	100–800
Ileum	140	100	5	15–30	2000–3000
Diarrhea	50	40	35	45	—

Modified from Gomella LG, ed. Clinician's Pocket Reference. *6th ed. Norwalk, Conn: Appleton and Lange; 1989. Used with permission.*

5 Blood Component Therapy

■ RED CELL TRANSFUSIONS

Prior to transfusion of any red cell products, three things must be considered: (1) the absolute level of hemoglobin (HGB) or hematocrit (HCT); (2) the patient's symptoms; and (3) the physiologic capabilities. Transfusion should not be undertaken strictly to achieve a specific HCT.

GENERAL GUIDELINES

1. Hemoglobin greater than 10 g/dL: No transfusion.
2. Hemoglobin 8–10 g/dL: Avoid transfusion unless a therapeutic trial shows a marked improvement in symptoms.
3. Hemoglobin 6–8 g/dL: Try to avoid transfusion by reducing activity and treating underlying disease.
4. Hemoglobin less than 6 g/dL: Transfusion almost always indicated.

ANEMIA

When confronted with a chronic anemia, one must consider whether the HGB and HCT accurately reflect the red blood cell (RBC) mass. The RBC mass is more important with respect to oxygen transport than the measured HCT or HGB; however, a low HGB or HCT usually reflect a low RBC mass. Instances in which plasma volume may be increased (congestive heart failure, splenomegaly, paraproteinemia) may lead to an apparently more severe anemia than is actually present; also, contraction of the plasma volume can lessen the apparent severity of an anemia and this must be considered prior to transfusion.

Acute Blood Loss. In the setting of acute blood loss, restoration of blood volume and tissue perfusion as well as improvement of oxygen-carrying capacity must be accomplished. Electrolyte solutions and/or colloids should be used initially. Blood losses of 500–1000 mL in an adult usually do not require blood transfusion unless there is an underlying anemia or there are other medical conditions that would be an indication for the added oxygen-carrying capacity.

RBC Products—Availability and Indications

1. **Whole blood.** There are few indications for transfusion of whole blood today except for transfusion of the massively bleeding patient where volume and oxygen-carrying capacity can be supplied in one

product. Stored whole blood is not adequate replacement for platelets or labile coagulation factors.

2. **Packed RBCs.** Basically a unit of whole blood with two thirds of the plasma removed. This has become the standard red cell product for most transfusions.
3. **Leukocyte-poor RBCs.** Seventy to ninety percent of leukocytes are removed by a variety of techniques. Leukocyte-poor red cells are used in patients with a history of repeated febrile reactions to standard packed RBC transfusions. These reactions are usually due to leukocyte antigens. Leukocyte-poor RBCs can be indicated in patients expected to receive large amounts of blood products including platelets in an effort to decrease the incidence of formation of alloantibodies. They also may be indicated for use in bone marrow transplant candidates.
4. **Washed RBCs.** Virtually all plasma and nonerythrocyte cellular elements are removed. Washed cells are indicated in patients with febrile reactions to leukocyte-poor RBCs, in patients with allergic reactions to plasma components (IgA deficiency), and in patients with paroxysmal nocturnal hemoglobinuria where exposure to complement may exacerbate the hemolytic process.
5. **Frozen stored RBCs.** Used mainly to store blood for autologous transfusion after elective surgery and to maintain availability of units for patients with alloantibodies to high-incidence blood group antigens.

Complications. See Transfusion Reaction. p 251.

■ GRANULOCYTE TRANSFUSIONS

Indications. Granulocyte transfusions are rarely used but are of benefit in very selected settings. Studies have shown the benefit of white blood cell (WBC) transfusions in patients with severe neutropenia and gram-negative bacteremia that is persistent despite appropriate antibiotic therapy for at least 48 hours. In this specific setting, daily transfusion of at least 10^{10} WBCs until infection resolves and/or the granulocyte count recovers to 500/mL are appropriate. The use of WBC transfusions prophylactically, for fever of unknown origin, or for nonbacterial infections in the neutropenic patient has not been shown to be effective and cannot be recommended.

Complications. White blood cell transfusions are associated with numerous possible adverse reactions. (See Transfusion Reaction, p 251.)

1. **Immediate febrile transfusion reaction.** Most common, occurring within a few hours of transfusion. Clinical signs include fever, chills, cyanosis, dyspnea, wheezing, nausea, vomiting, pruritus, urticaria, anxiety, and hypertension or hypotension. The etiology can be multifactorial, but one of the major factors is alloimmunization to granulocyte antigens. This can be reduced by human leukocyte antigen

(HLA) type-specific WBC transfusions. Symptoms can be treated with antihistamines, antipyretics, and steroids. The same measures may be undertaken as premedications in an effort to prevent the reaction.

2. **Pulmonary infiltrates and adult respiratory distress syndrome.** One of the most serious WBC posttransfusion hazards. The exact mechanism is unknown. Mortality can be significant.
3. **Other potential hazards**
   a. **Transmission of infectious agents.** Usually viral, the most serious being cytomegalovirus.
   b. **Graft-versus-host disease.** Occurring in patients who have severe underlying immune defects resulting from disease or therapy. Common in patients with leukemias and lymphomas. It would be reasonable to consider irradiation of all blood products in these patients, although firm recommendations cannot be made at this time.

■ PLATELET TRANSFUSIONS

(See also Chapter 1, Thrombocytopenia, p 246.)

Indications. Platelet transfusions are indicated for any patient with a major bleeding event having a qualitative or quantitative platelet disorder. Prophylactic platelet transfusions are most commonly indicated with radiation- or chemotherapy-induced bone marrow suppression. Studies done on leukemic patients have shown that spontaneous major bleeding increases dramatically with platelet counts below 5000. Minor bleeding increases as the platelet count falls below 20,000. Most centers transfuse prophylactically for platelet counts below 20,000. Patients with lifelong quantitative or qualitative platelet disorders should not be prophylactically transfused solely on the basis of platelet count, bleeding time, or other platelet function studies. Overutilization of platelets increases the risk of alloimmunization and subsequently, there will be an inadequate response to platelet transfusions when clearly needed for major bleeding episodes or invasive procedures. Likewise, patients with idiopathic thrombocytopenic purpura (ITP) should not be prophylactically transfused.

Complications

1. **Transmission of viral infections**
2. **Reactions to plasma components, RBCs, and WBCs.** Reactions to RBC antigens rarely cause a hemolytic transfusion reaction. They can cause alloimmunity and the potential for problems such as the use of Rh-positive platelets in an Rh-negative female. The patient should receive intravenous anti-D globulin (RhoGAM) if of childbearing age.
3. **Possible transmission of bacterial infections.** A potential problem because of the storage time and storage temperature of platelet concentrates.
4. **Development of alloimmunization.** Eventually occurs in two thirds

of multiply transfused patients. May necessitate the use of HLA-matched platelets to achieve adequate posttransfusion counts.

■ PLASMA COMPONENT THERAPY

The following is a list of commonly available plasma products and selected remarks about indications and complications.

Fresh-Frozen Plasma

1. Contains all factors, but titers of factors VIII and V decline with long-term storage. Can be used for replacement of other factor deficiencies, but problems include long turnaround time because of the need for thawing and the potential volume of plasma needed to correct certain factor deficiencies.
2. Other side effects include urticaria, fever, nausea, headaches, and pruritus. These can usually be treated and/or prevented with antihistamines and antipyretics.
3. Transmission of viral infections is less likely than with the factor concentrates.

Cryoprecipitate

1. Contains high levels of factor VIII, von Willebrand factor, and fibrinogen. Useful in factor VIII deficiency, von Willebrand disease, disorders of fibrinogen, and uremic bleeding.
2. Risk of transfusion-associated hepatitis is high.

Factor VIII Concentrate

1. Various preparations are available. Only heat-treated preparations should be used to minimize the risk of transmitting human immunodeficiency virus.
2. Use is limited to patients with factor VIII deficiency.

Vitamin K-Dependent Factor Concentrates (Konyne, Proplex)

1. Contains factors II, VII, IX, and X, protein C, and protein S. Useful in these specific factor deficiencies and in patients with factor VIII inhibitors.
2. Risk of hepatitis and thromboembolic disease exists because of the presence of activated factors in some preparations.

Single-Donor Plasma

1. Collected from one donor unit of whole blood. Levels of factors V and VIII decline appreciably with storage and single-donor plasma should not be used to replace these factors.
2. Risk of hepatitis and other infections equivalent to the risk associated with transfusing a unit of whole blood.

Gamma Globulin. There are many different forms of intravenous and intramuscular gamma globulins available with a wide variety of indications and reactions.

1. **Indications**
   - **a.** Nonspecific immunoglobulin for hepatitis A and non-A/non-B hepatitis prophylaxis. Hepatitis B immunoglobulin is used for prophylaxis for hepatitis B. Specific immunoglobulins can also be used for postexposure prophylaxis for varicella and rabies.
   - **b.** Prophylactic or therapeutic intravenous use in patients with inherited or acquired humoral immune deficiencies.
   - **c.** Therapy of acute and chronic immune thrombocytopenic purpura.
2. **Reactions.** The following are adverse effects that might result from the administration of gamma globulin.
   - **a. Anaphylactoid reaction.** An immediate reaction attributed to complement activation. Symptoms and signs may include flushing, chest tightness, dyspnea, fever, chills, nausea, vomiting, hypotension, and back pain. These are uncommon reactions with the currently available preparations but can occur with both intravenous and intramuscular administration. Therapy consists of discontinuation of the infusion and use of diphenhydramine (Benadryl), steroids, epinephrine, and vasopressors if necessary.
   - **b. Inflammatory reaction.** Characteristically a delayed reaction. Signs and symptoms may include headache, malaise, fever, chills, and nausea. The reaction disappears with discontinuation of gamma globulin therapy.

REFERENCES

Mollison PL, Engelfriet CP, Contreras M. The transfusion of platelets, leucocytes, haemopoietic cells and plasma components. In: *Blood Transfusion in Clinical Medicine.* 8th ed. Oxford: Blackwell Scientific; 1987:160–193.

Mollison PL, Engelfriet CP, Contreras M. The transfusion of red cells. In: *Blood Transfusion in Clinical Medicine.* 8th ed. Oxford: Blackwell Scientific; 1987:95–159.

6 Ventilator Management

- **Indications and Setup**
- **Routine Modifications of Settings**
- **Troubleshooting**
  - **a.** Agitation
  - **b.** Hypoxemia
  - **c.** Hypercarbia
  - **d.** High Peak Pressures
- **Weaning**

INDICATIONS AND SETUP

I. Indications

A. Ventilatory failure. Judged by the degree of hypercarbia. A $PaCO_2 > 50$ Torr indicates ventilatory failure; however, many patients will have chronic ventilatory failure with renal compensation (retaining HCO_3^-) to adjust the pH toward normal. Thus, absolute pH is often a better guide to determine the need for ventilatory assistance than $PaCO_2$. A respiratory acidosis with a rapidly falling pH or an absolute pH < 7.24 is an indication for ventilatory support.

The prototype of pure ventilatory failure is the drug overdose patient in whom there is a sudden loss of central respiratory drive with uncontrolled hypercarbia. Patients with sepsis, neuromuscular disease, and chronic obstructive pulmonary disease (COPD) may also have hypercarbic ventilatory failure.

B. Hypoxemic respiratory failure. Inability to oxygenate is an important indication for ventilatory support. A $PaO_2 < 60$ Torr on $\geq 50\%$ inspired fraction of oxygen (FiO_2) constitutes hypoxemic respiratory failure. Although these patients can sometimes be managed with higher FiO_2 delivery systems, such as partial or nonrebreather masks or continuous positive airway pressure (CPAP) delivered by mask, they are at high risk for respiratory arrest and should be closely monitored in an intensive care unit (ICU). Worsening of the respiratory status necessitates prompt intubation and ventilatory support.

The prototype disease for hypoxemic respiratory failure is adult respiratory distress syndrome (ARDS) in which the high shunt fraction leads to refractory hypoxemia.

C. Mixed respiratory failure. Most patients actually have failure of both ventilation and oxygenation. The indications for ventilatory support remain the same as listed earlier. The threshold for initiating ventilatory support will be even lower with these patients as oxygen management may further compound hypercarbia.

An example of mixed respiratory failure is COPD with acute bronchitis. Bronchospasm alters the ventilation-perfusion ratio ($\dot{V}/\dot{Q}$) relationships leading to worsening hypoxemia. Bronchospasm and accumulated secretions lead to a high work of breathing and consequent hypercarbia.

D. Neuromuscular failure. This is actually a category of ventilatory failure but deserves special mention because of differing management. Hypercarbia occurs just before arrest and thus criteria other than arterial blood gases (ABGs) are needed.

1. In progressive tachypnea, breath rates higher than 24/min are an early sign of respiratory failure. A progressive rise in the breath rate or sustained breath rates higher than 35/min are an indication for ventilatory support.
2. Abdominal paradox indicates dyssynergy of chest wall muscles and diaphragms and impending respiratory failure. It is manifested by inward movement of the abdominal wall during inspiration rather than the normal outward motion.
3. A vital capacity < 15 mL/kg (1000 mL for a normal body-sized person) is associated with acute respiratory arrest as well as an inability to clear secretions. Similarly, a negative inspiratory force less negative than −25 cm H_2O implies impending respiratory arrest.

Guillain-Barré syndrome is the prototype of a neuromuscular disease in which the preceding criteria need strict attention. A patient with Guillain-Barré syndrome should be closely observed and followed with frequent vital capacity (VC). A rapidly falling VC or VC < 1000 mL requires initiation of respirator support.

II. Tracheal Intubation (See Chapter 3, Endotracheal Intubation, p 324.) Endotracheal intubation is actually the most difficult and most complication-ridden part of ventilator initiation. Skill and experience are required for correct placement. Aspiration, esophageal intubation, and right mainstem bronchus intubation are common complications. Bilateral breath sounds always need to be confirmed by chest auscultation in each axilla. An immediate postintubation portable chest x-ray should be obtained. Intubation can be accomplished by three routes.

A. Nasotracheal intubation. This can be accomplished blindly and in an awake patient. It requires experience and adequate local anesthesia. Complications include esophageal intubation, nosebleeds, kinking of the endotracheal tube (ETT), and postobstructive sinusitis. A smaller ETT is usually required for nasotracheal versus orotracheal intubation; ; this leads to a higher work of breathing because of increased resistance, difficulties with adequate suctioning, and higher ventilation pressures. Nasotracheal ETTs are more comfortable than orotracheal ETTs and are less damaging to the larynx because of better stabilization in the airway.

B. Orotracheal intubation. Placement of orotracheal tubes requires normal neck mobility to allow hyperextension of the neck for direct visualization of the vocal cords. Larger ETTs can be placed by this route. Adequate local anesthesia or sedation is necessary for safe placement without aspiration.

C. Tracheostomy. Tracheostomy is a surgical procedure most often done acutely for upper airway obstruction; however, in patients who require more than 14–21 days of ventilatory support, a tracheostomy is recommended. Tracheostomy tubes facilitate the weaning process by decreasing tube resistance as the tube is shorter and of greater radius. Patients are able to eat and find the tubes more comfortable.

III. Ventilator Setup

A. The ventilator. Almost all modern ventilators are time- and volume-cycled. Elaborate alarm systems are present to alert personnel to inadequate ventilation, high pressure, disconnection of the ETT, and so forth.

Effective ventilation is measured by changes in $PaCO_2$. Minute ventilation ($\dot{V}_e$) is tidal volume × breath rate. Thus, ventilation may be adjusted by changing the breath rate, the tidal volume, or both. Tidal volumes above 12 mL/kg may cause overdistension of alveoli and increase the risk of pneumothorax. Most initial tidal volumes are therefore set at 10–12 mL/kg.

Oxygenation is adjusted by changing FiO_2. Prolonged FiO_2 higher than 60% may cause pulmonary fibrosis. Thus, down-adjustment to "safe levels" sufficient to maintain O_2 saturation > 90% should be attempted if indicated by ABGs. If an O_2 saturation > 90% cannot be maintained when decreasing the FiO_2 < 60%, other means such as positive end-expiratory pressure (PEEP) can be used.

The mode of ventilation should be specified.

1. Control mode delivers a set rate and tidal volume irrespective of patient efforts.
2. Assist control (AC) mode allows patient triggering of machine breaths once a threshold of inspiratory flow or effort is made. It also supplies a backup rate in case of apnea or paralysis.
3. Intermittent mandatory ventilation (IMV) provides a set number of machine breaths per minute and allows the patient to make spontaneous breaths as well. Synchronized intermittent mandatory ventilation (SIMV) allows synchronization of the IMV

breaths with patient efforts. As the rate is turned down, the patient assumes more and more of the work of breathing.

4. Continuous positive airway pressure (CPAP) allows completely spontaneous respirations while the patient is still connected to the ventilator. A set amount of continuous pressure may be applied as well (from 0 to 30 cm H_2O).

Initial ventilator settings should be dictated by the underlying condition as well as previous blood gas results. An example of settings for a patient status postrespiratory arrest would be

- FiO_2 1.0
- Assist control mode
- Rate 14
- Tidal volume 800 mL

An attempt should be made to supply the patient with at least as much minute ventilation as was required prior to intubation. Thus, patients with pulmonary edema, ARDS, or neuromuscular disease may require minute ventilation rates of 14–22 L/min. The AC mode will generally be more comfortable and will alleviate the work of breathing to a large extent. Sample settings might be

- FiO_2 1.0
- Assist control mode
- Rate 18
- Tidal volume 750 mL

The patient with COPD, on the other hand, should not be overventilated initially. Such patients may have a chronically high bicarbonate because of renal compensation, and overventilation could cause a severe alkalosis. Sample settings might be

- FiO_2 0.5
- SIMV mode
- Pressure support 15 cm
- Rate 12
- Tidal volume 800 mL

B. Additional setup requirements

1. Restrain the patient's hands as a natural reaction to the ETT upon awakening is to pull it out.

2. Place a nasogastric tube to decompress the stomach and/or to continue essential oral medications.

3. Obtain a stat portable chest x-ray to confirm ETT placement and to reassess any underlying pulmonary disease.

4. Treat any underlying pulmonary disease (maximize bronchodilators in status asthmaticus or vasodilators and diuretics in pulmonary edema).

5. Consider prophylactic measures. Heparin 5000 U subcutaneously every 12 hours may reduce the incidence of pulmonary embolism while the patient is on bed rest. Stress ulceration bleeding can be prevented by the use of any of the following: antacids, ranitidine (Zantac), sucralfate (Carafate).

6. Order other medications as needed such as morphine for pain, lorazepam (Ativan) for restlessness, and haloperidol (Haldol) for agitation.

■ ROUTINE MODIFICATION OF SETTINGS

Arterial blood gases should be monitored and adjusted to a normal pH (7.37–7.44) and a $PaO_2 > 60$ Torr on less than 60% O_2. Tachypnea should be investigated for adequacy of ventilation or for any new cause, such as a fever, prior to sedating the patient.

I. Adjusting PaO_2

- **A. To decrease:** FiO_2 should be decreased in increments of 10% to 20% with either ABGs or oximetry checked in between. The rule of 7s states that there will be a 7-Torr fall in PaO_2 for each 1% decrease in FiO_2.
- **B. To increase**
  1. Ventilation has some effect on PaO_2 (as shown by the alveolar air equation); therefore, correction of the respiratory acidosis will improve oxygenation.
  2. Positive end-expiratory pressure can be added in increments of 2 to 4 cm H_2O. PEEP recruits previously collapsed alveoli, holds them open, and restores functional residual capacity (FRC) to a more physiologic level. It counteracts pulmonary shunts and will raise PaO_2. PEEP increases intrathoracic pressure and may thus impede venous return and decrease cardiac output. This is particularly true in the presence of volume depletion and shock. If PEEP levels > 12–14 cm H_2O are needed, the placement of a Swan-Ganz catheter is recommended to monitor mixed venous oxygen levels and cardiac output.

II. Adjusting $PaCO_2$

- **A. To decrease**
  1. Increase the rate.
  2. Check for leaks in the system.
- **B. To increase**
  1. Decrease the rate.
  2. You may have to switch from AC mode to SIMV mode to eliminate patient-driven central hyperventilation.
  3. An old (but tried and true!) method is to place increased exhalation tubing to increase deadspace and actually have the patient rebreathe CO_2.

■ TROUBLESHOOTING

Agitation

I. **Problem.** The ventilator patient may become agitated, constantly struggling, trying to pull out all tubes, and actively fighting the respirator.

II. **Immediate Questions**

- A. **Is the patient still properly connected?** Hypoxemia and/or hypercarbia resulting from the patient's becoming disconnected from the respirator may result in agitation.
- B. **What were the most recent arterial blood gases?** Again, hypoxemia and/or hypercarbia can cause agitation. Adjusting the settings can correct either problem.
- C. **What does the chest x-ray show?** Atelectasis from mucous plugging or pneumothorax, which can occur spontaneously in asthmatics or as a result of barotrauma, can result in hypoxemia or hypercarbia.
- D. **What is the underlying diagnosis? What are the current medications and intravenous fluids?** Agitation may be related to the underlying diagnosis or a medication and unrelated to the respiratory status. Cimetidine (Tagamet) and narcotics can cause confusion, especially in the elderly. Multiple metabolic disturbances such as hyponatremia and hypernatremia can lead to confusion and possibly agitation.
- E. **What are the ventilator settings?** The ventilator setting may have been set incorrectly, resulting in hypoxemia or hypercarbia. Barotrauma resulting in pneumothorax is associated with high PEEP settings.

III. **Differential Diagnosis**

- A. **Causes of respiratory decompensation**
  1. **Worsening of underlying pulmonary disease**
  2. **Pneumothorax**
  3. **Endotracheal tube displacement.** Out of trachea, high in the glottis, or down the right mainstem bronchus.
  4. **Mucous plugs.** May result in atelectasis and hypoxemia.
  5. **Ventilator malfunction**
  6. **Pulmonary embolism.** Immobilization is a major risk for PE.
  7. **Aspiration**
  8. **Inadequate oxygenation and/or respiratory muscle fatigue**
- B. **Sepsis**
- C. **ICU psychosis**
- D. **Medications.** Multiple medications such as digoxin (Lanoxin), lidocaine, theophylline, imipenem-cilastatin (Primaxin), diazepam (Valium), and cimetidine may cause psychosis, especially in high doses or with decreased clearance states.
- E. **Electrolyte imbalance.** Hyponatremia, hypernatremia, hyper-

calcemia, hypocalcemia, and hypophosphatemia can cause confusion which can lead to agitation.

IV. Database

A. Physical examination key points

1. **Endotracheal tube.** Carefully check the patency, position, and function of the endotracheal tube (ETT).
2. **Vital signs.** Tachypnea may suggest hypoxemia. Tachycardia and hypertension can result from agitation or be associated with respiratory failure or an underlying problem such as myocardial infarction. Hypotension implies sepsis, cardiogenic shock, or possibly tension pneumothorax or massive pulmonary embolism. An elevated temperature suggests sepsis or possibly a pulmonary infection. Tachycardia, tachypnea, and fever may be associated with PE. A pulsus paradoxus > 20 mm Hg implies severe respiratory distress or pericardial tamponade.
3. **HEENT.** Check for distended neck veins which can result from pericardial tamponade. Tracheal deviation may be caused by a tension pneumothorax.
4. **Chest.** Auscultate for bilateral breath sounds. Absent breath sounds on one side suggest pneumothorax or an improperly placed ETT. Bilateral absent breath sounds can be secondary to either bilateral pneumothoraces or severe respiratory failure.
5. **Extremities.** Check for cyanosis.
6. **Skin.** Palpate for subcutaneous emphysema which can result from a very high PEEP or may be seen in asthmatics.

B. Laboratory data

1. **Arterial blood gases.** To rule out hypoxemia and hypercarbia as well as a severe acidosis and alkalosis.
2. **Electrolyte panel.** Including calcium and phosphorus.

C. Radiologic and other studies.

A chest x-ray to rule out atelectasis and pneumothorax and to evaluate underlying pulmonary pathology.

V. Plan

A. Emergency management

1. Examine the patient as outlined earlier. Carefully check the ETT function, ventilator connections, and chart.
2. Suction the patient vigorously. This confirms tube patency and clears out any mucous plugs.
3. Manually bag the patient to check for ease of ventilation. Marked difficulty can be seen with tension pneumothorax.
4. Obtain ABGs, electrolyte panel, and stat chest x-ray.
5. If the patient appears cyanotic or "air hungry," turn the inspired fraction of oxygen (FiO_2) to 1.0 and the ventilator mode to assist control.
6. If hypotension and unilateral breath sounds are found concomitantly, consider chest tube insertion for tension pneu-

mothorax. Patients on ventilators can rapidly die of tension pneumothoraces.

7. If ICU psychosis is suspected, reassure the patient. Have the family members help to reorient the patient. Often a familiar voice will work wonders! Ask the nurses to move the patient to a room with a window; this has been show to reduce ICU psychosis.
8. Check the ventilator settings. Perhaps too much effort is required to open the valves or to initiate a breath.
9. If everything else is stable and the patient is endangering himself or herself, sedate the patient. Haloperidol (Haldol) 0.5–2.0 mg IM or IV and lorazepam (Ativan) 0.5–2.0 mg IV are the currently recommended agents.

HYPOXEMIA

I. **Problem.** The respirator patient requires $\geq$ 60% FiO_2 to maintain a $PaO_2 > 60$ Torr.

II. **Immediate Questions**

A. **What is the sequence of arterial blood gases? In other words, is this an acute or a slowly developing change?** A rapid deterioration implies an immediate life-threatening process such as a tension pneumothorax or a massive pulmonary embolism.

B. **What is the underlying diagnosis?** A patient with long-bone fractures may develop fat embolus syndrome, a patient with sepsis may develop adult respiratory distress syndrome, or a patient with head injury might develop neurogenic pulmonary edema.

C. **What are the ventilator settings? Has a change been made recently?** An error may have been made with the ventilator settings or recent changes may have been made too aggressively in an attempt to wean the patient from the ventilator.

III. **Differential Diagnosis**

A. **Shunts secondary to alveolar filling or by obstructed bronchi with consequent collapse**
   1. **Pneumonia**
   2. **Pulmonary contusion**
   3. **Atelectasis.** The endotracheal tube may be too far in the right mainstem bronchus or there may be mucous plugs.
   4. **ARDS or cardiogenic pulmonary edema**

B. **Cardiac level shunt.** An acute ventricular septal defect, especially in the setting of an acute myocardial infarction (MI), may develop. Sudden pulmonary hypertension may occasionally lead to a patent foramen ovale and physiologic shunt at the atrial level. A tip-off to this is a worsening shunt and PaO_2 as positive end-expiratory pressure (PEEP) is increased.

C. **Shunts secondary to pneumothorax**

D. Ventilation/perfusion ($\dot{V}/\dot{Q}$) mismatch

1. **Bronchospasm**
2. **Pulmonary embolism**
3. **Aspiration.** Still possible, even when an ETT is in place.

E. Inadequate ventilation

1. **Ventilator disconnection or malfunction**
2. **Wrong settings.** Has the patient recently been changed to IMV which has resulted in hypoventilation?
3. **Sedatives.** Can result in hypoxemia secondary to hypoventilation. Sedatives should be used cautiously, especially during weaning.
4. **Neuromuscular disease.** Hypophosphatemia or aminoglycosides can cause neuromuscular weakness, which can cause hypoxemia secondary to hypoventilation and lack of sighing.

IV. Database

A. Physical examination key points

1. **Endotracheal tube.** Confirm proper ETT position and listen for any leaks.
2. **Vital signs.** Tachypnea implies worsening of the respiratory status. Tachycardia can be associated with a variety of conditions including PE, sepsis, MI, and worsening of underlying pulmonary pathology. Fever can be seen with PE or an infection.
3. **Neck.** Stridor suggests upper airway obstruction.
4. **Chest.** Check for bilateral breath sounds, signs of consolidation, or new onset of wheezing. Unilateral breath sounds suggest a pneumothorax or possibly displacement of the ETT in one of the mainstem bronchi. Palpate the chest for new subcutaneous emphysema, which can occur in asthmatics or as a result of high PEEP.
5. **Heart.** New murmurs or a new third heart sound (S_3) or fourth heart sound (S_4) may be seen with an MI.
6. **Extremities.** Check nailbeds for cyanosis from worsening of the pulmonary status. Also check legs for unilateral edema or other signs of phlebitis, which point to PE.
7. **Skin.** Check for new rashes to suggest a drug or anaphylactic reaction.

B. Laboratory data

1. Repeat ABGs or check oximetry to assess accuracy of initial ABGs and progression of deterioration.
2. Sputum appearance and gram stain may direct antibiotic therapy if pneumonia is present.
3. A Swan-Ganz catheter will have to be in place to measure mixed venous oxygen saturation ($M\dot{V}O_2$). $M\dot{V}O_2$ is a direct reflection of oxygen delivery to the tissues and extraction of oxygen. It can be used to determine the presence of an intracardiac shunt.

C. Radiologic and other studies

1. **Stat chest x-ray.** To rule out atelectasis and pneumothorax, and to evaluate underlying pulmonary disease.
2. **Electrocardiogram.** An evolving MI may be evident. New right-axis deviation, right bundle branch block, P pulmonale, or an S wave in lead I, a Q wave in lead III, and a T wave in lead III ($S_1Q_3T_3$) imply PE; however, these characteristic findings are often absent. Sinus tachycardia is the most common electrocardiographic finding with PE.
3. **$\dot{V}/\dot{Q}$ scan.** To be obtained if clinical suspicion is high for PE.
4. **Swan-Ganz catheter.** To measure PaO_2 and to exclude a cardiac shunt as well as to measure cardiac output and $M\dot{V}O_2$.

V. Plan

A. Suction. Vigorously suction the patient to prove patency of the ETT and dislodge mucous plugs.

B. Correct anemia. Oxygen delivery to tissue depends on the hemoglobin as well as the cardiac output and PaO_2.

C. Treat underlying disorders.

1. Insert chest tube for pneumothorax.
2. Reassess antibiotic choices. A pneumonia secondary to *Legionella* requires erythromycin.
3. Consider more vigorous chest physical therapy or even bronchoscopy for recalcitrant mucous plugging or atelectasis.
4. Maximize bronchodilators if bronchospasm is the problem. Corticosteroids such as hydrocortisone 125–500 mg or methylprednisolone 60–200 mg should be added and dosed every 4 hours. Aerosolized albuterol (Ventolin) or metaproterenol (Alupent) should likewise be given at least every 4 hours.
5. Cardiogenic pulmonary edema should be vigorously treated with afterload reduction and diuresis.

D. Optimize ventilator settings

1. Correct any hypoventilation. This may mean giving up on weaning and using the AC mode with the patient essentially controlled on a high minute ventilation.
2. Increase FiO_2 to 100%. Your first priority is to prevent anoxic brain or cardiac damage. You may then reduce the FiO_2 as other maneuvers further improve the pO_2.
3. PEEP will recruit unused, collapsed, or partially collapsed alveoli to overcome pulmonary shunts. It should be added in 2- to 4-cm increments while monitoring cardiac output and blood pressure.
4. As a last resort, oxygen consumption ($\dot{V}O_2$) can be markedly reduced by administering a muscular blocking agent. Vercuronium bromide (Norcuron) may be given as a bolus of 5–15 mg and then a continuous drip of 4–12 mg/h. Norcuron is preferred over pavulon as it has a shorter half-life and does not cause tachycardia. Remember to continue to give pain and

sedation medications as these agents do not block sensations.

E. Optimize hemodynamics.

1. Consider Swan-Ganz placement when high levels of PEEP are in use, when shock of unclear cause is present, when a cardiac shunt is suspected, or when volume status is unclear.
2. Correct volume excess because it will obviously make congestive heart failure and ARDS much worse.
3. Likewise, volume depletion will alter both cardiac output and $\dot{V}/\dot{Q}$ ratios and may adversely affect oxygen delivery. A fall in blood pressure with the addition of PEEP almost always means volume depletion.
4. Correct anemia so as to maximize O_2 delivery. If ARDS is present, red blood cell transfusions should either be washed or given through leukocyte removal filters to prevent an exacerbation of the disease from the transfusion.
5. Correct low cardiac output to maximize O_2 delivery. Administer positive inotropic agents such as dobutamine and agents for afterload reduction such as intravenous nitroglycerin or nitroprusside.

HYPERCARBIA

I. Problem. $PaCO_2$ remains > 40 Torr. $PaCO_2$ is a direct reflection of both CO_2 production and alveolar ventilation. $PaCO_2$ increases when ventilation/perfusion ($\dot{V}/\dot{Q}$) mismatch worsens or deadspace increases.

II. Immediate Questions

A. What is the sequence of arterial blood gases? In other words, is this an acute or a slowly developing change? Rapid deterioration implies an immediate life-threatening process such as a tension pneumothorax or a massive pulmonary embolism.

B. What is the underlying diagnosis? Worsening of underlying pulmonary disease (pneumonia, atelectasis, or bronchospasm) can cause hypoventilation. Long-bone fractures may be complicated by fat emboli. A patient with sepsis may develop adult respiratory distress syndrome, and head injury may be complicated by neurogenic pulmonary edema.

III. Differential Diagnosis

A. Inadequate minute ventilation ($\dot{V}_e$)

1. **Too low a rate, inadequate tidal volume, or both**
2. **Patient tiring during synchronized intermittent mandatory ventilation or weaning**
3. **Endotracheal tube leak**
4. **Worsening bronchospasm**
5. **Pulmonary embolism.** Remember, immobilization is a major risk factor.

B. Increased CO_2 production

1. High-carbohydrate feedings

2. Increased metabolism. Includes hyperthyroidism, fever, sepsis, and high work of breathing as well as rewarming after surgical procedures, a common but frequently overlooked cause of CO_2 production.

C. Oversedation. Decreases central ventilatory drive.

IV. Database

A. Physical examination key points

1. Endotracheal tube. Check ETT position and look for a leak.

2. Vital signs. Tachycardia can be associated with fever, sepsis, worsening bronchospasm, PE, and hyperthyroidism. Tachypnea can be seen with PE, worsening bronchospasm, or sepsis. Fever suggests infection but can also be seen with hyperthyroidism and PE.

3. Chest. Auscultate looking for new onset of wheezes or a change in the equality of breath sounds.

4. Heart. Listen for a new loud P_2 which suggests a PE.

5. Extremities. Check the legs for unilateral edema or other signs of phlebitis.

6. Musculoskeletal exam. Check for signs of respiratory fatigue: abdominal paradox or accessory muscle use seen with severe respiratory failure.

B. Laboratory data

1. Arterial blood gases. Repeat ABGs or check oximetry to assess accuracy of initial ABGs and progression of deterioration.

2. Complete blood count with differential. An increased white count with an increase in banded neutrophils suggests an infection or sepsis.

C. Radiologic and other studies. With a chest x-ray, proper ETT position can be ensured and new pulmonary infiltrates can be ruled out.

V. Plan

A. Check the position and function of the ETT. If there is a persistent leak, replace the tube.

B. Verify proper ventilator function. Especially check for leaky connections.

C. Drugs. Verify that the ordered sedation medications are those that have been given and note when they were last given. If the patient is oversedated, you can either increase the minute ventilation or reverse sedation from narcotics with naloxone (Narcan) 0.4 mg IV.

D. Look for a source of sepsis. Adjust antibiotics as indicated. Lower $\dot{V}O_2$ by treating fever with Tylenol or a cooling blanket.

E. Review ventilator settings. If the tidal volume is too low, dead-space ventilation will be present. Correct this by raising the tidal volume. If the patient is tiring on a low SIMV rate, switch to either a higher rate or back to assist control mode.

F. **Review the nutrition regimen in use.** If the patient is critically ill with bronchospasm or ARDS, you may be forced to reduce CO_2 production. To do this, reduce the D25W in hyperalimentation fluids to D15W or D10W. The caloric difference can be made up with lipids; as much as 500 mL 20% intralipids can be given IV daily.

HIGH PEAK PRESSURES

I. **Problem.** The ventilator peak pressures remain consistently above 50 cm H_2O.

II. **Immediate Questions**

A. **Is this a new problem or has it developed progressively?** The answer to this question will be readily available on the respiratory therapy bedside flow sheet.

B. **What is the underlying diagnosis?** Severe underlying pulmonary disease can cause high ventilatory peak pressures.

C. **What are the most recent arterial blood gases?** A decrease in the pO_2 and/or an increase in the pCO_2 may point to a worsening of the underlying pulmonary disease.

D. **Has endotracheal tube function or position changed? Is it possible to suction the patient?** The tube could be kinked or plugged with secretions.

III. **Differential Diagnosis**

A. **ETT**

1. Too small or obstructed with secretions.
2. Kinked, especially if nasotracheally placed.
3. Migration down the right mainstem so that the entire tidal volume is going into one lung. This also increases coughing and anxiety.

B. **Incorrect ventilator settings**

1. **High tidal volume.** Tidal volumes > 12 mL/kg may tremendously increase distension pressure.
2. **High positive end-expiratory pressure.** The PEEP should always be used at the lowest possible level.
3. **High minute ventilation.** A high minute ventilation may lead to the phenomenon of "auto PEEP," whereby there is inadequate time to exhale leading to "stacked breaths."

C. **Worsening lung disease.** All of these conditions show concomitant falls in lung compliance.

1. **Severe status asthmaticus**
2. **Adult respiratory distress syndrome**
3. **Cardiogenic pulmonary edema**
4. **Interstitial lung disease**

D. Uncooperative or agitated patient

1. **Biting the ETT**
2. **Fighting the ventilator**
3. **Coughing**

E. Abdominal distension

F. Tension pneumothorax. It is always imperative to exclude this as a cause of new onset of high peak pressures because death can occur quickly.

IV. Database

A. Physical examination key points

1. **Endotracheal tube.** Check position to rule out migration down the right mainstem bronchus and patency of the ETT.
2. **Vital signs.** Tachycardia and tachypnea can occur with worsening of the underlying pulmonary disease and with agitation. Hypotension and tachycardia suggest tension pneumothorax.
3. **HEENT.** An increase in jugular venous distension (JVD) implies congestive heart failure. Tracheal deviation can be seen with tension pneumothorax.
4. **Chest.** Absent breath sounds, especially with hypotension, and unilateral hyperresonance to percussion point to tension pneumothorax. Rales suggest congestive heart failure.
5. **Heart.** A third heart sound (S_3) implies left ventricular dysfunction/congestive heart failure.
6. **Abdomen.** Examine for tenderness and distension.
7. **Extremities.** New cyanosis is consistent with worsening of the underlying pulmonary disease. Edema will be seen with biventricular or right-sided heart failure.
8. **Skin.** Check for subcutaneous emphysema which can be associated with barotrauma or seen with severe asthma.

B. Laboratory data

1. **Arterial blood gases.** Repeat ABGs or check oximetry to assess accuracy of initial AGBs and progression of deterioration.
2. **Complete blood count with differential.** An increased white count with an increase in banded neutrophils suggests an infection or sepsis.

C. Radiologic and other studies. Use a stat portable chest x-ray to check position, rule out kinking of ETT, rule out pneumothorax, and assess any change in underlying pulmonary disease.

V. Plan

A. Try to suction the patient. If the patient is biting down, insert an oral airway or sedate the patient. If the patient is not biting down on the ETT but the suction tube will not go down, the tube is kinked or blocked and must be replaced.

B. Ambu bag the patient and confirm equal breath sounds. Unequal breath sounds could result from a tension pneumothorax or from improper positioning of the ETT. Reposition the ETT if necessary. On an average-sized person, an oral ETT should not be in farther than 24 cm at the lip; however, there is considerable variability among patients and the chest x-ray should always be reviewed. If there is a lot of resistance to bagging, a tension pneumothorax may be present.

C. Place a chest tube if a pneumothorax is present.

D. Adjust the ventilator. Try to reduce PEEP to the minimum needed for adequate oxygenation. Try reducing high tidal volumes to 10 mL/kg body weight. Increase FiO_2 as needed to ensure adequate oxygenation.

E. Sedation may have to be increased.

F. Adjustment of alarms. If all possibilities have been evaluated, alarms may be increased to higher levels; however, the risk of an acute tension pneumothorax will increase with higher peak pressures.

■ WEANING

I. Requirements. Once the underlying cause of respiratory failure has been corrected, it is time for the most arduous task of all: weaning the patient from the respirator.

A. Stabilization. The underlying disease is under optimum control.

B. Initiation of weaning. The process is begun in the early morning. Patients like to rest rather than work all night—just like doctors!

1. $PaO_2 \geq 60$ Torr on no PEEP and $FiO_2 \leq 0.5$.
2. Minute ventilation < 10 L/min.
3. Negative inspiratory force more negative than -20 cm H_2O.
4. Vital capacity > 800 mL.
5. Tidal volume > 300 mL.

II. Techniques

A. T-Piece (or T-tube bypass). The patient is taken off the respirator for a limited period of time and the ETT is connected to a constant flow of O_2 (usually 40%). If the patient tolerates breathing independently, the length of time off the respirator is progressively increased. This is a tried and true method. It is particularly easy to use in patients with no underlying lung disease such as in a recovering drug overdose.

There are several drawbacks to this technique. No alarms are available as the patient is totally disconnected from the ventilator. It is time consuming for the respiratory therapists and nurses. Perhaps most importantly, it is much more work than spontaneously breathing without an ETT. This is due to the relatively small diameter of the tube. Remember, resistance increases by the fourth power of the radius.

B. Synchronized intermittent mandatory ventilation. In this method, fewer and fewer machine breaths are given as the patient begins taking spontaneous breaths in between. For example, a patient breathing at a rate of 14 in AC mode is switched to SIMV mode, rate 14. The rate is then decreased to 10, to 6, to 4, and then to 0. Most physicians either place the patient on continuous positive airway pressure mode at this juncture or observe the patient briefly on a T-piece.

This method has several theoretical advantages over T-piece weaning. Backup alarms including automatic rates in case of apnea are in place. A graded assumption of work is done allowing respiratory muscle "retraining"; however, this method has never been proven clearly superior to T-piece weaning. Moreover, there is still a high work of breathing because of the ETT resistance as well as the inherent resistance of the SIMV circuit valves.

One way to decrease the work of breathing with the SIMV weaning technique is to add pressure support (PS) to the system. Pressure support is a positive pressure boost that is initiated when a certain liter flow rate during inspiration is sensed by the respirator. It then supplies a set amount of positive pressure (and by Boyle's law, it also supplies some tidal volume). A PS level of 10–15 cm will overcome the increased work caused by the ETT resistance.

C. Continuous positive airway pressure and pressure support. In this method, the patient is switched to the spontaneous breathing mode, which in modern ventilators is the CPAP mode. In current usage, CPAP is equivalent to PEEP except it is used exclusively in spontaneously breathing mode. Anywhere from 0 to 30 cm pressure may be used, but generally the lowest level possible (usually 0–5 cm) is preferred. Pressure support may be used concomitantly to augment patient spontaneous breaths. It can then be progressively decreased as the patient increases tidal volumes. For example, PS levels of 25, then 20, then 15, and finally 10 can be used while monitoring the patient's breath rate, tidal volumes, and ABGs.

This method requires an alert, cooperative patient who is spontaneously breathing and if you do not have that, why wean anyway? Machine backup functions remain in place in case of apnea or other inadequate parameters.

III. Timing. Deciding when to extubate the patient is part of the art of medicine. Still, fulfilling certain criteria ensures success. Weaning parameters (as discussed earlier) are acceptable:

A. Breath rate is < 30/min.
B. ABGs show a pH > 7.35 and adequate oxygenation.
C. The patient is awake and alert.
D. A normal gag reflex is present.
E. The stomach is not distended.

IV. Postextubation. After extubation, it is important that the patient be encouraged to cough frequently and forcefully. Respiratory therapy treatments should be continued. Incentive spirometry should be used several times an hour while awake to encourage deep breathing. The patient must be carefully observed for stridor, respiratory muscle fatigue, or other signs of failure. Oxygen should be given at the same level or at a level slightly higher than was given via the respirator prior to intubation. The ABGs should be checked 2–4 hours after extubation to confirm adequate ventilation and oxygenation.

REFERENCES

Burns DM. Mechanical ventilation: Devices and methods. In: Bordow RA, Moser KM, eds. *Manual of Clinical Problems in Pulmonary Medicine,* 2nd ed. Boston: Little, Brown; 1985:238–241.

Burns DM. Mechanical ventilation: Weaning and complications. In: Bordow RA, Moser KM, eds. *Manual of Clinical Problems in Pulmonary Medicine,* 2nd ed. Boston: Little, Brown; 1985:241–244.

Glauser FL, Polatty C, Sessler CN. Worsening oxygenation in the mechanically ventilated patient: Causes, mechanisms and early detection. *Am Rev Respir Dis* 1988;138:458–465.

Luce JM, et al. Intermittent mandatory ventilation. *Chest* 1981;79:678–685.

MacIntyre NR. Weaning from mechanical ventilatory support: Volume-assisting intermittent breaths versus pressure-assisting every breath. *Respir Care* 1988; 33:121–125.

Spragg RC, Krieger BP. Airway control. In: Bordow RA, Moser KM, eds. *Manual of Clinical Problems in Pulmonary Medicine,* 2nd ed. Boston: Little, Brown; 1985:235–238.

7 Commonly Used Medications

This section is designed to serve as a quick reference to the medications commonly used in medical patients. You should be familiar with all the indications, contraindications, and side effects of any medicines that you prescribe. Such detailed information is beyond the scope of this manual and can be found in the package insert, *Physician's Desk Reference (PDR)*, or American Hospital Formulary Service.

Drugs in this section are listed in alphabetical order by generic names. Some of the more common trade names are listed for each medication. Drugs under the control of the Drug Enforcement Agency (Schedule 2–5 controlled drugs) are indicated by the symbol [C].

CLASSES OF GENERIC DRUGS

Analgesic/Anti-inflammatory/Antipyretic Agents

Acetaminophen
Acetaminophen with butalbital
Acetaminophen with codeine
Aspirin
Aspirin with butalbital and caffeine
Aspirin with codeine
Buprenorphine
Butorphanol
Codeine
Diclofenac sodium
Diflunisal
Fenoprofen
Flurbiprofen
Hydromorphone
Ibuprofen
Indomethacin
Ketoprofen
Levorphanol
Meperidine
Methadone
Morphine sulfate
Nalbuphine
Naproxen
Oxycodone
Pentazocine
Piroxicam
Propoxyphene
Sulindac
Tolmetin

Antacid/Antigas Agents

Aluminum carbonate
Aluminum hydroxide
Aluminum hydroxide with magnesium hydroxide
Aluminum hydroxide with magnesium hydroxide and simethicone
Aluminum hydroxide with magnesium trisilicate
Calcium carbonate
Dihydroxyaluminum sodium carbonate
Magaldrate
Simethicone

Antianxiety Agents

Alprazolam
Buspirone
Chlordiazepoxide
Clorazepate
Diazepam
Doxepine
Hydroxyzine
Lorazepam
Meprobamate
Oxazepam
Prazepam

Antiarrhythmic Agents

Amiodarone
Bretylium
Disopyramide
Lidocaine
Mexiletine
Procainamide
Quinidine
Tocainide

Antibiotics

Amikacin
Amoxicillin
Amoxicillin/potassium clavulanate
Ampicillin
Ampicillin/sulbactam
Azlocillin
Aztreonam
Carbenicillin
Cefaclor
Cefadroxil
Cefamandole
Cefazolin
Cefixime
Cefmetazole
Cefonicid
Cefoperazone
Ceforanide
Cefotaxime
Cefotetan
Cefoxitin
Ceftazidime
Ceftizoxime
Ceftriaxone
Cefuroxime
Cefuroxime axetil
Cephalexin
Cephalothin
Cephapirin
Cephradine
Chloramphenicol
Ciprofloxacin
Clindamycin
Cloxacillin
Cortisporin, otic and ophthalmic
Demeclocycline
Dicloxacillin
Doxycycline
Erythromycin
Ethambutol
Gentamicin

Imipenem-cilastatin
Isoniazid
Methicillin
Metronidazole
Mezlocillin
Minocycline
Moxalactam
Nafcillin
Neomycin sulfate
Norfloxacin
Oxacillin
Penicillin G aqueous
Penicillin G benzathine
Penicillin G procaine
Penicillin V potassium
Pentamidine
Piperacillin
Rifampin
Silver sulfadiazine
Streptomycin
Sulfamethoxazole
Sulfasalazine
Sulfisoxazole
Tetracycline
Ticarcillin
Ticarcillin/potassium clavulanate
Tobramycin
Trimethoprim-sulfamethoxazole
Vancomycin

Anticoagulant/Thrombolytic and Related Agents

Alteplase, recombinant
Aminocaproic acid
Anistreplase
Antihemophilic factor (factor VIII)
Dipyridamole
Heparin
Pentoxifylline
Protamine sulfate
Streptokinase
Urokinase
Warfarin

Anticonvulsants

Carbamazepine
Clonazepam
Diazepam
Ethosuximide
Lorazepam
Pentobarbital
Phenobarbital
Phenytoin
Valproic acid

Antidepressants

Amitriptyline
Amoxapine
Desipramine
Doxepin
Fluoxetine
Imipramine
Maprotiline
Nortriptyline
Protriptyline
Trazodone

Antidiabetic Agents

Acetohexamide
Chlorpropamide
Glipizide
Glyburide
Insulins
Tolazamide
Tolbutamide

Antidiarrheal Agents

Diphenoxylate with atropine
Kaolin and pectin
Lactobacillus
Loperamide
Opium, camphorated tincture
Opium, tincture

Antiemetics/Emetics

Benzquinamide
Chlorpromazine
Dimenhydrinate
Dronabinol
Droperidol
Ipecac syrup
Meclizine
Metoclopramide
Nabilone
Prochlorperazine
Promethazine
Trimethobenzamide

Antifungal Agents

Amphotericin B
Clotrimazole
Econazole
Fluconazole
Flucytosine
Griseofulvin
Ketoconazole
Miconazole
Nystatin

Antigout Agents

Allopurinol
Colchicine
Probenecid
Sulfinpyrazone

Antihistamines

Astemizole
Azatadine
Brompheniramine
Chlorpheniramine
Clemastine fumarate
Cyproheptadine
Diphenhydramine
Promethazine
Terfenadine
Trimeprazine
Triprolidine

Antihyperlipidemic Agents

Cholestyramine
Colestipol
Gemfibrozil
Lovastatin
Niacin
Probucol

Antihypertensive Agents

Acebutolol
Atenolol
Captopril
Clonidine
Diazoxide
Diltiazem
Enalapril
Guanabenz
Guanadrel
Guanethidine

Guanfacine
Hydralazine
Labetalol
Lisinopril
Methyldopa
Metoprolol
Minoxidil
Nadolol
Nicardipine
Nifedipine
Nitroglycerin
Nitroprusside
Penbutolol
Pindolol
Prazosin
Propranolol
Terazosin
Timolol
Trimethaphan camsylate
Verapamil

Antiparkinsonian Agents

Amantadine
Benztropine
Bromocriptine
Carbidopa/levodopa
Trihexyphenidyl

Antipsychotic Agents

Chlorpromazine
Fluphenazine
Haloperidol
Lithium carbonate
Mesoridazine
Molindone
Perphenazine
Prochlorperazine
Thioridazine
Thiothixene
Trifluoperazine

Antitussives, Decongestants, Expectorants, and Mucolytic Agents

Acetylcysteine
Benzonatate
Codeine
Dextromethorphan
Guaifenesin
Pseudoephedrine

Antiviral Agents

Acyclovir
Amantadine
Ganciclovir
Vidarabine
Zidovudine

Bronchodilators

Albuterol
Aminophylline
Bitolterol
Ephedrine
Epinephrine
Isoetharine
Isoproterenol
Metaproterenol
Oxytriphylline
Terbutaline
Theophylline

Cardiovascular Agents

Acebutolol
Amrinone
Atenolol
Atropine
Carteolol
Digoxin
Diltiazem
Dipyridamole
Dobutamine
Dopamine
Edrophonium
Ephedrine
Epinephrine
Esmolol
Isoproterenol
Isosorbide dinitrate
Labetalol
Metoprolol
Nadolol
Nicardipine
Nifedipine
Nitroglycerin
Norepinephrine
Penbutolol
Phenylephrine
Pindolol
Propranolol
Sodium polystyrene sulfonate
Timolol
Verapamil

Cathartics/Laxatives

Bisacodyl
Docusate calcium
Docusate sodium
Glycerin suppositories
Lactulose
Magnesium citrate
Magnesium hydroxide
Mineral oil
Polyethylene glycol-electrolyte solution
Psyllium
Sorbitol

Diuretics

Acetazolamide
Amiloride
Bumetanide
Chlorothiazide
Chlorthalidone
Ethacrynic acid
Furosemide
Hydrochlorothiazide
Hydrochlorothiazide and amiloride
Hydrochlorothiazide and spironolactone
Hydrochlorothiazide and triamterene
Indapamide
Mannitol
Metolazone
Spironolactone
Triamterene

Emetics (see **Antiemetics/Emetics**)

Gastrointestinal Agents

Belladonna, tincture
Cimetidine
Dicyclomine
Famotidine
Mesalamine enema
Metoclopramide
Misoprostol
Nizatidine
Omeprazole
Pancreatin
Pancrealipase
Propantheline
Ranitidine
Sucralfate
Vasopressin

Hormones/Synthetic Substitutes

Cortisone
Desmopressin
Desoxycorticosterone acetate (DOCA)
Dexamethasone
Estradiol transderm
Estrogen, conjugated
Fludrocortisone acetate
Glucagon
Hydrocortisone
Medroxyprogesterone
Methylprednisolone
Metyrapone
Prednisone
Prednisolone
Vasopressin

Immunosupressive Agents

Antithymocyte globulin (ATG)
Azathioprine
Cyclosporine
Steroids

Local Anesthetic Agents

Anusol
Lidocaine
Lidocaine with epinephrine

Muscle Relaxants

Baclofen
Carisoprodol
Chlorzoxazone
Cyclobenzaprine
Diazepam
Methocarbamol
Pancuronium
Vecuronium

Narcotic Antagonist

Naloxone

Plasma Volume Expanders

Albumin
Dextran 40
Hetastarch
Plasma protein fraction

Respiratory Inhalants

Acetylcysteine
Atropine
Beclomethasone
Cromolyn sodium
Flunisolide
Ipratropium bromide

Sedatives/Hypnotics

Diphenhydramine
Flurazepam
Hydroxyzine
Lorazepam
Pentobarbital
Phenobarbital
Secobarbital
Temazepam
Triazolam

Supplements

Calcium salts
Cholecalciferol
Cyanocobalamin
Ferrous sulfate
Folic acid
Iron dextran
Magnesium sulfate
Phytonadione (vitamin K)
Potassium supplements
Pyridoxine
Sodium bicarbonate
Thiamine

Thyroid/Antithyroid Agents

Levothyroxine
Liothyronine
Methimazole
Propylthiouracil
SSKI (saturated solution of potassium iodide)

Toxoids/Vaccines/Sera

Hepatitis B immune globulin
Hepatitis B vaccine
Immune globulin, intravenous
Pneumococcal vaccine, polyvalent
Tetanus immune globulin
Tetanus toxoid

Urinary Tract Agents

Belladonna and opium suppositories
Bethanechol
Flavoxate
Methenamine mandelate and hippurate
Nalidixic acid
Neomycin-polymixin B irrigant
Nitrofurantoin
Oxybutynin
Phenazopyridine
Trimethoprim

Miscellaneous Agents

α-Proteinase inhibitor
Charcoal
Dantrolene
Disulfiram
Epoetin (α erythropoietin)
Lindane (γ benzene hexachloride)
Midazolam
Physostigmine

INDICATIONS AND DOSAGES OF GENERIC DRUGS

■ Acebutolol (Sectral)

See Table 7–7, p 492.

■ Acetaminophen (Tylenol, Others)

Indications: Mild pain; headache; fever.

Actions: Nonnarcotic analgesic, antipyretic.

Dosage: *Adult:* 650–1000 mg PO or rectally every 4–6 hours.

Supplied: Tablets 325 mg, 500 mg; elixir 120 mg/5 mL; suppositories 325 mg, 650 mg.

Notes: Overdose causes hepatotoxicity, treated with *N*-acetylcysteine, charcoal not usually recommended; unlike aspirin, has no anti-inflammatory or platelet-inhibiting action.

■ Acetaminophen with Butalbital and Caffeine (Fioricet)

Indications: Mild pain; headache, especially with associated stress.

Actions: Nonnarcotic analgesic.

Dosage: 1 or 2 tablets or capsules PO every 4–6 hours prn.

Supplied: Each tablet or capsule contains 325 mg acetaminophen, 40 mg caffeine, and 50 mg butalbital.

■ Acetaminophen with Codeine (Tylenol #1, #2, #3, #4) [C]

Indications: Relief of mild to moderate pain.

Actions: Combined effects of acetaminophen and a narcotic analgesic.

Dosage: 1 or 2 tablets every 3–4 hours prn.

Supplied: Tablets, capsules, elixir (5 mL = acetaminophen 120 mg and codeine 12mg).

Notes: Codeine in #1 = 7.5 mg, #2 = 15 mg, #3 = 30 mg, #4 = 60 mg.

■ Acetazolamide (Diamox)

Indications: Diuresis; glaucoma; alkalinization of urine.

Actions: Carbonic anhydrase inhibitor.

Dosage: *Diuretic:* 250–375 mg IV or PO QD.
Glaucoma: 250 mg PO QD–QID; maximum of 1000 mg/d.

Supplied: Tablets 125 mg, 250 mg; sustained-release capsules 500 mg; injection 500 mg/vial.

Notes: Contraindicated in renal failure and sulfa hypersensitivity. Follow Na^+ and K^+. Watch for metabolic acidosis.

■ Acetohexamide (Dymelor)

See Table 7–10, p 497.

■ Acetylcysteine (Mucomyst)

Indications: Mucolytic agent as adjuvant therapy for chronic bronchopulmonary diseases and cystic fibrosis; as antidote to acetaminophen hepatotoxicity within 24 hours of ingestion.

Actions: Splits disulfide linkages between mucoprotein molecular complexes; protects liver by restoring glutathione levels in acetaminophen overdose.

Dosage: *Nebulizer:* 3–5 mL of 20% solution diluted with equal volume of water or normal saline administered TID–QID.
Antidote: PO through a nasogastric tube, 140 mg/kg diluted 1:4 in carbonated beverage as loading dose, then 70 mg/kg every 4 hours for 17 doses.

Supplied: Solution 10%, 20%.

Notes: Watch for bronchospasm when used by inhalation in asthmatics; activated charcoal will adsorb acetylcysteine when given orally for acute acetaminophen ingestion/toxicity.

■ Acyclovir (Zovirax)

Indications: Treatment and prevention of herpes simplex and varicella zoster viral infections.

Actions: Inhibits viral DNA replication.

Dosage: *Topical:* Apply 0.5-in. ribbon every 3 hours.
Oral: Initial genital herpes—200 mg PO every 4 hours while awake, for a total of 5 capsules per day for 10 days.

- Chronic suppression: 200 mg PO TID for up to 6 months.
- Intermittent therapy: as for initial treatment, except treat for 5 days initiated at the earliest prodrome.
- Herpes zoster (shingles): 800 mg 5 times per day for 7 days.

Intravenous: Recommended for herpes simplex encephalitis, and systemic infection. With normal renal function (creatinine clearance > 50 mL/min) 5 mg/kg IV every 8 hours for 5–7 days.

Supplied: Ointment 5%; capsules 200 mg; injection 500 mg/vial.

Notes: Adjust dose in renal failure.

■ Albumin (Albuminar, Albutein, Buminate, Others)

Indications: Plasma volume expansion for shock resulting from burns, surgery, hemorrhage, or other trauma.

Actions: Maintenance of plasma colloid oncotic pressure.

Dosage: 25 g IV initially; subsequent infusions should depend on clinical situation and response.

Supplied: Solution 5%, 25%.

Note: Contains 130–160 mEq Na^+/L.

■ Albuterol (Proventil, Ventolin)

Indications: Treatment of bronchospasm in reversible obstructive airway disease; prevention of exercise-induced bronchospasm.

Actions: Beta-adrenergic sympathomimetic bronchodilator.

Dosage: 2–4 inhalations every 4–6 hours; 1 rotocap every 4–6 hours; 2–4 mg PO TID–QID.

Supplied: Tablets 2 mg, 4 mg; syrup 2 mg/5 mL; metered dose inhaler; solution for nebulization 0.08%, 0.5%; rotocap 200 μg.

■ Allopurinol (Zyloprim, Lopurin, Others)

Indications: Gout; treatment of hyperuricemia of malignancies; uric acid urolithiasis.

Actions: Xanthine oxidase inhibitor.

Dosage: Initial 100 mg PO QD; usual 300 mg PO QD.

Supplied: Tablets 100 mg, 300 mg.

Notes: Aggravates acute gouty attack, do not begin until acute attack resolves.

■ Alprazolam (Xanax) [C]

Indications: Management of anxiety disorders; anxiety associated with depression.

Actions: Benzodiazepine.

Dosage: 0.25–0.5 mg PO TID, maximum 4 mg/d.

Supplied: Tablets 0.25 mg, 0.5 mg, 1.0 mg.

Notes: Reduce dose in elderly and debilitated patients.

■ Alteplase, Recombinant (Activase)

Indications: Treatment of acute myocardial infarction.

Actions: A tissue plasminogen activator resulting in thrombolysis.

Dosage: 100 mg IV over 3 hours.

Supplied: Powder for injection 20 mg, 50 mg.

Notes: Bleeding as adverse effect.

■ Aluminum Carbonate (Basaljel)

Indications: Hyperacidity (peptic ulcer, hiatal hernia, etc); supplement to management of hyperphosphatemia.

Actions: Neutralizes gastric acid.

Dosage: 2 capsules or tablets or 10 mL (in water) every 2 hours prn.

Supplied: Capsules, tablets, suspension.

■ Aluminum Hydroxide (Amphojel, Alternagel)

Indications: Hyperacidity (peptic ulcer, hiatal hernia, etc); supplement to management of hyperphosphatemia.

Actions: Neutralizes gastric acid.

Dosage: 10–30 mL or 1 or 2 tablets (0.6 g) PO 4–6 times daily.

Supplied: Tablets 300 mg, 600 mg; chewable tablets 500 mg; suspension 320 mg/5 mL, 600 mg/5 mL.

Notes: Can be used in renal insufficiency; can cause constipation.

■ Aluminum Hydroxide with Magnesium Hydroxide (Maalox)

Indications: Hyperacidity (peptic ulcer, hiatal hernia, etc).

Actions: Neutralizes gastric acid.

Dosage: 10–60 mL or 2–4 tablets PO QID or prn.

Supplied: Tablets, suspension.

Notes: Doses QID best given after meals and at bedtime; caution in renal failure, can cause hypermagnesemia, especially with renal insufficiency.

■ Aluminum Hydroxide with Magnesium Hydroxide and Simethicone (Mylanta, Mylanta II, Maalox Plus)

Indications: Hyperacidity with bloating (peptic ulcer, etc).

Actions: Neutralizes gastric acid.

Dosage: 10–60 mL or 2–4 tablets PO QID or prn.

Supplied: Tablets, suspension.

Notes: Caution in renal insufficiency (can cause hypermagnesemia); Mylanta II contains twice the amount of aluminum and magnesium hydroxide as Mylanta.

■ Aluminum Hydroxide, Magnesium Trisilicate, and Alginic Acid (Gaviscon)

Indications: Symptomatic relief of heartburn; hiatal hernia.

Actions: Neutralizes gastric acid.

Dosage: 2–4 tablets or 15–30 mL PO QID followed by water.

Supplied: Tablets, suspension.

■ α-Proteinase Inhibitor (Prolastin)

Indications: Congenital α_1-antitrypsin deficiency.

Actions: Replacement of α_1-antitrypsin.

Dosage: 60 mg/kg IV once weekly.

Supplied: Check vial for mg/mL present in vial.

Notes: May cause delayed fever up to 12 hours after administration.

■ Amantadine (Symmetrel)

Indications: Influenza A viral infection or prophylaxis; Parkinsonism.

Actions: Prevents release of infectious viral nucleic acid into the host cell; releases dopamine from intact dopaminergic terminals.

Dosage: *Influenza A:* 200 mg PO QD or 100 mg PO BID.
Parkinsonism: 100 mg PO BID; 100 mg PO QD if patient is taking other anti-Parkinsonian drugs.

Supplied: Capsules 100 mg; syrup 50 mg/5 mL.

Notes: Reduce dose in renal failure.

■ Amikacin (Amikin)

Indications: Short-term therapy of serious infections caused by gram-negative aerobes and staphylococci.

Actions: Aminoglycoside antibiotic.

Dosage: 15 mg/kg/24 h divided every 8–12 hours or based on renal function; refer to aminoglycoside dosing in Tables 7–13 and 7–14, p 499.

Supplied: Injection 100 mg/2 mL; 500 mg/2 mL.

Notes: Not a first-line drug; may be effective against gram-negative bacteria resistant to gentamicin or tobramycin. Monitor renal function and drug levels carefully for dosage adjustments. See Table 7–12, p 498.

■ Amiloride (Midamor)

Indications: Hypertension; congestive heart failure.

Actions: Potassium-sparing diuretic.

Dosage: 5 mg PO QD; increase to 10 mg QD if needed.

Supplied: Tablets 5 mg.

Notes: Hyperkalemia may occur. Monitor serum potassium.

■ Aminocaproic Acid (Amicar)

Indications: Treatment of excessive bleeding resulting from systemic hyperfibrinolysis and urinary fibrinolysis.

Actions: Inhibits fibrinolysis via inhibition of plasminogen activator substances.

Dosage: 100 mg/kg IV then 1 g/m^2/h to maximum dose of 18 g/m^2/d or 100 mg/kg/dose every 8 hours.

Supplied: Injection 250 mg/mL; tablets 500 mg; syrup 250 mg/mL.

Note: Administer for 8 hours or until bleeding is controlled. Contraindicated in disseminated intravascular coagulation. NOT FOR UPPER URINARY TRACT BLEEDING.

■ Aminophylline

Indications: Asthma, bronchospasm.

Actions: Relaxes the smooth muscle of the bronchi and pulmonary blood vessels.

Dosage: *Acute asthmatic attack:* Load 6 mg/kg IV, then 0.4–0.9 mg/kg/h IV.
Chronic asthma: 24 mg/kg/d divided every 6 hours.

Supplied: Injection 25 mg/mL; tablets 100 mg, 200 mg; solution 105 mg/5 mL; suppositories 250 mg, 500 mg.

Notes: Individualize dosage. Signs of toxicity include nausea, vomiting, irritability, tachycardia, ventricular arrhythmias, and seizures. Following serum levels is necessary (see Table 7–11, p 498). Aminophylline is about 85% theophylline. Erratic absorption of rectal doses.

■ Amiodarone (Cordarone)

Indications: Treatment of recurrent ventricular fibrillation or hemodynamically unstable ventricular tachycardia.

Actions: Class III antiarrhythmic.

Dosage: *Loading dose:* 800–1600 mg/d for 1–3 weeks.
Maintenance: 600–800 mg/d for 1 month, then 200–400 mg/d.

Supplied: Tablets 200 mg.

Notes: Average half-life is 53 days. Potentially toxic effects leading to pulmonary fibrosis, liver failure, ocular opacities, as well as exacerbation of arrhythmias. PATIENT MUST BE HOSPITALIZED DURING LOADING and response requires 1 month as a rule.

■ Amitriptyline (Elavil, Others)

Indications: Depression; peripheral neuropathy; chronic pain; cluster and migraine headaches.

Actions: Tricyclic antidepressant.

Dosage: Initially 50–100 mg PO QHS; can increase to 300 mg QHS

Supplied: Tablets 10 mg, 25 mg, 50 mg, 75 mg, 100 mg, 150 mg; injection 10 mg/mL.

Notes: Strong anticholinergic side effects; can cause urinary retention, sedation.

■ Amoxapine (Asendin)

Indications: Depression; anxiety.

Actions: Tricyclic antidepressant.

Dosage: Initially 150 mg PO HS or 50 mg PO TID; increase to 300 mg daily.

Supplied: Tablets 25 mg, 50 mg, 100 mg, 150 mg.

Notes: Reduce dose in elderly. Taper slowly when discontinuing therapy.

■ Amoxicillin (Amoxil, Larotid, Polymox, Others)

Indications: Treatment of susceptible gram-negative bacteria (*Hemophilus influenzae, Escherichia coli, Proteus mirabilis, Neisseria gonorrhoeae*) and gram-positive bacteria (streptococci).

Actions: Inhibits cell wall synthesis.

Dosage: 250–500 mg PO every 8 hours.

Supplied: Capsules 250 mg, 500 mg; suspension 50 mg/5 mL, 125 mg/5 mL, 250 mg/5 mL.

Notes: Cross-hypersensitivity with penicillin. Can cause diarrhea, but less than with ampicillin. Skin rash is common. Many hospital strains of *E. coli* are now resistant.

■ Amoxicillin/Potassium Clavulanate (Augmentin)

Indications: Antibiotic effective against β-lactamase–producing strains of *H. influenzae, Staphylococcus aureus, E. coli,* and *Klebsiella pneumoniae.*

Actions: Combination of a β-lactam antibiotic and a β-lactamase inhibitor.

Dosage: 250–500 mg as amoxicillin PO every 8 hours.

Supplied: Tablets (amoxicillin/potassium clavulanate) 250/125 mg, 500/125 mg; suspension 125/31.25 mg per 5 mL, 250/62.5 mg per 5 mL.

Notes: DO NOT SUBSTITUTE two 250-mg tablets for one 500-mg tablet or an overdose of clavulanic acid will occur. GI intolerance is most common side effect.

■ Amphotericin B (Fungizone)

Indications: Severe, systemic fungal infections.

Actions: Binds to the sterols in the fungal membrane, altering membrane permeability.

Dosage: Test dose of 1 mg, then gradually increase dose as tolerated up to 0.25–0.5 mg/kg/24 h IV over 6 hours. Total dose varies with indications. Doses often range from 35 to 50 mg QD or QOD.

Supplied: Powder for injection 50 mg/vial.

Notes: Severe side effects with IV infusion. Monitor liver and renal function. Hypokalemia and hypomagnesemia may be seen from renal wasting. Pretreatment with aspirin or acetaminophen and antihistamines (Benadryl, etc) helps minimize adverse effects such as fever. Small amounts of heparin (1 U/mL) and hydrocortisone (1 mg/mg amphotericin) added to the infusate may help minimize phlebitis.

■ Ampicillin (Amcil, Omnipen, Others)

Indications: Treatment of susceptible gram-negatives (*Shigella, Salmonella, E. coli, H. influenzae, P. mirabilis, N. gonorrhoeae*) and gram-positives (streptococci).

Actions: β-Lactam antibiotic; inhibits cell wall synthesis.

Dosage: 500 mg–2 g IM/IV every 6 hours or 250–500 mg PO QID.

Supplied: Capsules 250 mg, 500 mg; suspension 100 mg/mL, 125 mg/5 mL, 250 mg/5 mL, 500 mg/5 mL. Powder for injection.

Notes: Cross-hypersensitivity with penicillin. Can cause diarrhea and skin rash. Many hospital strains of *E. coli* are now resistant.

■ Ampicillin/Sulbactam (Unasyn)

Indications: β-Lactamase–producing strains of *Staph. aureus, H. influenzae, Klebsiella* species, *P. mirabilis,* and *Bacteroides* species.

Actions: Combination of a β-lactam antibiotic and a β-lactamase inhibitor.

Dosage: 1.5–3.0 g (2:1 ampicillin sodium:sulbactam) IM/IV every 6 hours.

Supplied: Powder for injection 1.5 g, 3.0-g vials.

Notes: Ampicillin and sulbactam are in a 2:1 ratio.

■ Amrinone (Inocor)

Indications: Short-term management of congestive heart failure.

Actions: Positive inotrope with vasodilating activity.

Dosage: Initially give IV bolus of 0.75 mg/kg over 2–3 minutes, followed by a maintenance dose of 5–10 μg/kg/min.

Supplied: Injection 5 mg/mL.

Notes: Not to exceed 10 mg/kg/d. Incompatible with dextrose-containing solutions. Monitor for fluid and electrolyte changes and renal function during therapy.

■ Anistreplase (Eminase)

Indications: Acute myocardial infarction.

Actions: Thrombolytic agent.

Dosage: 30 U IV over 2–5 minutes.

Supplied: Vials containing 30 U.

Notes: Clearance is approximately 90 minutes after rapid infusion. May cause bleeding.

■ Antihemophilic Factor (Factor VIII) (Monoclate)

Indications: Treatment of classical hemophilia A.

Actions: Replaces missing clotting factor VIII.

Dosage: 1 AHF U/kg increases factor VIII concentration in the body by approximately 2%. Units required = (kg) (desired factor VIII increase as % normal level) (0.5).

Supplied: Check each vial for the number of units contained within the vial.

Notes: Patient's percentage of normal level of factor VIII concentration must be ascertained prior to dosing for these calculations. Not effective in controlling bleeding of patients with von Willebrand's disease.

■ Antithymocyte Globulin (ATG) (Atgam)

Indications: Management of allograft rejection in renal transplant patients.

Actions: Reduces the number of circulating, thymus-dependent lymphocytes.

Dosage: Adults: 10–30 mg/kg/d.

Supplied: Injection 50 mg/mL.

Notes: Do not administer to any patient with a prior history of severe systemic reaction to any other equine gamma-globulin preparation. Discontinue treatment if severe unremitting thrombocytopenia or leukopenia occurs.

■ Anusol, Anusol-HC

Indications: Symptomatic relief of pain from external and internal hemorrhoids.

Actions: Local anesthetic.

Dosage: 1 suppository every morning, every night, HS, and after each bowel movement. Apply cream freely to anal area every 6–12 hours.

Supplied: Suppository, cream, ointment.

Note: Anusol-HC also contains hydrocortisone for anti-inflammatory effect.

■ Aspirin (Bayer, Others)

Indications: Mild pain; headache; fever; inflammation; prevention of emboli; prevention of myocardial infarction.

Actions: Prostaglandin inhibitor.

Dosage: *Pain, fever:* 325–360 mg every 4–6 hours PO or rectally.
Rheumatoid arthritis: 3–6 g/d.
Platelet inhibitory action: 325 mg QD.
Prevention of MI: 325 mg QD.

Supplied: Tablets 325 mg, 500 mg; enteric-coated tablets 325 mg, 500 mg, 650 mg, 975 mg; sustained-release tablets 650 mg, 800 mg; suppositories 60 mg, 120 mg, 125 mg, 130 mg, 195 mg, 200 mg, 300 mg, 325 mg, 600 mg, 650 mg, 1.2 g.

Notes: GI upset and erosion are common adverse reactions. May be prevented by ingestion with food. Enteric-coated forms are available. See drug levels for salicylate, Table 7–11, p 498.

■ Aspirin with Butalbital and Caffeine (Fiorinal) [C]

Indications: Mild pain; headache, especially as associated with stress.

Actions: Nonnarcotic analgesic.

Dosage: 1 or 2 tablets (capsules) PO every 4–6 hours prn.

Supplied: Each capsule or tablet contains 325 mg aspirin, 40 mg caffeine, 50 mg butalbital.

Notes: Also available with codeine: #1 = 7.5 mg; #2 = 15 mg; #3 = 30 mg. Significant drowsiness associated with use.

■ Aspirin with Codeine (Empirin #1, #2, #3, #4) [C]

Indications: Relief of mild to moderate pain.

Actions: Combined effects of aspirin and a narcotic analgesic.

Dosage: 1 or 2 tablets PO every 3–4 hours prn.

Supplied: Tablets 325 mg and codeine as below.

Notes: Codeine in #1 = 7.5 mg, #2 = 15 mg, #3 = 30 mg, #4 = 60 mg.

■ Astemizole (Hismanal)

Indications: Allergic rhinitis.

Actions: Antihistamine.

Dosage: 10 mg daily.

Supplied: Tablet 10 mg.

Notes: Nonsedating. Take on an empty stomach. May affect allergy skin testing for weeks after one dose. May cause ventricular arrhythmias.

■ Atenolol (Tenormin)

See Table 7–7, p 492.

■ Atropine

Indications: Symptomatic bradycardia, Parkinsonism, relief of pylorospasm.

Actions: Antimuscarinic agent.

Dosage: *Emergency cardiac care*: 0.5 mg IV every 15 minutes up to 2.0 mg total.

Supplied: Tablets 0.3 mg, 0.4 mg, 0.6 mg; injection 0.05 mg/mL, 0.1 mg/mL, 0.3 mg/mL, 0.4 mg/mL, 0.5 mg/mL, 0.8 mg/mL, 1.0 mg/mL.

Notes: Can cause blurred vision, urinary retention, dried mucous membranes.

■ Azatadine (Optimine)

Indications: Hay fever; allergic rhinitis; chronic urticaria.

Actions: Antihistamine.

Dosage: 1–2 mg PO BID.

Supplied: Tablets 1 mg.

Notes: Has many anticholinergic side effects.

■ Azathioprine (Imuran)

Indications: Adjunct for the prevention of rejection in renal transplantation; rheumatoid arthritis; systemic lupus erythematosus.

Actions: Immunosuppressive agent.

Dosage: 1–3 mg/kg/d.

Supplied: Tablets 50 mg; injection 100 mg/20 mL.

Notes: May cause GI intolerance. Injection should be handled as with any antineoplastic agent.

■ Azlocillin (Azlin)

See Table 7–6, p 490.

■ Aztreonam (Azactam)

Indications: Specific for aerobic gram-negative bacteria including *Pseudomonas aeruginosa*.

Actions: Monobactam antibiotic. Inhibits cell wall synthesis.

Dosage: 1–2 g IV/IM every 6–12 hours.

Supplied: Powder for injection 500 mg, 1 g, 2 g.

Notes: Not effective against gram-positive or anaerobic bacteria. Can be given to penicillin-allergic patients.

■ Baclofen (Lioresal)

Indications: Management of spasticity secondary to chronic disorders such as multiple sclerosis or spinal cord lesions.

Actions: Centrally acting skeletal muscle relaxant.

Dosage: 5 mg PO TID initially; increase every 3 days to maximum effect; maximum 80 mg/d.

Supplied: Tablets 10 mg, 20 mg.

Notes: Caution in epileptics; neuropsychiatric disturbances.

■ Beclomethasone (Beconase, Vancenase Nasal Inhalers)

Indications: Allergic rhinitis refractory to conventional therapy with antihistamines and decongestants.

Actions: Inhaled corticosteroid.

Dosage: 1 spray intranasally BID–QID.

Supplied: Nasal inhaler.

Notes: Nasal spray delivers 42 μg/dose.

■ Beclomethasone (Beclovent, Vanceril Oral Inhaler)

Indications: Chronic asthma.

Actions: Inhaled corticosteroid.

Dosage: 2 inhalations TID–QID (maximum 20 per day)

Supplied: Oral inhaler.

Notes: NOT effective for acute asthmatic attacks. An anti-inflammatory topical steroid. Can cause oral thrush.

■ Belladonna and Opium Suppositories (B&O Suppositories) [C]

Indications: Treatment of bladder spasms; moderate to severe pain.

Actions: Antispasmodic agent.

Dosage: Insert 1 suppository rectally every 4–6 hours prn.

Supplied: Suppositories 15A, 16A. 15A = 30 mg powdered opium, 16.2

mg belladonna extract; 16A = 60 mg powdered opium, 16.2 mg belladonna extract.

Notes: Anticholinergic side effects. Caution subjects about sedation, urinary retention, constipation.

■ Belladonna Tincture

Indications: Adjunctive therapy in peptic ulcer disease, spastic colon, diarrhea.

Actions: Antimuscarinic/antispasmodic agent.

Dosage: 0.6–1.0 mL PO 3 or 4 times daily.

Supplied: Liquid with 27–33 mg of belladona alkaloids/100 mL.

Notes: Liquid contains 65%–70% alcohol. Anticholinergic side effects. Use with caution in patients with narrow-angle glaucoma.

■ Benzonatate (Tessalon, Perles)

Indications: Symptomatic relief of nonproductive cough.

Actions: Anesthetizes the stretch receptors in the respiratory passages.

Dosage: 100 mg PO TID.

Supplied: Capsule 100 mg.

Notes: May cause sedation.

■ Benzquinamide (Emete-Con)

Indications: Nausea and vomiting.

Actions: Antiemetic.

Dosage: 50 mg IM every 3–4 hours prn.

Supplied: Powder for injection 50 mg/vial.

Notes: Alternative antiemetic when phenothiazines or antihistamine is contraindicated.

■ Benztropine (Cogentin)

Indications: Parkinsonism; drug-induced extrapyramidal disorders.

Actions: Antimuscarinic agent.

Dosage: 1–6 mg PO, IM, or IV in divided doses.

Supplied: Tablets 0.5 mg, 1.0 mg, 2.0 mg; injection 1 mg/mL.

Notes: Anticholinergic side effects.

■ Bethanechol (Urecholine, Duvoid, Others)

Indications: Neurogenic atony of the bladder with urinary retention.

Actions: Stimulates the parasympathetic nervous system.

Dosage: 10–50 mg PO TID–QID or 5 mg SC TID–QID and prn.

Supplied: Tablets 5 mg, 10 mg, 25 mg, 50 mg; injection 5 mg/mL.

Notes: Contraindicated in bladder outlet obstruction, asthma, heart disease. DO NOT administer IM or IV.

■ Bisacodyl (Dulcolax)

Indications: Constipation; bowel prep.

Actions: Stimulant laxative.

Dosage: 5–10 mg PO or 10 mg rectally prn.

Supplied: Enteric-coated tablets 5 mg; suppository 10 mg.

Notes: DO NOT use with an acute abdomen or bowel obstruction. DO NOT chew tablets. DO NOT give within 1 hour of antacids or milk.

■ Bitolterol (Tornalate)

Indications: Prophylaxis and treatment of asthma and reversible bronchospasm.

Actions: Sympathomimetic bronchodilator.

Dosage: 2 inhalations every 8 hours.

Supplied: Aerosol 0.8%.

■ Bretylium (Bretylol)

Indications: Acute treatment of ventricular arrhythmias unresponsive to conventional therapy.

Actions: Class III antiarrhythmic.

Dosage: 5 mg/kg IV over 1 minute; may repeat every 15–30 minutes with 10 mg/kg (maximum of 30 mg/kg); maintenance 1–2 mg/min IV infusion.

Supplied: Injection 50 mg/mL.

Notes: Nausea and vomiting are associated with rapid IV push. Should gradually reduce dose and discontinue in 3–5 days. Effects are seen within first 10–15 minutes. Transient rise in blood pressure seen initially. Hypotension is most frequent adverse effect and occurs within the first hour of treatment.

■ Bromocriptine (Parlodel)

Indications: Parkinson's syndrome.

Actions: Acts directly on the striatal dopamine receptors.

Dosage: 1.25 mg PO BID initially, titrated to effect.

Supplied: Tablets 2.5 mg; capsules 5 mg.

Notes: Nausea and vertigo are common side effects.

■ Brompheniramine (Dimetane, Others)

Indications: Allergic reactions.

Actions: Antihistamine.

Dosage: 4–8 mg PO TID–QID or 10 mg IM every 6–12 hours.

Supplied: Tablets 4 mg; sustained-release tablets 8 mg, 12 mg; elixir 2 mg/5 mL; injection 10 mg/mL, 100 mg/mL.

Notes: Anticholinergic side effects.

■ Bumetanide (Bumex)

Indications: Edema from congestive heart failure, hepatic cirrhosis, and renal disease.

Actions: Loop diuretic.

Dosage: 0.5–2.0 mg PO daily; 0.5–1.0 mg IV every 8–24 hours.

Supplied: Tablets 0.5 mg, 1.0 mg; injection 0.25 mg/mL.

Notes: Monitor fluid and electrolyte (K^+) status during treatment.

■ Buprenorphine (Buprenex)

Indications: Relief of moderate to severe pain.

Actions: Narcotic agonist-antagonist.

Dosage: 0.3 mg IM or slow IVP every 6 hours prn.

Supplied: Injection 0.324 mg/mL (equal to 0.3 mg of buprenorphine).

Notes: May induce withdrawal syndrome in opioid dependent subjects.

■ Buspirone (BuSpar)

Indications: Short-term relief of anxiety.

Actions: Antianxiety agent.

Dosage: 5–10 mg TID.

Supplied: Tablets 5 mg, 10 mg.

Notes: NO abuse potential. NO physical or psychological dependence.

■ Butorphanol (Stadol)

Indications: Analgesic for moderate to severe pain.

Actions: Narcotic agonist-antagonist.

Dosage: 2 mg IM or 1 mg IV every 3–4 hours prn.

Supplied: Injection 1 mg/mL, 2 mg/mL.

Notes: May induce withdrawal syndrome in opioid-dependent subjects.

■ Calcium Carbonate (Tums, Alka-mints)

Indications: Hyperacidity (peptic ulcer, hiatal hernia, etc).

Actions: Neutralizes gastric acid.

Dosage: 500 mg–1.5 g prn.

Supplied: Chewable tablets 350 mg, 420 mg, 500 mg, 550 mg, 750 mg, 850 mg; suspension.

■ Calcium Salts (Chloride, Gluconate, Others)

Indications: Calcium replacement, ventricular fibrillation, electromechanical dissociation.

Actions: Dietary supplement; increased myocardial contractility.

Dosage: *Replacement*: 1–2 g PO QD.
Cardiac emergencies: Calcium chloride 0.5–1.0 g IV every 10 minutes OR calcium gluconate 1.0–2.0 g IV every 10 minutes.

Supplied: Oral; injections of the various salts.

Notes: Calcium chloride contains 270 mg (13.6 mEq) elemental calcium per gram. Calcium gluconate contains 90 mg (4.5 mEq) elemental calcium per gram.

■ Captopril (Capoten)

Indications: Hypertension; congestive heart failure.

Actions: Angiotension-converting enzyme inhibitor.

Dosage: *Hypertension*: Initially 25 mg PO BID or TID; titrate to a maintenance dose every 1–2 weeks by 25-mg increments per dose (maximum 450 mg/d) to desired effect.
Congestive heart failure: Initially 6.25–12.5 mg TID; titrate to desired effect.

Supplied: Tablets 12.5 mg, 25 mg, 50 mg, 100 mg.

Notes: Use with caution in renal failure. Give 1 hour before meals. Can cause rash, proteinuria, and cough.

■ Carbamazepine (Tegretol)

Indications: Epilepsy; trigeminal neuralgia.

Actions: Anticonvulsant.

Dosage: 200 mg BID initially; increase by 200 mg/d; usual 800–1200 mg/d.

Supplied: Tablets 200 mg; chewable tablets 100 mg; suspension 100 mg/5 mL.

Notes: Can cause severe hematologic side effects; monitor CBC; monitor serum levels (see Table 7–11, p 498). Generic products are NOT interchangeable.

■ Carbenicillin (Geocillin, Geopen, Pyopen)

See Table 7–6, p 490.

■ Carbidopa/Levodopa (Sinemet)

Indications: Parkinson's disease.

Actions: Raises CNS levels of dopamine.

Dosage: Start at 10/100 BID–TID; titrate as needed.

Supplied: Tablets (mg carbidopa/mg levodopa) 10/100, 25/100, 25/250.

Notes: May cause psychiatric disturbances, orthostatic hypotension, dyskinesias, and cardiac arrhythmias.

■ Carisoprodol (Soma)

Indications: Adjunct to sleep and physical therapy for relief of painful musculoskeletal conditions.

Actions: Centrally acting muscle relaxant.

Dosage: 350 mg PO QID.

Supplied: Tablets 350 mg.

Notes: Avoid alcohol and other CNS depressants.

■ Carteolol (Cartrol)

See Table 7–7, p 492.

■ Cefaclor (Ceclor)

See Table 7–8A, p 493.

■ Cefadroxil (Duricef, Ultracef)

See Table 7–8A, p 493.

■ Cefamandole (Mandol)

See Table 7–8B, p 494.

■ Cefazolin (Ancef, Kefzol)

See Table 7–8A, p 493.

■ Cefixime (Suprax)

See Table 7–8C, pp 494–495.

■ Cefmetazole (Zefazone)

See Table 7–8B, p 494.

■ Cefonicid (Monicid)

See Table 7–8B, p 494.

■ Cefoperazone (Cefobid)

See Table 7–8C, pp 494–495.

■ Ceforanide (Precef)

See Table 7–8B, p 494.

■ Cefotaxime (Claforan)

See Table 7–8C, pp 494–495.

■ Cefotetan (Cefotan)

See Table 7–8B, p 494.

■ Cefoxitin (Mefoxin)

See Table 7–8B, p 494.

■ Ceftazidime (Fortaz, Tazidime, Tazicef)

See Table 7–8C, pp 494–495.

■ Ceftizoxime (Cefizox)

See Table 7–8C, pp 494–495.

■ Ceftriaxone (Rocephin)

See Table 7–8C, pp 494–495.

■ Cefuroxime (Ceftin, Zinacef)

See Table 7–8B, p 494.

■ Cephalexin (Keflex)

See Table 7–8A, p 493.

■ Cephalothin (Keflin)

See Table 7–8A, p 493.

■ Cephapirin (Cefadyl)

See Table 7–8A, p 493.

■ Cephradine (Velosef, Anspor)

See Table 7–8A, p 493.

■ Charcoal, Activated (Superchar, Actidose, Liqui-char)

Indications: Emergency treatment in poisoning by most drugs and chemicals.

Actions: Adsorbent detoxicant.

Dosage: *Acute intoxication*: 30–100 g.
Gastrointestinal dialysis: 25–50 g every 4–6 hours.

Supplied: Powder, liquid.

Notes: Administer with a cathartic. Liquid dosage forms are in sorbitol base. Protect airway in lethargic or comatose patient.

■ Chloramphenicol (Chloromycetin)

Indications: Serious infections caused by gram-positive and gram-negative aerobic and anaerobic bacteria.

Actions: Interferes with protein synthesis.

Dosage: 50–100 mg/kg/d PO or IV in four divided doses.

Supplied: Capsules 250 mg, 500 mg; suspension 150 mg/5 mL; powder for injection.

Notes: Aplastic anemia has been associated with the use of this agent. Monitor hematology labs carefully. Reduce dose with hepatic impairment. Oral agents should be used whenever possible as the oral products are more bioavailable than the injection. *Pseudomonas aeruginosa* is almost always resistant.

■ Chlordiazepoxide (Librium) [C]

Indications: Anxiety; tension; alcohol withdrawal.

Actions: Benzodiazepine, sedative, antianxiety.

Dosage: *Mild anxiety, tension*: 5–10 mg PO TID–QID or prn.
Severe anxiety, tension: 25–50 mg IM or IV TID–QID or prn.
Alcohol withdrawal: 50–100 mg IM or IV; repeat in 2–4 hours if needed, up to 300 mg in 24 hours; gradually taper daily dosage.

Supplied: Capsules and tablets 5 mg, 10 mg, 25 mg; powder for injection 100 mg/ampoule.

Notes: Reduce dosage in the elderly; absorption of IM doses can be erratic.

■ Chlorothiazide (Diuril)

Indications: Hypertension; edema; congestive heart failure.

Actions: Thiazide diuretic.

Dosage: 500 mg–1.0 g PO or IV QD–BID.

Supplied: Tablets 250 mg, 500 mg; suspension 250 mg/5 mL; powder for injection 500 mg/vial.

Notes: Contraindicated in anuria.

■ Chlorpheniramine (Chlor-Trimeton, Others)

Indications: Allergic reactions.

Actions: Antihistamine.

Dosage: 4 mg PO every 4–6 hours prn; 8–12 mg PO BID sustained-release.

Supplied: Tablets 4 mg; chewable tablets 2 mg; sustained-release tablets 8 mg, 12 mg; syrup 2 mg/5 mL; injection 10 mg/mL, 100 mg/mL.

Notes: Anticholinergic side effects, sedation.

■ Chlorpromazine (Thorazine)

Indications: Psychotic disorders; apprehension; intractable hiccups; control of nausea and vomiting.

Actions: Phenothiazine antipsychotic, antiemetic.

Dosage: *Acute anxiety, agitation*: 10–25 mg PO or rectally BID–TID.
Severe symptoms: 25 mg IM; can repeat in 1 hour, then 25–50 mg PO or rectally TID.
Outpatient antipsychotic: 10–25 mg PO BID–TID.
Hiccups: 25–50 mg PO BID–TID.

Supplied: Tablets 10 mg, 25 mg, 50 mg, 100 mg, 200 mg; capsules sustained-release 30 mg, 75 mg, 150 mg, 200 mg, 300 mg; syrup 10 mg/5 mL; concentrate 30 mg/mL, 100 mg/mL; suppositories 25 mg, 100 mg; injection 25 mg/mL.

Notes: Beware of extrapyramidal side effects; sedation; has alpha-adrenergic blocking properties.

■ Chlorpropamide (Diabinese)

See Table 7–10, p 497.

■ Chlorthalidone (Hygroton, Others)

Indications: Hypertension; edema associated with congestive heart failure; steroid and estrogen therapy.

Actions: Thiazide diuretic.

Dosage: 50–100 mg PO QD.

Supplied: Tablets 25 mg, 50 mg, 100 mg.

Notes: Contraindicated in anuric patients.

■ Chlorzoxazone (Paraflex, Parafon Forte DSC)

Indications: Adjunct to rest and physical therapy for the relief of discomfort associated with acute, painful musculoskeletal conditions.

Actions: Centrally acting skeletal muscle relaxant.

Dosage: 250–500 mg TID–QID.

Supplied: Tablets 250 mg; caplets 500 mg.

■ Cholecalciferol (Vitamin D_3, Delta D)

Indications: Dietary supplement for treatment of vitamin D deficiency.

Actions: Enhances intestinal calcium absorption.

Dosage: 400–1000 IU PO daily.

Supplied: Tablets 400 IU, 1000 IU.

Notes: 1 mg cholecalciferol = 40,000 IU of vitamin D activity.

■ Cholestyramine (Questran)

Indications: Adjunctive therapy for the reduction of serum cholesterol in patients with primary hypercholesterolemia; relief of pruritis associated with partial biliary obstruction.

Actions: Binds bile acids in the intestine to form insoluble complexes.

Dosage: Individualized to 4 g 1–6 times daily.

Supplied: 4 g cholestyramine resin/9 g of powder.

Notes: Mix 4 g cholestyramine in 2–6 oz of noncarbonated beverage.

■ Cimetidine (Tagamet)

Indications: Duodenal ulcer; ulcer prophylaxis in hypersecretory states such as trauma, burns, surgery, Zollinger-Ellison syndrome, etc.

Actions: Histamine-2 receptor antagonist.

Dosage: *Active ulcer*: 300 mg IV every 6–8 hours; 400 mg PO BID or 800 mg QHS.
Maintenance therapy: 400 mg PO QHS.

Supplied: Tablets 200 mg, 300 mg, 400 mg, 800 mg; liquid 300 mg/5 mL; injection 300 mg/2 mL.

Notes: Extend dosing interval to every 12 hours with creatinine clearance <30 mL/min; decrease dose in elderly, may cause confusion; drug interactions with theophylline, digoxin, and possibly others.

■ Ciprofloxacin (Cipro)

Indications: Broad-spectrum activity against a variety of gram-positive and gram-negative aerobic bacteria.

Actions: DNA gyrase inhibitor, interferes with DNA synthesis.

Dosage: 250–750 mg PO every 12 hours.

Supplied: Tablets 250 mg, 500 mg, 750 mg.

Notes: Not active against streptococci. Drug interaction with theophylline, increases theophylline serum levels. Absorption inhibited by antacids; nausea, diarrhea, vomiting, and abdominal discomfort are common side effects. CONTRAINDICATED IN PREGNANCY.

■ Clemastine Fumarate (Tavist)

Indications: Allergic rhinitis.

Actions: Antihistamine.

Dosage: 1.34 mg BID to 2.68 mg TID, maximum 8.04 mg/d.

Supplied: Tablets 1.34 mg, 2.68 mg; syrup 0.67 mg/5 mL.

■ Clindamycin (Cleocin)

Indications: Susceptible strains of streptococci, pneumococci, staphylococci, and gram-positive and gram-negative anaerobes; no activity against gram-negative aerobes.

Actions: Bacteriostatic; interferes with protein synthesis.

Dosage: 150–450 mg PO QID; 300–600 mg IV every 6 hours or 900 mg IV every 8 hours.

Supplied: Capsules 75 mg, 150 mg; suspension 75 mg/5 mL; injection 300 mg/2 mL.

Notes: Beware of severe diarrhea that may represent pseudomembranous colitis caused by *Clostridium difficile.*

■ Clonazepam (Klonopin) [C]

Indications: Lennox-Gastaut syndrome; akinetic and myoclonic seizures; absence seizures.

Actions: Benzodiazepine anticonvulsant.

Dosage: 1.5 mg/d in 3 divided doses; increase by 0.5–1.0 mg/d every 3 days prn up to 20 mg/d.

Supplied: Tablets 0.5 mg, 1.0 mg, 2.0 mg.

Notes: CNS side effects including sedation.

■ Clonidine (Catapres)

Indications: Hypertension; opioid and tobacco withdrawal.

Actions: Centrally acting alpha-adrenergic stimulant.

Dosage: 0.10 mg PO BID adjusted daily by 0.10 to 0.20-mg increments (maximum 2.4 mg/d).

Supplied: Tablets 0.1 mg, 0.2 mg, 0.3 mg.

Notes: Dry mouth, drowsiness, and sedation occur frequently. More effective for hypertension when combined with diuretic. Rebound hypertension can occur with abrupt cessation with doses above 0.2 mg BID.

■ Clonidine Transdermal (Catapres TTS)

Indications: Hypertension.

Actions: Centrally acting alpha-adrenergic stimulant.

Dosage: Apply one patch every 7 days to a hairless area on the upper arm or torso; titrate according to individual therapeutic requirements.

Supplied: TTS-1, TTS-2, TTS-3 (programmed to deliver 0.1, 0.2, 0.3 mg of clonidine per day, for 1 week).

Notes: Doses above two TTS-3 are usually not associated with increased efficacy.

■ Clorazepate (Tranxene) [C]

Indications: Acute anxiety disorders; acute alcohol withdrawal symptoms; adjunctive therapy in partial seizures.

Actions: Benzodiazepine.

Dosage: 15–60 mg/d PO in single or divided doses.

Supplied: Capsules and tablets 3.75 mg, 7.5 mg, 15 mg.

Notes: Monitor patients with renal and hepatic impairment as drug may accumulate. CNS depressant effects.

■ Clotrimazole (Lotrimin, Mycelex)

Indications: Treatment of candidiasis and tinea infections.

Actions: Antifungal; alters cell membrane permeability.

Dosage: *Orally*: one troche dissolved slowly in the mouth 5 times a day for 14 days.
Vaginally: *Cream*—one applicatorful HS for 7–14 days. *Tablets*—100 mg vaginally HS for 7 days or 200 mg (2 tablets) vaginally HS for 3 days or 500-mg tablet vaginally HS X 1.
Topically: Apply 3 or 4 times daily for 10–14 days.

Supplied: Cream 1%; solution 1%; lotion 1%; troche 10 mg; vaginal tablets 100 mg, 500 mg; vaginal cream 1%.

Notes: Oral prophylaxis common in immunosuppressed patients.

■ Cloxacillin (Cloxapen, Tegopen)

See Table 7–5, p 489.

■ Codeine [C]

Indications: Mild to moderate pain; symptomatic relief of cough.

Actions: Narcotic analgesic; depresses cough reflex.

Dosage: *Analgesic*: 15–60 mg PO or IM QID prn.
Antitussive: 5–15 mg PO every 4 hours prn.

Supplied: Tablets 15 mg, 30 mg, 60 mg; injection 30 mg/mL, 60 mg/mL.

Notes: Most often used in combination with acetaminophen or other agents such as terpin hydrate or guaifenesin; 120 mg is equivalent to 10 mg morphine IM.

■ Colchicine

Indications: Acute gout.

Actions: Inhibits migration of leukocytes and reduces production of lactic acid by leukocytes.

Dosage: Initially 0.5–1.2 mg, then 0.5–1.2 mg every 1–2 hours until GI side effects develop (maximum 8 mg/d).

Supplied: Tablets 0.5 mg, 0.6 mg; injection 1 mg/2 mL.

Notes: Use with caution in elderly and patients with renal impairment. Colchicine 1–2 mg IV within 24–48 hours of an acute attack can be diagnostic and therapeutic in a monoarticular arthritis.

■ Colestipol (Colestid)

Indications: Adjunctive therapy for the reduction of serum cholesterol in patients with primary hypercholesterolemia.

Actions: Binds bile acids in the intestine to form an insoluble complex.

Dosage: 15–30 g per day divided into 2–4 doses.

Supplied: 5-g packets; 500-g bottles.

Notes: Do not use dry powder; mix with beverages, soups, cereals, etc.

■ Cortisporin Ophthalmic

Indications: Treatment of superficial ocular infections by organisms susceptible to neomycin, polymyxin, and bacitracin (ointment only).

Actions: Antibiotic combination.

Dosage: *Suspension*: Instill 1 or 2 drops into affected eye(s) every 3–4 hours.
Ointment: Insert $\frac{1}{2}$ in. of ointment into conjunctival sac 3 or 4 times daily.

Supplied: Ophthalmic suspension; ophthalmic ointment.

Notes: If no improvement in symptoms in 3–4 days, reconsider diagnosis (e.g., viral or fungal etiology).

■ Cortisporin Otic

Indications: Treatment of superficial bacterial infections of the external auditory canal by organisms sensitive to neomycin or polymyxin. Suspension may also be used in the treatment of infections in mastoidectomy and fenestration cavities.

Actions: Antibiotic combination.

Dosage: 4 drops instilled into external auditory canal 3 or 4 times daily.

Supplied: Otic solution; otic suspension.

Notes: Use suspension form only in case of ruptured ear drum.

■ Corticosteroids

See Steroids in Table 7–4, p 476.

■ Cortisone

See Steroids in Table 7–4, p 476.

■ Cromolyn Sodium (Intal, Nasalcrom, Opticrom)

Indications: Adjunct to the treatment of asthma; NOT for acute attack; prevention of exercise-induced asthma; allergic rhinitis; ophthalmic allergic manifestations.

Actions: Antiasthmatic, antiallergic, and mast cell stabilizer.

Dosage: *Inhalation*: 20 mg (as powder in capsule) inhaled QID; aerosol, 2 puffs inhaled QID.
Nasal instillation: Spray once in each nostril 2–6 times daily.
Ophthalmic: 1 or 2 drops in each eye 4–6 times daily.

Supplied: Capsules for inhalation 20 mg; solution for nebulization 20 mg/2 mL; metered dose inhaler; nasal solution 40 mg/mL; ophthalmic solution 4%.

Notes: Inhalation of dry powder can cause cough and bronchospasm; may need to switch to metered dose inhaler. May require 2–4 weeks for maximal effect in perennial allergic disorders.

■ Cyancobalamin/Vitamin B_{12}

Indications: Pernicious anemia and other B_{12} deficiency states.

Actions: Dietary replacement of vitamin B_{12}.

Dosage: 100 μg, IM or SC QD for 1 week, then 100 μg IM twice a week for 1 month, then 100 μg IM monthly.

Supplied: Tablets 25 μg, 50 μg, 100 μg, 250 μg, 500 μg, 1000 μg; injection 30 g/mL, 100 g/mL, 1000 g/mL.

Notes: Oral absorption highly erratic, altered by many drugs and not recommended.

■ Cyclobenzaprine (Flexeril)

Indications: Adjunct to rest and physical therapy for relief of muscle spasm associated with acute painful musculoskeletal conditions.

Actions: Centrally acting skeletal muscle relaxant.

Dosage: 10 mg PO TID.

Supplied: Tablets 10 mg.

Notes: Do not use for longer than 2–3 weeks. Has sedative and anticholinergic properties.

■ Cyclosporine (Sandimmune)

Indications: Prophylaxis of organ rejection in kidney, liver, and heart allogeneic transplants in conjunction with adrenal corticosteroids.

Actions: Reversible inhibition of immunocompetent lymphocytes.

Dosage: *Oral*: 15 mg/kg/d beginning 12 hours prior to transplant; after 2 weeks, taper dose by 5% per week to 5–10 mg/kg/d.
Intravenous: If patient unable to take orally, give one-third oral dose IV.

Supplied: Oral solution 100 mg/mL; injection 50 mg/mL.

Notes: Should NOT be administered with any other immunosuppressive agents except adrenal corticosteroids. May elevate BUN and creatinine, which may be confused with renal transplant rejection. Has many drug interactions. Should be administered in glass containers.

■ Cyproheptadine (Periactin)

Indications: Allergic reactions; especially good for itching.

Actions: Phenothiazine antihistamine.

Dosage: 4 mg PO TID, maximum 0.5 mg/kg/d.

Supplied: Tablets 4 mg; syrup 2 mg/5 mL.

Notes: Anticholinergic side effects and drowsiness common. May stimulate appetite in some patients.

■ Dantrolene Sodium (Dantrium)

Indications: Treatment of clinical spasticity resulting from upper motor neuron disorders such as spinal cord injuries, strokes, cerebral palsy, or multiple sclerosis; treatment of malignant hyperthermic crisis.

Actions: Skeletal muscle relaxant.

Dosage: *Spasticity*: Initially 25 mg PO QD, titrate to effect by 25 mg up to maximum dose of 100 mg PO QID prn.

Malignant hyperthermia: *Treatment*: rapid IV push beginning at 1 mg/kg until symptoms subside or 10 mg/kg reached. *Postcrisis follow-up*: 4–8 mg/kg/d in 3 or 4 divided doses for 1–3 days to prevent recurrence.

Supplied: Capsules 25 mg, 50 mg, 100 mg; powder for injection 20 mg/vial.

Notes: Monitor liver function tests (ALT and AST) closely.

■ Demeclocycline (Declomycin)

Indications: Treatment of SIADH; antimicrobial agent of the tetracycline familv

Actions: Bacteriostatic; inhibits protein synthesis.

Dosage: *SIADH*: 300–600 mg PO every 12 hours.
Antimicrobial: 150 mg every 6 hours or 300 mg PO every 12 hours.

Supplied: Capsules 150 mg; tablets 150 mg, 300 mg.

Notes: Reduce dose in renal failure. May cause diabetes insipidus.

■ Desipramine (Norpramine)

Indications: Endogenous depression.

Actions: Tricyclic antidepressant.

Dosage: 25–200 mg/d in single or divided doses; usually as a single HS dose.

Supplied: Tablets 25 mg, 50 mg, 75 mg, 100 mg, 150 mg; capsules 25 mg, 50 mg.

Notes: Many anticholinergic side effects including blurred vision, urinary retention, dry mouth.

■ Desmopressin (DDAVP, Stimate)

Indications: Diabetes insipidus (intranasal and parenteral); bleeding resulting from hemophilia A and type I von Willebrand's disease (parenteral).

Actions: Synthetic analog of vasopressin, a naturally occurring human antidiuretic hormone; increases factor VIII.

Dosage: *Diabetes insipidus*: *Intranasal*—0.1–0.4 mL (10–40 μg) daily as a single dose or in 2 or 3 divided doses. *Parenterally*—0.5–1 mL (2–4 g) daily in 2 divided doses; if converting from intranasal to parenteral dosing, use one-tenth intranasal dose.

Hemophilia A and von Willebrand's Disease: 0.3 μg/kg diluted to 50 mL with normal saline solution infused slowly over 15–30 minutes.

Supplied: Injection 4 g/mL; nasal solution 0.1 g/mL.

Notes: In the elderly, adjust fluid intake to avoid water intoxication and hyponatremia.

■ Desoxycorticosterone Acetate (DOCA, Percorten)

Indications: Partial treatment for adrenocortical insufficiency.

Actions: Adrenal cortical steroid with potent mineralocorticoid activity.

Dosage: *Injection*: 2–5 mg/d IM into upper outer quadrant of gluteal region.
Pellets: By surgical implantation.

Supplied: Injection 5 mg/mL; repository injection 25 mg/mL; pellets 125 mg.

Notes: Must be used in conjunction with a glucocorticoid.

■ Dexamethasone (Decadron)

See Steroids in Table 7–4, p 476.

■ Dextran 40 (Rheomacrodex)

Indications: Plasma expander for adjunctive therapy in shock.

Actions: Plasma volume expander.

Dosage: *Shock*: 10 mL/kg infused rapidly with maximum dose of 20 mL/kg in the first 24 hours; total daily dosage beyond 24 hours should not exceed 10 mL/kg and should be discontinued after 5 days.

Supplied: 10% Dextran 40 in 0.9% sodium chloride or 5% dextrose; Dextran 70 can be used for prophylaxis for deep vein thrombosis.

Notes: Observe for hypersensitivity reactions: monitor renal function and electrolytes.

■ Dextromethorphan (Mediquell, Benylin DM)

Indications: To control nonproductive cough.

Actions: Depresses the cough center.

Dosage: 10–20 mg PO every 4 hours prn.

Supplied: Chewy squares 15 mg; lozenges 5 mg; syrup 15 mg/5 mL, 10 mg/5 mL, 7.5 mg/5 mL, 5 mg/5 mL; liquid, sustained action 30 mg/5 mL.

■ Diazepam (Valium) [C]

Indications: Anxiety, alcohol withdrawal, muscle spasm, status epilepticus, preoperative sedation.

Actions: Benzodiazepine.

Dosage: *Status epilepticus*: 0.2–0.5 mg/kg/dose IV every 15–30 minutes to maximum dose of 30 mg.
Anxiety, muscle spasm: 2–10 mg PO or IM every 3–4 hours prn.
Preoperative: 5–10 mg PO or IM 20–30 minutes before procedure; can be given IV just prior to procedure.
Alcohol withdrawal: Initially 2–5 mg IV, may require up to 1000–2000 mg in 24-hour period for major withdrawal symptoms.

Supplied: Sustained-release capsules 15 mg; tablets 2 mg, 5 mg, 10 mg; solution 5 mg/5 mL, 5 mg/mL; injection 5 mg/mL.

Notes: Do not exceed 5 mg/min IV as respiratory arrest can occur. Absorption of IM dose can be erratic.

■ Diazoxide (Hyperstat, Proglycem)

Indications: Hypertensive emergencies; management of hypoglycemia resulting from hyperinsulinism.

Actions: Relaxes smooth muscle in the peripheral arterioles; inhibits pancreatic insulin release.

Dosage: *Hypertensive crisis*: 1–3 mg/kg/dose IV up to maximum of 150 mg IV; may repeat at 15-minute intervals until desired effect is achieved.
Hyperinsulinemic hypoglycemia: 3–8 mg/kg/24 hr PO divided every 8–12 hours.

Notes: Cannot be titrated.

■ Diclofenac Sodium (Voltaren)

See Table 7–9, p 496.

■ Dicloxacillin (Dynapen, Dycill)

See Table 7–5, p 489.

■ Dicyclomine (Bentyl)

Indications: Treatment of functional/irritable bowel syndromes.

Actions: Smooth muscle relaxant.

Dosage: 20 mg PO QID initially, increase to 160 mg/d or 20 mg IM every 6 hours.

Supplied: Capsules 10 mg, 20 mg; tablets 20 mg; syrup 10 mg/5 mL; injection 10 mg/mL.

Notes: Anticholinergic effects may limit dosage.

■ Digoxin (Lanoxin, Lanoxicaps)

Indications: Congestive heart failure; atrial fibrillation and flutter; paroxysmal atrial tachycardia.

Actions: Positive inotrope, increases refractory period of atrioventricular node.

Dosage: *Oral digitalization*: 0.50–0.75 mg PO; then 0.25 mg PO every 6–8 hours to a total dose between 1.0 and 1.5 mg.
Intravenous or intramuscular digitalization: 0.25–0.50 mg IM or IV; then 0.25 mg every 4–6 hours to a total dose of about 1 mg.
Daily maintenance: 0.125–0.500 mg PO, IM, or IV QD (average daily dose 0.125–0.250 mg).

Supplied: Capsules 0.05 mg, 0.1 mg, 0.2 mg; tablets 0.125 mg, 0.25 mg, 0.5 mg; elixir 0.05 mg/mL; injection 0.1 mg/mL, 0.25 mg/mL.

Notes: Can cause heart block. Low potassium can potentiate toxicity. Reduce dose in renal failure. Symptoms of toxicity include nausea, vomiting, headache, fatigue, visual disturbances (yellow-green halos around lights), and cardiac arrhythmias (see Table 7–11, p 498). IM injection can be painful and have erratic absorption.

■ Dihydroxyaluminum Sodium Carbonate (Rolaids)

Indications: Heartburn; gastroesophageal reflux; acid ingestion.

Actions: Neutralizes gastric acid.

Dosage: 1 or 2 tablets prn.

Supplied: Chewable tablets 334 mg.

■ Diltiazem (Cardizem)

Indications: Angina pectoris; prevention of reinfarction; hypertension.

Actions: Calcium channel blocker.

Dosage: 30 mg PO QID initially; titrate to 180–360 mg/d in divided doses as needed. Sustained-release: 60–120 mg PO BID, titrate to effect, maximum dose 360 mg/d.

Supplied: Tablets 30 mg, 60 mg, 90 mg, 120 mg; sustained-release tablets 60 mg, 90 mg, 120 mg.

Notes: Contraindicated in sick-sinus syndrome, atrioventricular block, and hypotension.

■ Dimenhydrinate (Dramamine)

Indications: Prevention and treatment of nausea, vomiting, dizziness, or vertigo of motion sickness.

Actions: Antiemetic.

Dosage: 50–100 mg PO every 4–6 hours, maximum of 400 mg/d; 50 mg IM/IV prn.

Supplied: Tablets; chewable tablets; capsules 50 mg; injection 50 mg/mL.

Notes: Anticholinergic side effects.

■ Diphenhydramine (Benadryl, Others)

Indications: Allergic reactions; motion sickness; potentiation of narcotics; sedation; cough suppression; treatment of extrapyramidal reactions.

Actions: Antihistamine, antiemetic.

Dosage: 25–50 mg PO or IM BID–TID.

Supplied: Tablets and capsules 25 mg, 50 mg; elixir 12.5 mg/5 mL; syrup 12.5 mg/5 mL; injection 10 mg/mL, 50 mg/mL.

Notes: Anticholinergic side effects including dry mouth, urinary retention. Causes sedation. Increase dosing interval in moderate to severe renal failure.

■ Diphenoxylate with Atropine (Lomotil) [C]

Indications: Diarrhea.

Actions: A constipating meperidine congener.

Dosage: Initially 5 mg PO TID or QID until under control; then 2.5–5.0 mg PO BID.

Supplied: Tablets 2.5 mg diphenoxylate/0.025 mg atropine; liquid 2.5 mg diphenoxylate/0.025 mg atropine per 5 mL.

Notes: Atropine-type side effects.

■ Dipyridamole (Persantin)

Indications: Prevention of postoperative thromboembolic disorders; chronic angina pectoris.

Actions: Dilates coronary arteries; antiplatelet activity.

Dosage: *Antiplatelet effect*: 75–100 mg PO TID–QID.
Angina: 50 mg PO TID.

Supplied: Tablets 25 mg, 50 mg, 75 mg.

Notes: Aspirin potentiates the antiplatelet effects, may cause nausea and vomiting.

■ Disopyramide (Norpace, Napamide)

Indications: Suppression and prevention of premature ventricular contractions.

Actions: Class 1A antiarrhythmic.

Dosage: 400–800 mg/d divided every 6 hours for regular-release products and every 12 hours for sustained-release products.

Supplied: Capsules 100 mg, 150 mg; sustained-release capsules 100 mg, 150 mg.

Notes: Has anticholinergic side effects (urinary retention). Negative inotropic properties may induce congestive heart failure. Decrease dose in impaired hepatic function.

■ Disulfiram (Antabuse)

Indications: Alcohol consumption deterrent.

Actions: Blocks oxidation of alcohol to produce unpleasant reaction when alcohol is consumed.

Dosage: 500 mg PO QD for 1–2 weeks, then 250 mg PO QD.

Supplied: Tablets 250 mg, 500 mg.

Notes: Patients must avoid all hidden forms of alcohol (cough syrup, sauces etc.); CBC and liver function tests should be checked periodically.

■ Dobutamine (Dobutrex)

Indications: Short-term use in patients with cardiac decompensation secondary to depressed contractility.

Actions: Positive inotropic agent.

Dosage: Continuous IV infusion of 2.5–10 μg/kg/min; rarely 40 μg/kg/min may be required; titrate according to response.

Supplied: 250 mg/20 mL.

Notes: Monitor ECG for increase in heart rate, blood pressure, and increased ectopic activity. Monitor pulmonary wedge pressure and cardiac output if possible.

■ Docusate Calcium (Surfak, Others) Docusate Sodium (DOSS, Colace, Others)

Indications: Constipation-prone patient; adjunct to painful anorectal conditions (hemorrhoids).

Actions: Stool softener.

Dosage: 240 mg PO QD.

Supplied: Capsules 50 mg, 240 mg.

Notes: No significant side effects, no laxative action.

■ Dopamine (Intropin, Dopastat)

Indications: Short-term use in patients with cardiac decompensation secondary to decreased contractility; increase organ perfusion.

Actions: Positive inotropic agent.

Dosage: 5 μg/kg/min by continuous infusion titrated by increments of 5 μg/kg/min to maximum of 50 μg/kg/min based on effect.

Supplied: Injection 40 mg/mL, 80 mg/mL, 160 mg/mL.

Notes: Dosage greater than 10 μg/kg/min may decrease renal perfusion. Monitor urinary output. Monitor ECG for increase in heart rate, blood pressure, and increased ectopic activity. Monitor pulmonary capillary wedge pressure and cardiac output if possible.

■ Doxepin (Sinequan, Adapin)

Indications: Depression or anxiety.

Actions: Tricyclic antidepressant.

Dosage: 50–150 mg PO QD usually QHS but can be in divided doses.

Supplied: Capsules 10 mg, 25 mg, 50 mg, 75 mg, 100 mg, 150 mg; oral concentrate 10 mg/mL.

Notes: Anticholinergic, central nervous system, and cardiovascular side effects.

■ Doxycycline (Vibramycin)

Indications: Broad-spectrum antibiotic including activity against *Rickettsiae, Chlamydia,* and *Mycoplasma pneumoniae.*

Actions: Tetracycline; interferes with protein synthesis.

Dosage: 100 mg PO every 12 hours first day, then 100 mg PO QD or BID or 100 mg IV every 12 hours.

Supplied: Tablets 50 mg, 100 mg; capsules 50 mg, 100 mg; syrup 50 mg/5 mL; powder for oral suspension 25 mg/5 mL; powder for injection 100 mg, 200 mg per vial.

Notes: Useful for chronic bronchitis and prostatitis. Tetracycline of choice for patients with renal impairment. Contraindicated in pregnancy.

■ Dronabinol (Marinol) [C]

Indications: Nausea and vomiting associated with cancer chemotherapy.

Actions: Antiemetic.

Dosage: 5–15 mg/m^2 every 4–6 hours prn.

Supplied: Capsules 2.5 mg, 5 mg, 10 mg.

Notes: Principal psychoactive substance present in marijuana. Many CNS side effects.

■ Droperidol (Inapsine)

Indications: Nausea and vomiting.

Actions: Tranquilization, sedation, and antiemetic.

Dosage: 1.25–2.5 mg IV prn.

Supplied: Injection 2.5 mg/mL.

Notes: May cause drowsiness, moderate hypotension, and occasionally tachycardia.

■ Econazole (Spectazole)

Indications: Treatment of most tinea, cutaneous *Candida*, and tinea versicolor infections.

Actions: Topical antifungal.

Dosage: Apply to affected areas BID (QD for *tinea versicolor* for 2–4 weeks.

Supplied: Topical cream 1%.

Notes: Relief of symptoms and clinical improvement may be seen early in treatment, but course of therapy should be carried out to avoid recurrence.

■ Edrophonium (Tensilon)

Indications: Diagnosis of myasthenia gravis; acute myasthenic crisis; curare antagonist; paroxysmal atrial tachycardia.

Actions: Anticholinesterase.

Dosage: *Test for myasthenia gravis*: 2 mg IV in 1 minute; if tolerated, give 8 mg IV; a positive test is a brief increase in strength.
Paroxysmal atrial tachycardia: 10 mg IV to a maximum of 40 mg.

Supplied: Injection 10 mg/mL.

Notes: Can cause severe cholinergic effects; keep atropine available.

■ Enalapril (Vasotec)

Indications: Hypertension; congestive heart failure.

Actions: Angiotension-converting enzyme inhibitor.

Dosage: 2.5–5 mg/d PO titrated by effect to 10–40 mg/d as 1 or 2 divided doses, or 1.25 mg IV every 6 hours.

Supplied: Tablets 2.5 mg, 5 mg, 10 mg, 20 mg; injection 1.25 mg/mL.

Notes: Initial dose could produce symptomatic hypotension, especially with diuretics. Discontinue diuretic for 2–3 days prior to initiation of therapy with enalapril if possible. Monitor closely for increases in serum potassium. Can cause nonproductive cough.

■ Ephedrine

Indications: Acute bronchospasm; nasal congestion; hypotension; narcolepsy; enuresis; myasthenia gravis.

Actions: Sympathomimetic that stimulates both alpha and beta receptors.

Dosage: 25–50 mg IM/IV every 10 minutes to maximum 150 mg/d or 25–50 mg PO every 3–4 hours prn.

Supplied: Injection 25 mg/mL, 50 mg/mL; capsules 25 mg, 50 mg; syrup 11 mg/5 mL, 20 mg/5 mL.

■ Epinephrine (Adrenalin, Sus-Phrine, Others)

Indications: Cardiac arrest; anaphylactic reactions; acute asthma.

Actions: Beta-adrenergic agonist with alpha effects.

Dosage: *Emergency cardiac care*: 0.5–1.0 mg (5–10 mL of 1:10,000) IV every 5 minutes to response.
Anaphylaxis: 0.3–0.5 mL of 1:1000 dilution SC; may repeat every 10–15 minutes to maximum of 1 mg/dose and 5 mg/d.
Asthma: 0.3–0.5 mL of 1:1000 dilution SC repeated at 20-minute to 4-hour intervals OR 1 inhalation (metered dose) repeated in 1–2 minutes OR suspension 0.1–0.3 mL SC for extended effect.

Supplied: Injection 1:1000, 1:10,000, 1:100,000; suspension for injection 1:200; aerosol; solution for nebulization.

Notes: Sus-Phrine offers sustained action. In acute cardiac settings can be given via endotracheal tube if a central line is not available.

■ Epoetin Alpha (Epogen)

Indications: Anemia associated with chronic renal failure.

Actions: Erythropoietin supplementation.

Dosage: 50–100 U/kg 3 times weekly.

Supplied: Injection 2000 U, 4000 U, 10,000 U.

Notes: May cause hypertension, headache, tachycardia, nausea, and vomiting.

■ Erythromycin (E-Mycin, Ilosone, Erythrocin, ERYC, Others)

Indications: Group A streptococci (*Streptococcus pyrogenes*); alpha-hemolytic streptococci and *Neisseria gonorrhoeae* infections in penicillin-sensitive patients; *S. pneumoniae*; *Mycoplasma pneumoniae*; Legionnaire's disease; and soft tissue infection caused by *S. aureus.*

Actions: Bacteriostatic, interferes with protein synthesis.

Dosage: 250–500 mg PO QID or 500 mg–1 g IV QID.

Supplied: *Powder for injection as lactobionate and gluceptate salts*: 250 mg, 500 mg, 1 g.
Base: tablets 250 mg, 333 mg, 500 mg; capsules 125 mg, 250 mg.
Estolate: chewable tablets 125 mg, 250 mg; capsules 125 mg, 250 mg; drops 100 mg/mL; suspension 125 mg/5 mL, 250 mg/5 mL.
Stearate: tablets 250 mg, 500 mg.
Ethylsuccinate: chewable tablets 200 mg; tablets 400 mg; suspension 200 mg/5 mL, 400 mg/5 mL.

Notes: Frequent mild GI disturbances. Estolate salt is associated with cholestatic jaundice. Erythomycin base not well absorbed from the GI tract. Some forms such as ERYC are better tolerated with respect to GI irritation.

■ Esmolol (Brevibloc)

Indications: Supraventricular tachycardia; noncompensatory sinus tachycardia.

Actions: Beta-adrenergic blocking agent.

Dosage: Initiate treatment with 500 μg/kg load over 1 minute, then 50 μg/kg/min for 4 minutes; if inadequate response, repeat loading dose and follow with maintenance infusion of 100 μg/kg/min for 4 minutes; continue titration process by repeating loading dose followed by incremental increases in the maintenance dose of 50 μg/kg/min for 4 minutes until desired heart rate is reached or a decrease in blood pressure occurs; average dose is 100 μg/kg/min.

Supplied: Injection 10 mg/mL, 250 mg/mL.

Notes: Monitor closely for hypotension; decreasing or discontinuing infusion will reverse hypotension in approximately 30 minutes.

■ Estradiol Transdermal (Estraderm)

Indications: Severe vasomotor symptoms associated with menopause; female hypogonadism.

Actions: Hormonal replacement.

Dosage: 0.05 system twice weekly, adjust dose as necessary to control symptoms.

Supplied: Transdermal patches 0.05 mg, 0.1 mg (delivers 0.05 mg or 0.1 mg per 24 hours).

■ Estrogen, Conjugated (Premarin)

Indications: Moderate to severe vasomotor symptoms associated with menopause; atrophic vaginitis; palliative therapy of advanced prostatic carcinoma; prevention of estrogen deficiency–induced osteoporosis.

Actions: Hormonal replacement.

Dosage: 0.3–1.25 mg/d PO cyclically; prostatic carcinoma requires 1.25–2.5 mg PO TID.

Supplied: Tablets 0.3 mg, 0.625 mg, 0.9 mg, 1.25 mg, 2.5 mg; injection 25 mg/mL.

Notes: Do not use in pregnancy; associated with an increased risk of endometrial carcinoma, gallbladder disease, thromboembolism, and possibly breast cancer.

■ Ethacrynic Acid (Edecrin)

Indications: Edema; congestive heart failure; ascites; any time rapid diuresis is desired.

Actions: Loop diuretic.

Dosage: 50–200 mg PO QD or 50 mg IV prn.

Supplied: Tablets 25 mg, 50 mg; powder for injection 50 mg.

Notes: Contraindicated in anuria; many severe side effects.

■ Ethambutol (Myambutol)

Indications: Pulmonary tuberculosis.

Actions: Inhibits cellular metabolism.

Dosage: 15 mg/kg PO daily as single dose.

Supplied: Tablets 100 mg, 400 mg.

Notes: May cause vision changes and GI upset.

■ Ethosuximide (Zarontin)

Indications: Absence (petit mal) seizures.

Actions: Anticonvulsant.

Dosage: 500 mg QD PO initially; increase by 250 mg/d every 4–7 days as needed.

Supplied: Capsules 250 mg; syrup 250 mg/5 mL.

Notes: Blood dyscrasias and CNS and GI side effects may occur. Use with caution in patients with renal or hepatic impairment (see Table 7–11, p 498.).

■ Famotidine (Pepcid)

Indications: Short-term treatment of active duodenal ulcer and benign gastic ulcer; maintenance therapy for duodenal ulcer; hypersecretory conditions.

Actions: H_2 antagonist.

Dosage: *Ulcer*: 40 mg PO HS or 20 mg IV every 12 hours.
Hypersecretory: 20–160 mg PO every 6 hours.
Maintenance: 20 mg PO QHS.

Supplied: Tablets 20 mg, 40 mg; suspension 40 mg/5 mL; injection 10 mg/mL.

Notes: Decrease dose in severe renal failure. Increased effectiveness with antacids.

■ Fenoprofen (Nalfon)

See Table 7–9, p 496.

■ Ferrous Sulfate

Indications: Iron deficiency anemia; iron supplementation.

Actions: Dietary supplementation.

Dosage: 100–200 mg/d of elemental iron divided TID–QID.

Supplied: Tablets 195 mg, 300 mg, 325 mg; sustained-release capsules 150 mg, 250 mg; drops 75 mg/0.6 mL, 125 mg/mL; elixir 220 mg/5 mL; syrup 90 mg/5 mL.

Notes: Will turn stools and urine dark. Can cause GI upset, constipation. Vitamin C taken with ferrous sulfate will increase the absorption of iron especially in patients with atropic gastritis.

■ Flavoxate (Urispas)

Indications: Symptomatic relief of dysuria, urgency, nocturia, suprapubic pain, urinary frequency, and incontinence.

Actions: Counteracts smooth muscle spasm of the urinary tract.

Dosage: 100–200 mg 3 or 4 times daily.

Supplied: Tablets 100 mg.

Notes: May cause drowsiness, blurred vision, and dry mouth.

■ Fluconazole (Diflucan)

Indications: Oropharyngeal and esophageal candidiasis; cryptococcal meningitis.

Actions: Inhibits fungal cytochrome P-450 sterol demethylation.

Dosage: 100–400 mg PO or IV QD.

Supplied: Tablets 50 mg, 100 mg, 200 mg; injection 2 mg/mL.

Notes: Adjust dose in renal insufficiency.

■ Flucytosine (Ancobon)

Indications: Serious infections caused by susceptible strains of *Candida* or *Cryptococcus*.

Actions: Antifungal.

Dosage: 50–150 mg/kg/d divided every 6 hours.

Supplied: Capsules 250 mg, 500 mg.

Notes: May cause nausea, vomiting, and diarrhea; take capsules a few at a time over 15 minutes.

■ Fludrocortisone Acetate (Florinef)

Indications: Partial treatment for adrenocortical insufficiency.

Actions: Mineralocorticoid replacement.

Dosage: 0.05–0.1 mg/24h.

Supplied: Tablets 0.1 mg.

Notes: Must be used in conjunction with a glucocorticoid supplement; dose changes based on plasma renin activity; can cause congestive heart failure.

■ Flunisolide (Aerobid)

Indications: Bronchial asthma in patients requiring chronic corticosterioid therapy.

Actions: Topical corticosteroid.

Dosage: 2–4 inhalations twice daily.

Supplied: Aerosol delivers 250 mg/actuation.

Notes: May cause thrush. NOT for acute asthmatic attack.

■ Fluoxetine (Prozac)

Indications: Depression.

Actions: Selective serotonin reuptake inhibitor.

Dosage: 20 mg/24 h PO QD initially; titrate to maximum dose of 80 mg/24 h.

Supplied: Capsules 20 mg.

Notes: May cause nausea, nervousness, and weight loss.

■ Flurbiprofen (Ansaid)

See Table 7–9, p 496.

■ Fluphenazine (Prolixin, Permitil)

Indications: Psychotic disorders.

Actions: Phenothiazine antipsychotic.

Dosage: 0.5–10 mg/day in divided doses PO q6–8h; average maintenance 5.0 mg/d or 1.25 mg IM initially then 2.5–10 mg/d in divided doses q6–8h PRN.

Supplied: Tablets 1 mg, 2.5 mg, 5 mg, 10 mg; concentrate 5 mg/mL; elixir 2.5 mg/5mL; injection 2.5 mg/mL.

Notes: Reduce dose in elderly; monitor liver functions; may cause drowsiness; do not administer concentrate with caffeine, tannic acid, or pectin-containing products.

■ Flurazepam (Dalmane) [C]

Indications: Insomnia.

Actions: Benzodiazepine.

Dosage: 15–30 mg PO QHS prn.

Supplied: Capsules 15 mg, 30 mg.

Notes: Reduce dose in elderly.

■ Folic Acid

Indications: Macrocytic (folate deficiency) anemia.

Actions: Dietary supplementation.

Dosage: *Supplement*: 0.4 mg PO QD.
Folate deficiency: 1.0 mg PO QD–TID.

Supplied: Tablets 0.1 mg, 0.4 mg, 0.8 mg, 1.0 mg; injection 5 mg/mL, 10 mg/mL.

■ Furosemide (Lasix)

Indications: Edema; hypertension; congestive heart failure.

Actions: Loop diuretic.

Dosage: 20–80 mg PO or IV QD or BID.

Supplied: Tablets 20 mg, 40 mg, 80 mg; solution 10 mg/mL, 40 mg/5 mL; injection 10 mg/mL.

Notes: Monitor for hypokalemia. Use with caution in hepatic disease.

■ Ganciclovir (Cytovene)

Indications: Cytomegalovirus retinitis.

Actions: Inhibits viral DNA synthesis.

Dosage: 5 mg/kg IV every 12 hours for 14–21 days, then 5 mg/kg IV QD or 6 mg/kg/d IV for 5 days of every week.

Supplied: Powder for injection 500 mg.

Notes: NOT a cure for cytomegalovirus. Granulocytopenia and thrombocytopenia are the major toxic effects. Potential carcinogen.

■ Gemfibrozil (Lopid)

Indications: Hypertriglyceridemia (type IV and V hyperlipoproteinemia).

Actions: Lipid-regulating agent.

Dosage: 1200 mg/d PO in 2 divided doses 30 minutes before the morning and evening meals.

Supplied: Capsules 300 mg; tablets 600 mg.

Notes: Monitor liver function tests and serum lipids during therapy. Cholelithiasis may occur secondary to treatment. May enhance effect of warfarin.

■ Gentamicin (Garamycin)

Indications: Serious infections caused by susceptible *Pseudomonas, Proteus, E. coli, Klebsiella, Enterobacter, Serratia,* and for initial treatment of gram-negative sepsis.

Actions: Bactericidal; interferes with protein synthesis.

Dosage: Based on renal function and serum concentration desired; refer to aminoglycoside dosing in Tables 7–13 and 7–14, p 499.

Supplied: Injection 40 mg/mL, 10 mg/mL, 2 mg/mL.

Notes: Nephrotoxic and ototoxic. Decrease dose with renal insufficiency. Monitor creatinine clearance and serum concentration for dosage adjustments. See Table 7–12, p 498.

■ Glipizide (Glucotrol)

See Table 7–10, p 497.

■ Glucagon

Indications: Treatment of severe hypoglycemic reactions in diabetic patients with sufficient liver glycogen stores.

Actions: Accelerates liver glycogenolysis.

Dosage: 0.5–1.0 mg SC, IM, or IV repeated after 20 minutes as needed.

Supplied: Powder for injection 1 mg, 10 mg.

Notes: Administration of glucose IV is necessary if patient fails to respond to glucagon. Ineffective in state of starvation, adrenal insufficiency, or chronic hypoglycemia.

■ Glyburide (Diabeta, Micronase)

See Table 7–10, p 497.

■ Glycerin Suppository

Indications: Constipation.

Actions: Hyperosmolar laxative.

Dosage: 1 suppository rectally prn.

Supplied: Suppositories adult, pediatric; liquid 4 mL/applicatorful.

■ Griseofulvin (Fulvicin, Grisactin, Gris-PEG, Grifulvin)

Indications: Treatment of ringworm infections of the skin, hair, and nails that will not respond to topical agents alone.

Actions: Inhibits fungal cell division.

Dosage: *Tinea corporis*: 330–375 mg PO QD for 2–4 weeks.
Tinea cruris: 330–375 mg PO QD for 2–4 weeks.
Tinea capitis: 330–375 mg PO QD for 4–6 weeks.
Tinea pedis: 660–750 mg PO QD for 4–8 weeks.
Tinea unguium: 660–750 mg PO QD for 4–8 months.

Supplied: *Microsize*: capsules 125 mg, 250 mg; tablets 250 mg, 500 mg; suspension 125 mg/5 mL.
Ultramicrosize: tablets 125 mg, 165 mg, 250 mg, 330 mg.

Notes: Patients on extended therapy should be monitored for renal, hepatic, and hematopoietic function. Beneficial effect may not be apparent for some time. Patient should continue entire course of therapy. GI absorption improved when taken with food.

■ Guaifenesin (Robitussin, Others)

Indications: Symptomatic relief of dry, nonproductive cough.

Actions: Expectorant.

Dosage: 100–400 mg PO every 3–6 hours prn.

Supplied: Tablets 100 mg, 200 mg; tablets sustained-release 600 mg; capsules 200 mg; capsules sustained-release 300 mg; syrup 67 mg/5 mL, 100 mg/5 mL, 200 mg/5 mL.

■ Guanabenz (Wytensin)

Indications: Hypertension.

Actions: Central alpha-adrenergic agonist.

Dosage: Initially 4 mg PO BID; increase by 4 mg/d increments at 1- to 2-week intervals up to maximum of 32 mg BID.

Supplied: Tablets 4 mg, 8 mg.

Notes: Sedation, dry mouth, dizziness, and headache are common.

■ Guanadrel (Hylorel)

Indications: Hypertension.

Actions: Inhibits norepinephrine release from peripheral storage sites.

Dosage: 5 mg PO BID initially; increase by 10 mg/d increments at 1-week intervals up to maximum of 75 mg PO BID.

Supplied: Tablets 10 mg, 25 mg.

Notes: Interactions with tricyclic antidepressants. Fewer orthostatic changes and less impotence than with guanethidine.

■ Guanethidine (Ismelin)

Indications: Hypertension.

Actions: Inhibits release of norepinephrine peripherally.

Dosage: Initially 10–25 mg PO QD; increase dose based on response.

Supplied: Tablets 10 mg, 25 mg.

Notes: May produce profound orthostatic hypotension especially with diuretic use. May potentiate effects of vasopressor agents. Interaction with tricyclic antidepressants reduces the effectiveness of guanethidine. Increased bowel movements and explosive diarrhea possible.

■ Guanfacine (Tenex)

Indications: Hypertension.

Actions: Centrally acting alpha-adrenergic agonist.

Dosage: 1 mg QHS initially; increase by 1 mg/24 hr increments to maximum dose of 3 mg/24 hr; split dose BID if increase in BP at end of dosing interval.

Supplied: Tablets 1 mg.

Notes: Use with thiazide diuretic is recommended. Sedation and drowsiness are common. Rebound hypertension may occur with abrupt cessation of therapy.

■ Haloperidol (Haldol)

Indications: Management of psychotic disorders; agitation.

Actions: Antipsychotic, neuroleptic.

Dosage: *Moderate symptoms*: 0.5–2.0 mg PO BID–TID.
Severe symptoms or agitation: 3–5 mg PO BID–TID or 1–5 mg IM every 4 hours prn (maximum 100 mg/d).

Supplied: Tablets 0.5 mg, 1 mg, 2 mg, 5 mg, 10 mg, 20 mg; liquid concentrate 2 mg/mL; injection 5 mg/mL, decanoate 50 mg/mL.

Notes: Can cause extrapyramidal symptoms and hypotension. Reduce dose in elderly patients.

■ Heparin Sodium

Indications: Venous thrombosis; prevention of venous thrombosis and pulmonary emboli; atrial fibrillation with embolus formation; acute arterial occlusion.

Actions: Acts with antithrombin III to inactivate thrombin and to inhibit thromboplastin formation.

Dosage: *Prophylaxis*: 3000–5000 U SC every 8–12 hours.
Treatment of thrombosis: Loading dose of 50–75 U/kg IV, then about 10–20 U/kg IV every hour (adjust based on partial thromboplastin time [PTT]).

Supplied: Injection 10 U/mL, 100 U/mL, 1000 U/mL, 5000 U/mL, 10,000 U/mL, 20,000 U/mL, 40,000 U/mL.

Notes: Follow PTT, thrombin time, or activated clotting time to assess effectiveness. Heparin has little effect on the prothrombin time. For full anticoagulation PTT should be 1½ to 2 times the control. Can cause thrombocytopenia; follow platelet counts.

■ Hepatitis B Immune Globulin (HyperHep, H-BIG, Hep-B-Gammagee)

Indications: Exposure to HB_SAg-positive patients through blood, plasma, or serum (accidental needlestick, mucous membrane contact, oral ingestion).

Actions: Passive immunization.

Dosage: 0.06 mL/kg IM to maximum of 5 mL; within 24 hours of exposure; repeat 1 month after exposure.

Supplied: Injection in 1-mL, 4-mL, and 5-mL vials.

Notes: Administered in gluteal or deltoid muscle. If exposure continues should receive hepatitis B vaccine.

■ Hepatitis B Vaccine (Recombivax HB, Engerix-B)

Indications: Prevention of type B hepatitis.

Actions: Active immunization.

Dosage: 3 IM doses of 1 mL each, the first two given 1 month apart, the third 6 months after the first.

Supplied: Heptavax-B injection 20 μg/mL; Recombivax HB injection 10 μg/mL.

Notes: IM injections for ADULTS to be administered in the deltoid. May cause fever and injection site soreness.

■ Hetastarch (Hespan)

Indications: Plasma volume expansion as an adjunct in treatment of shock resulting from hemorrhage, surgery, burns, other trauma.

Actions: Synthetic colloid with properties similar to albumin.

Dosage: 500 to 1000 mL (do not usually exceed 1500 mL/d) IV at a rate not to exceed 20 mL/kg/h.

Supplied: Injection 30 g/500 mL in 0.9% sodium chloride.

Notes: NOT a substitute for blood or plasma. Contraindicated in patients with severe bleeding disorders, severe congestive heart failure, or renal failure with oliguria or anuria.

■ Hydralazine (Apresoline)

Indications: Moderate to severe hypertension.

Actions: Peripheral vasodilator.

Dosage: Begin at 10 mg PO QID, then increase to 25 mg QID to a maximum of 300 mg/d; for rapid control of pressure, 10 to 40 mg IM prn.

Supplied: Tablets 10 mg, 25 mg, 50 mg, 100 mg; injection 20 mg/mL.

Notes: Use with caution with impaired hepatic function, coronary artery disease. Compensatory sinus tachycardia can be eliminated with addition of propranolol. Chronically high doses can cause systemic lupus erythematosus–like syndrome. Supraventricular tachycardia can occur after IM administration.

■ Hydrochlorothiazide (HydroDIURIL, Esidrix, Others)

Indications: Edema; hypertension; congestive heart failure.

Actions: Thiazide diuretic.

Dosage: 25–100 mg PO QD in single or divided doses.

Supplied: Tablets 25 mg, 50 mg, 100 mg; oral solution 50 mg/5 mL, 100 mg/mL.

Notes: Hypokalemia is frequent. Hyperglycemia, hyperuricemia, hyperlipidemia, and hyponatremia are common.

■ Hydrochlorothiazide and Amiloride (Moduretic)

Indications: Hypertension; adjunctive therapy for congestive heart failure.

Actions: Combined effects of a thiazide diuretic and a potassium-sparing diuretic.

Dosage: 1 or 2 tablets PO QD.

Supplied: Tablets (amiloride/hydrochlorothiazide) 5 mg/50 mg.

Notes: Should not be given to diabetics or patients with renal failure.

■ Hydrochlorothiazide and Spironolactone (Aldactazide)

Indications: Edema (congestive heart failure, cirrhosis); hypertension.

Actions: Combined effects of a thiazide diuretic and a potassium-sparing diuretic.

Dosage: 25–200 mg each component per day in divided doses.

Supplied: Tablets (hydrochlorothiazide/spironolactone) 25 mg/25 mg, 50 mg/50 mg.

■ Hydrochlorothiazide and Triamterene (Dyazide, Maxzide)

Indications: Edema; hypertension.

Actions: Combined effects of a thiazide diuretic and a potassium-sparing diuretic.

Dosage: *Dyazide*: 1 or 2 capsules PO QD–BID.
Maxzide: 1 tablet per day.

Supplied: *Dyazide capsule*: 50 mg triamterene/25 mg hydrochlorothiazide.
Maxzide—25 mg tablet: 37.5 mg triamterene/25 mg hydrochlorothiazide.
Maxzide tablet: 75 mg triamterene/50 mg hydrochlorothiazide.

Notes: Hydrochlorothiazide component in maxzide more bioavailable than dyazide. Can cause hyperkalemia as well as hypokalemia. Follow serum potassium.

■ Hydrocortisone

See Steroids in Table 7–4, p 476.

■ Hydromorphone (Dilaudid) [C]

Indications: Moderate to severe pain.

Actions: Narcotic analgesic.

Dosage: 1–4 mg PO, IM, IV, or rectally every 4–6 hours prn.

Supplied: Tablets 1 mg, 2 mg, 3 mg, 4 mg; injection 1 mg/mL, 2 mg/mL, 3 mg/mL, 4 mg/mL, 10 mg/mL; suppositories 3 mg.

Notes: 1.5 mg IM equivalent to 10 mg morphine IM.

■ Hydroxyzine (Atarax, Vistaril)

Indications: Anxiety; tension; sedation; itching.

Actions: Antihistamine, anxiety.

Dosage: *Anxiety or sedation*: 50–100 mg PO or IM QID or prn (maximum of 600 mg/d).
Itching: 25–50 mg PO or IM TID–QID.

Supplied: Tablets 10 mg, 25 mg, 50 mg, 100 mg; capsules 25 mg, 50 mg, 100 mg; syrup 10 mg/5 mL; injection 25 mg/mL, 50 mg/mL.

Notes: Useful in potentiating the effects of narcotics. NOT for IV use. Drowsiness and anticholinergic effects are common.

■ Ibuprofen (Motrin, Rufen, Advil, Others)

See Table 7–9, p 496.

■ Imipenem-Cilastatin (Primaxin)

Indications: Treatment of serious infections caused by a wide variety of susceptible bacteria; inactive against *Staph. aureus*, group A and B streptococci, and others.

Actions: Bactericidal; interferes with cell wall synthesis.

Dosage: 250–500 mg (imipenem) IV every 6 hours.

Supplied: Injection (imipenem-cilastatin) 250 mg/250 mg, 500 mg/500 mg.

Notes: Seizures may occur if drug accumulates. Adjust dosage for renal failure to avoid drug accumulation if calculated creatinine clearance is <70 mL/min.

■ Imipramine (Tofranil)

Indications: Depression.

Actions: Tricyclic antidepressant.

Dosage: *Hospitalized*: Start at 100 mg/24 h in divided doses; can increase over several weeks to 250–300 mg/24 h.
Outpatient: Maintenance of 50–150 mg QHS not to exceed 200 mg/24 h.

Supplied: Tablets 10 mg, 25 mg, 50 mg; capsules 75 mg, 100 mg, 125 mg, 150 mg; injection 12.5 mg/mL.

Notes: Do not use with monoamine oxidase inhibitors. Less sedation than with amitriptyline.

■ Immune Globulin Intravenous (Gamimune N, Sandoglobulin, Gammagard)

Indications: IgG antibody deficiency diseases such as congenital agammaglobulinemia and common variable hypogammaglobulinemia; idiopathic thrombocytopenic purpura.

Actions: IgG supplementation.

Dosage: *Immunodeficiency*: 100–200 mg/kg IV monthly at rate of 0.01–0.04 mL/kg/min up to maximum of 400 mg/kg per dose.
Idiopathic thrombocytopenic purpura: 400 mg/kg per dose IV QD × 5 days.

Supplied: Injection 50 mg/mL; powder for injection 0.5-g, 1-g, 2.5-g, 3-g, 5-g, 6-g, 10-g vials.

Notes: Adverse effects are associated mostly with rate of infusion.

■ Indapamide (Lozol)

Indications: Hypertension; congestive heart failure.

Actions: Thiazide diuretic.

Dosage: 2.5–5.0 mg PO QD.

Supplied: Tablets 2.5 mg.

Notes: Doses greater than 5 mg do not have additional effects on lowering blood pressure.

■ Indomethacin (Indocin)

See Table 7–9, p 496.

■ Insulin

Indications: Diabetes mellitus that cannot be controlled by diet and/or oral hypoglycemic agents.

Actions: Insulin supplementation.

Dosage: Based on serum glucose levels; usually given SC; can also be given IV or IM.

Supplied: See Tables 7–1 and 7–2.

Notes: The highly purified insulins provide an increase in free insulin. Monitor patients closely for several weeks when changing doses.

TABLE 7–1. COMPARISON OF STANDARD INSULINS

Type of Insulin	Onset (h)	Peak (h)	Duration (h)
■ **RAPID**			
Regular	0.5–1.0	2–4	6–8
Semilente	1.0–2.0	5–10	12–16
■ **INTERMEDIATE**			
NPH	1.0–1.5	4–12	24
Lente	1.0–2.5	7–15	24
■ **PROLONGED**			
PZI	4.0–8.0	14–24	36+
Ultralente	4.0–8.0	10–30	36+

Modified from Gomella LG, ed. Clinician's Pocket Reference. *Norwalk, Conn: Appleton & Lange; 1989. Used with permission.*

TABLE 7–2. COMPARISON OF NEW HIGHLY PURIFIED INSULINS

Type of Insulin	Onset (h)	Peak (h)	Duration (h)
■ **RAPID**			
Regular Iletin II	0.25–0.5	2.0–4.0	5–7
Humulin R	0.5	2.0–4.0	6–8
Novolin R	0.5	2.5–5.0	5–8
■ **INTERMEDIATE**			
NPH Iletin II	1.0–2.0	6–12	18–24
Lente Iletin II	1.0–2.0	6–12	18–24
Humulin N	1.0–2.0	6–12	14–24
Novulin L	2.5–5.0	7–15	18–24
Novulin 70/30	0.5	7–12	24
■ **PROLONGED**			
Ultralente	4.0–6.0	14–24	28–36
Humulin U	4.0–6.0	8–20	24–28

Modified from Gomella LG, ed. Clinician's Pocket Reference. *6th ed. Norwalk, Conn: Appleton & Lange; 1989. Used with permission.*

■ Ipecac Syrup

Indications: Treatment of drug overdose and certain cases of poisoning.

Actions: Irritation of GI mucosa and stimulation of chemoreceptor trigger zone.

Dosage: 15–30 mL PO followed by 200–300 mL water; if no emesis occurs in 20 minutes, may repeat once.

Supplied: Syrup 15 mL, 30 mL.

Notes: Do not use for ingestion of petroleum distillates, strong acid, base, or other corrosive or caustic agents. Not for use in comatose or unconscious patients. Use caution in CNS depression and depressant overdose.

■ Ipratropium Bromide Inhalant (Atrovent)

Indications: Bronchospasm associated with chronic obstructive pulmonary disease.

Actions: Synthetic anticholinergic agent similar to atropine.

Dosage: 2–4 puffs QID.

Supplied: Metered dose inhaler 18 μg/dose.

Notes: NOT for initial treatment of acute episodes of bronchospasm.

■ Iron Dextran (Imferon)

Indications: Iron deficiency when oral supplementation is not possible.

Actions: Parenteral iron supplementation.

Dosage: Based on estimate of iron deficiency (see package insert).

Supplied: Injection 50 mg (Fe)/mL.

Notes: Must give a test dose because anaphylaxis is common. May be given deep IM using "Z-track" technique although IV route is most preferred.

■ Isoetharine (Bronkosol, Bronkometer)

Indications: Bronchial asthma and reversible bronchospasm.

Actions: Sympathomimetic bronchodilator.

Dosage: *Nebulization*: 0.25–1.0 mL diluted 1:3 with saline every 4–6 hours.
Metered dose inhaler: 1 or 2 inhalations every 4 hours.

Supplied: Metered dose inhaler 340 μg/dose; solution for inhalation.

■ Isoniazid (INH)

Indications: Active tuberculosis and the prevention of tuberculosis.

Actions: Bactericidal; interferes with lipid and nucleic acid biosynthesis.

Dosage: *Active tuberculosis*: 5 mg/kg/24 h PO QD (usually 300 mg/d).
Prophylaxis: 300 mg/kg/24 h PO for 6–12 months.

Supplied: Tablets 50 mg, 100 mg, 300 mg; syrup 50 mg/5 mL; injection 100 mg/mL.

Notes: Can cause severe hepatitis. Usually given with other antituberculous drugs for active tuberculosis. IM and IV routes are rarely used. To prevent peripheral neuropathy can give pyridoxine 50–100 mg/d.

■ Isoproterenol (Isuprel, Medihaler-Iso)

Indications: Shock, cardiac arrest, atrioventricular (AV) nodal block, antiasthmatic.

Actions: Beta-1 and beta-2 receptor stimulant.

Dosage: *Emergency cardiac care*: 2–20 μg/min IV infusion, titrated to effect.
Shock: 1–4 μg/min IV infusion, titrated to effect.
AV nodal block: 20–60 μg IV push; may repeat every 3–5 minutes; 1–5 μg/min IV infusion maintenance.
Nebulization: 1 or 2 inhalations 4–6 times daily.

Supplied: Aerosol 80 μg/dose, 125 μg/dose; solution for nebulization; injection 200 μg/mL.

Notes: Contraindications include tachycardia; pulse $>$ 130 beats per minute may induce ventricular arrhythmias.

■ Isosorbide Dinitrate (Isordil)

Indications: Angina pectoris.

Actions: Relaxation of vascular smooth muscle.

Dosage: *Acute angina*: 2.5–10.0 mg PO (chewable tablets) or sublingually every 5–10 minutes; $>$3 doses should not be given in 15- to 30-minute period.
Angina prophylaxis: 5–60 mg PO TID.

Supplied: Tablets 5 mg, 10 mg, 20 mg, 30 mg, 40 mg; sustained-release tablets 40 mg; sublingual tablets 2.5 mg, 5 mg, 10 mg; chewable tablets 5 mg, 10 mg; capsules 40 mg; sustained-release capsules 40 mg.

Notes: Nitrates should not be given on chronic every-6-hour or QID basis because of development of tolerance. Can cause headaches. Usually need to give a higher oral dose to achieve same results as with sublingual forms. Can be given with hydralazine to treat congestive heart failure.

■ Kaolin-Pectin (Kaopectate, Others)

Indications: Treatment of diarrhea.

Actions: Adsorbent demulcent.

Dosage: 60–120 mL PO after each loose stool or every 3–4 hours.

Supplied: Oral suspension.

■ Ketoconazole (Nizoral)

Indications: Treatment of systemic fungal infections: candidiasis, chronic mucocutaneous candidiasis, oral thrush, blastomycosis, coccidioidomycosis, histoplasmosis, and paracoccidioidomycosis; topical cream for localized fungal infections caused by dermatophytes and yeast.

Actions: Inhibits fungal cell wall synthesis.

Dosage: *Oral*: 200 mg PO QD; increase to 400 mg PO QD for very serious infections.
Topical: Apply to affected area once daily.

Supplied: Tablets 200 mg; suspension 100 mg/5 mL; topical cream 2%.

Notes: Associated with severe hepatotoxicity. Monitor liver function tests closely throughout course of therapy. DRUG INTERACTION with any agent increasing gastric pH, preventing absorption of ketoconazole. May enhance oral anticoagulants. May react with alcohol to produce disulfiram-like reaction.

■ Ketoprofen (Orudis)

See Table 7–9, p 496.

■ Labetalol (Trandate, Normodyne)

See Table 7–7, p 492.

Indications: Hypertension, hypertensive emergencies.

Actions: Alpha- and beta-adrenergic blocking agent.

Dosage: *Hypertension*: 100 mg PO BID initially; then 200–400 mg PO BID.
Hypertensive emergency: 20–80 mg IV bolus, then 2 mg/min IV infusion titrated to effect.

Supplied: Tablets 100 mg, 200 mg, 300 mg; injection 5 mg/mL.

■ *Lactobacillus* (Lactinex Granules)

Indications: Control of diarrhea, especially after antibiotic therapy.

Actions: Replacement of intestinal flora.

Dosage: 1 packet, 2 capsules, or 4 tablets with meals or liquids TID.

Supplied: Chewable tablets; capsules; powder in packets 1g.

■ Lactulose (Chronulac, Cephulac)

Indications: Hepatic encephalopathy, laxative.

Actions: Acidifies the colon, allowing ammonia to diffuse into the colon.

Dosage: *Acute hepatic encephalopathy*: 30–45 mL TID–QID.
Chronic laxative therapy: 30–45 mL PO TID–QID; adjust dosage every 1–2 days to produce 2 or 3 soft stools QD.

Supplied: Syrup 10 g/15 mL.

Notes: Can cause severe diarrhea resulting in hypernatremia.

■ Levorphanol (Levo-Dromoran) [C]

Indications: Moderate to severe pain.

Actions: Narcotic analgesic.

Dosage: 2 mg PO or SC prn.

Supplied: Tablets 2 mg; injection 2 mg/mL.

■ Levothyroxine (Synthroid)

Indications: Hypothyroidism.

Actions: Supplementation of T4.

Dosage: 25–50 μg/d initially; increase by 25–50 μg/d every month; usual dose 100–150 μg/d.

Supplied: Tablets 0.025 mg, 0.05 mg, 0.075 mg, 0.1 mg, 0.125 mg, 0.15 mg, 0.175 mg, 0.2 mg, 0.3 mg; injection 0.2 mg, 0.5 mg.

Notes: Titrate dosage based on clinical response and thyroid function tests. Dosage can be increased more rapidly in young to middle-aged patients. Elderly may require only 50–100 μg/d. In patients with possible coronary artery disease start with 12.5–25 μg/d.

■ Lidocaine (Xylocaine)

Indications: Treatment of cardiac arrhythmias, local anesthetic.

Actions: Class 1B antiarrhythmic.

Dosage: *Arrhythmias*: 1 mg/kg (50–100 mg) IV bolus, then 2–4 mg/min IV infusion; should repeat bolus after 5 minutes.
Local anesthetic: infiltrate a few milliliters of a 0.5–1.0% solution.

Supplied: Injection 0.5%, 1%, 2%, 4%, 10%, 20%.

Notes: Epinephrine is added to injectable forms for local anesthesia to prolong effect and help decrease bleeding. For IV forms, dosage reduction is required with liver disease and congestive heart failure. Dizziness, paresthesias, and convulsions are associated with toxicity. (See Table 7–11, p 498.)

■ Lindane (Gamma Benzene Hexachloride) (Kwell)

Indications: Head lice, crab lice, scabies.

Actions: An ectoparasiticide and ovicide.

Dosage: *Cream or lotion*: Apply thin layer after bathing and leave in place for 24 hours; pour on laundry.
Shampoo: Apply 30 mL and develop lather with warm water for 4 minutes; comb out nits.

Supplied: Cream 1%, lotion 1%; shampoo 1%.

Notes: Caution with overuse; may be absorbed into blood.

■ Liothyronine (Cytomel)

Indications: Hypothyroidism.

Actions: T3 replacement.

Dosage: Initial dose of 25 μg/24 h, then titration every 1–2 weeks according to clinical response and thyroid function tests to maintenance of 25–75 μg PO QD.

Supplied: Tablets 5 μg, 25 μg, 50 μg.

Notes: Reduce dose in elderly.

■ Lisinopril (Prinivil, Zestril)

Indications: Hypertension.

Actions: Angiotension-converting enzyme.

Dosage: 5–40 mg PO QD.

Supplied: Tablets 5 mg, 10 mg, 20 mg.

Notes: Dizziness, headache, and cough are common.

■ Lithium Carbonate (Eskalith, Others)

Indications: Manic episodes of manic-depressive illness; maintenance therapy in recurrent disease.

Actions: Effects a shift toward intraneuronal metabolism of catecholamines.

Dosage: *Acute mania*: 600 mg PO TID or 900 mg sustained-release BID. *Maintenance*: 300 mg PO TID–QID.

Supplied: Capsules 150 mg, 300 mg, 600 mg; tablets 300 mg; sustained-release tablets 300 mg, 450 mg; syrup 300 mg/5 mL.

Notes: Dosage must be titrated. Follow serum levels (see Table 7–11, p 498). Common side effects are polyuria and tremor. Contraindicated in patients with severe renal impairment. Sodium retention or diuretic use may potentiate toxicity.

■ Loperamide (Imodium)

Indications: Diarrhea.

Actions: Slows intestinal motility.

Dosage: 4 mg PO initially, then 2 mg after each loose stool, up to 16 mg/d.

Supplied: Capsules 2 mg; liquid 1 mg/5 mL.

Notes: Do not use in acute diarrhea caused by *Salmonella, Shigella*, or *C. difficile*.

■ Lorazepam (Ativan, Others) [C]

Indications: Anxiety and anxiety mixed with depression; insomnia; control of status epilepticus.

Actions: Benzodiazepine.

Dosage: *Anxiety*: 0.5–1 mg PO BID–TID.
Insomnia: 2–4 mg QHS.
Status Epilepticus: 2.5–10 mg/dose repeated at 15- to 20-minute interval × 2 prn.

Supplied: Tablets 0.5 mg, 1 mg, 2 mg; injection 2 mg/mL, 4 mg/mL.

Notes: Decrease dosage in elderly.

■ Lovastatin (Mevacor)

Indications: Adjunct to diet for the reduction of elevated total and low-density lipoprotein cholesterol levels in patients with primary hypercholesterolemia (types IIa and IIb).

Actions: Reduces production and increases catabolism of low-density lipoprotein cholesterol.

Dosage: 20 mg PO daily with the evening meal; may increase at 4-week intervals to maximum of 80 mg/d taken with meals.

Supplied: Tablets 20 mg.

Notes: Patient should be maintained on standard cholesterol-lowering diet throughout treatment. Monitor liver function tests every 6 weeks during first year of therapy. Annual ophthalmic exams for opacities. Headache and GI intolerance are common.

■ Magaldrate (Riopan, Lowsium)

Indications: Hyperacidity associated with peptic ulcer, gastritis, and hiatal hernia.

Actions: A low-sodium antacid.

Dosage: 1 or 2 tablets PO or 5–10 mL PO between meals and HS.

Supplied: Tablets; suspension.

Notes: Less than 0.3 mg sodium per tablet or teaspoon. Do not use in renal insufficiency.

■ Magnesium Citrate

Indications: Vigorous bowel prep; constipation.

Actions: Saline laxative.

Dosage: 120–240 mL PO prn.

Supplied: Effervescent solution.

Notes: Do not use in renal insufficiency or intestinal obstruction.

■ Magnesium Hydroxide (Milk of Magnesia)

Indications: Constipation.

Actions: Saline laxative.

Dosage: 15–30 mL OR 1 tablet PO prn.

Supplied: Suspension 8%; tablets 325 mg.

Notes: Do not use in renal insufficiency or intestinal obstruction.

■ Magnesium Sulfate

Indications: Replacement for low plasma levels (alcoholism, hyperalimentation); refractory hypocalcemia.

Actions: Magnesium supplementation.

Dosage: 1 to 2 g IM or IV; repeat dosing based on response and continued hypomagnesemia.

Supplied: Injection 100 mg/mL, 125 mg/mL, 500 mg/mL.

Notes: Do not use in renal insufficiency.

■ Mannitol

Indications: Osmotic diuresis (cerebral edema, oliguria, anuria, myoglobinuria, etc.).

Actions: Osmotic diuretic.

Dosage: *Test dose*: 0.2 g/kg/dose IV over 3–5 minutes; if no diuresis within 2 hours, discontinue.
Cerebral edema: 0.25 g/kg/dose IV push repeated at 5-minute intervals prn; increase incrementally to 1 g/kg/dose prn for intracranial hypertension.

Supplied: Injection 5%, 10%, 15%, 20%, 25%.

Notes: Caution with congestive heart failure or volume overload.

■ Maprotiline (Ludiomil)

Indications: Depressive neurosis; manic-depressive illness; major depressive disorder.

Actions: Tricyclic antidepressant.

Dosage: 75–150 mg/d QHS, maximum of 300 mg/d.

Supplied: Tablets 25 mg, 50 mg, 75 mg.

Notes: Contraindicated with monoamine oxidase inhibitors or seizure history. For patients > 60 years of age, give only 50–75 mg/d. Anticholinergic side effects.

■ Meclizine (Antivert)

Indications: Motion sickness; vertigo associated with diseases of the vestibular system.

Actions: Antiemetic, anticholinergic, and antihistaminic properties.

Dosage: 25 mg PO TID–QID prn.

Supplied: Tablets 12.5 mg, 25 mg, 50 mg; chewable tablets 25 mg; capsules 25 mg.

Notes: Drowsiness, dry mouth, and blurred vision commonly occur.

■ Medroxyprogesterone (Provera)

Indications: Secondary amenorrhea and abnormal uterine bleeding resulting from hormonal imbalance.

Actions: Progestin supplementation.

Dosage: *Secondary amenorrhea*: 5–10 mg PO QD for 5–10 days.
Abnormal uterine bleeding: 5–10 mg PO QD for 5–10 days beginning on the 16th or 21st day of menstrual cycle.

Supplied: Tablets 2.5 mg, 5.0 mg, 10 mg.

Notes: Contraindicated with past thromboembolic disorders, breast or gynecologic malignancy, or hepatic disease.

■ Meperidine (Demerol) [C]

Indications: Relief of moderate to severe pain.

Actions: Narcotic analgesic.

Dosage: 50–100 mg PO or IM every 3–4 hours prn.

Supplied: Tablets 50 mg, 100 mg; syrup 50 mg/5 mL; injection 10 mg/mL, 25 mg/mL, 50 mg/mL, 75 mg/mL, 100 mg/mL.

Notes: 75 mg IM equivalent to 10 mg morphine IM. Beware of respiratory depression.

■ Meprobamate (Equanil, Miltown)

Indications: Short-term relief of symptoms of anxiety.

Actions: Mild tranquilizer, antianxiety.

Dosage: 200–400 mg PO TID–QID; sustained-release 400–800 mg PO BID.

Supplied: Tablets 200 mg, 400 mg, 600 mg; sustained-release capsules 200 mg, 400 mg.

Notes: May cause drowsiness.

■ Mesalamine (Rowasa)

Indications: Treatment of mild to moderate distal ulcerative colitis, proctosigmoiditis, or proctitis.

Actions: Unknown; may topically inhibit prostoglandins.

Dosage: Retention enema daily at bedtime.

Supplied: Rectal suspension 4 g/60 mL.

■ Mesoridazine (Serentil)

Indications: Schizophrenia; acute and chronic alcoholism; chronic brain syndrome; psychoneurotic manifestations.

Actions: Phenothiazine antipsychotic.

Dosage: 25–50 mg PO TID initially; titrate to maximum of 300–400 mg/d.

Supplied: Tablets 10 mg, 25 mg, 50 mg, 100 mg; oral concentrate 25 mg/mL; injection 25 mg/mL.

Notes: Low incidence of extrapyramidal side effects.

■ Metaproterenol (Alupent, Metaprel)

Indications: Bronchodilator for asthma and reversible bronchospasm.

Actions: Sympathomimetic bronchodilator.

Dosage: *Inhalation*: 2 or 3 inhalations every 3–4 hours to maximum of 12 per 24 hours.
Oral: 20 mg PO every 6–8 hours.

Supplied: Metered dose inhaler 650 μg/dose; solution for inhalation 0.5%, 0.6%; tablets 10 mg, 20 mg; syrup 10 mg/5 mL.

Notes: Fewer beta-1 effects than with isoproterenol and longer acting.

■ Methadone (Dolophine) [C]

Indications: Severe pain; detoxification; maintenance of narcotic addiction.

Actions: Narcotic analgesic.

Dosage: 2.5–10 mg IM every 4 hours or 5–15 mg PO every 4 hours (titrate as needed).

Supplied: Tablets 5 mg, 10 mg; oral solution 5 mg/5 mL, 10 mg/5 mL; injection 10 mg/mL.

Notes: Equianalgesic with parenteral morphine. Long half-life. Increase dose slowly so as to avoid respiratory depression.

■ Methenamine Hippurate (Hiprex, Urex) Methenamine Mandelate (Mandelamine, Others)

Indications: Suppression of chronic urinary tract infection.

Actions: In acid urine converted to formaldehyde (bactericidal).

Dosage: 1 g PO BID.

Supplied: Tablets 1 g.

Notes: For maximum effect, urinary pH should be < 5.5. Use oral vitamin C or ammonium chloride to acidify urine. GI distress and urinary tract irritation are common.

■ Methicillin (Staphcillin)

See Table 7–5, p 489.

■ Methimazole (Tapazole)

Indications: Hyperthyroidism; preparation for thyroid surgery or radiation.

Actions: Blocks formation of T3 and T4.

Dosage: Initially 15–60 mg/d divided TID; maintenance of 5–15 mg PO QD.

Supplied: Tablets 5 mg, 10 mg.

Notes: Follow patient clinically and with thyroid function tests.

■ Methocarbamol (Robaxin)

Indications: Relief of discomfort associated with painful musculoskeletal conditions.

Actions: Centrally acting skeletal muscle relaxant.

Dosage: 1.5 g PO QID for 2–3 days, then 1 g PO QID maintenance therapy; IV form rarely indicated.

Supplied: Tablets 50 mg, 750 mg; injection 100 mg/mL.

Notes: Can discolor urine. May cause drowsiness or GI upset. Contraindicated with myasthenia gravis.

■ Methyldopa (Aldomet)

Indications: Essential hypertension.

Actions: Centrally acting antihypertensive agent.

Dosage: 250–500 mg PO BID–TID (maximum 2–3 g/d) OR 250 mg–1 g IV every 4–8 hours.

Supplied: Tablets 125 mg, 250 mg, 500 mg; oral suspension 250 mg/5 mL; injection 250 mg/5 mL.

Notes: Do not use in presence of liver disease. Can discolor urine. Initial transient sedation or drowsiness occurs frequently.

■ Methylprednisolone (Solu-Medrol)

See Table 7–4, p 476.

■ Metoclopramide (Reglan)

Indications: Relief of diabetic gastroparesis; symptomatic gastroesophageal reflux; relief of cancer chemotherapy-induced nausea and vomiting.

Actions: Stimulates motility of the upper GI tract.

Dosage: *Diabetic gastroparesis*: 10 mg PO 30 minutes AC and HS; or same dose given IV for 10 days, then switch to PO.
Gastroesophageal reflux: 10–15 mg 30 minutes AC and HS.
Antiemetic: 1–3 mg/kg slow IV 30 minutes prior to antineoplastic agent, then every 2 hours for 2 doses, then every 3 hours for 3 doses.

Supplied: Tablets 5 mg, 10 mg; syrup 5 mg/5 mL; injection 5 mg/mL.

Notes: Dystonic reactions common with high doses, and can be treated with IV Benadryl 50 mg. Can also be used to facilitate small bowel intubation and radiologic evaluation of the upper GI tract.

■ Metolazone (Diulo, Zaroxolyn)

Indications: Mild to moderate essential hypertension; edema secondary to renal disease or cardiac failure.

Actions: Thiazide-like diuretic.

Dosage: *Hypertension*: 2.5–5 mg PO daily.
Edema: 5–20 mg PO daily.

Supplied: Tablets 2.5 mg, 5 mg, 10 mg.

Notes: Monitor fluid and electrolytes.

■ Metoprolol IV (Lopressor)

Indications: Reduce the cardiovascular mortality in definite or suspected MI.

Dosage: 5 mg IV every 2 minutes × 3 doses.

Supplied: Injection 1 mg/mL.

Notes: Monitor blood pressure, heart rate, and electrocardiogram.

■ Metronidazole (Flagyl)

Indications: Amebiasis, trichomoniasis, *C. difficile*, and anaerobic infections.

Actions: Interferes with DNS synthesis.

Dosage: *Anaerobic infections*: 500 mg IV every 6–8 hours.
Amebic dysentery: 750 mg PO QD for 5–10 days.
Trichomoniasis: 2 g PO in one dose or 250 mg PO TID for 7 days.
C. difficile: 500 mg PO every 8 hours for 7–10 days.

Supplied: Tablets 250 mg, 500 mg; injection 500 mg.

Notes: For *Trichomonas* infections, also treat partner. Reduce dose in hepatic failure. No activity against aerobic bacteria. Use in combination in serious mixed infections or infections of unknown etiology.

■ Metyrapone (Metopirone)

Indications: Diagnostic test drug for hypothalamic-pituitary ACTH function.

Actions: Inhibits endogenous adrenal corticosteroid synthesis.

Dosage: *Day 1*: Control period—collect 24-hour urine to measure 17-hydroxycorticosteroids (17-OHCS) or 17-ketogenic steroids (17-KSG).
Day 2: ACTH test—50 U ACTH infused over 8 hours and measure 24-hour urinary steroids.
Days 3 and 4: Rest period.
Day 5: Administer metyrapone with milk or snack 750 mg PO every 4 hours for 6 doses.
Day 6: Determine 24-hour urinary steroids.

Supplied: Tablets 250 mg.

Notes: Normal 24-hour 17-OHCS is 3–12 mg; following ACTH it increases to 15–45 mg/24 h. Normal response to metyrapone is a twofold to fourfold increase in 17-OHCS excretion. Drug interactions with phenytoin, cyproheptadine, and estrogens may lead to subnormal response.

■ Mexiletine (Mexitil)

Indications: Suppression of symptomatic ventricular arrhythmias.

Actions: Class 1B antiarrhythmic.

Dosage: Administer with food or antacids; 200–300 mg every 8 hours; do not exceed 1200 mg/d.

Supplied: Capsules 150 mg, 200 mg, 250 mg.

Notes: Not to be used in cardiogenic shock or second- or third-degree atrioventricular block if no pacemaker. May worsen severe arrhythmias. Monitor liver function during therapy. Drug interactions with hepatic enzyme inducers and suppressors requiring dosage changes.

■ Mezlocillin (Mezlin)

See Table 7–6, p 490.

■ Miconazole (Monistat)

Indications: Severe systemic fungal infections including coccidioidomycosis, candidiasis, and cryptococcus, various tinea forms, cutaneous candidiasis, vulvovaginal candidiasis, tinea versicolor.

Actions: Fungicidal; alters permeability of the fungal cell membrane.

Dosage: *Systemic*: dosage range 200–3600 mg/24 h IV based on diagnosis, divided into 3 doses.
Topical: apply to affected area twice daily for 2–4 weeks.
Intravaginal: insert 1 applicatorful or suppository at bedtime for 7 days.

Supplied: Injection 10 mg/mL; topical cream 2%; lotion 2%; powder 2%; spray 2%; vaginal suppositories 200 mg; vaginal cream 2%.

Notes: Antagonistic to amphotericin B in vivo. Rapid IV infusion may cause tachycardia or arrhythmias. May potentiate coumadin drug activity.

■ Midazolam (Versed) [C]

Indications: Preoperative sedation; conscious sedation for short procedures.

Actions: Short-acting benzodiazepine.

Dosage: 1–5 mg IV/IM, titrate dose to effect.

Supplied: Injection 1 mg/mL, 5 mg/mL.

Notes: Monitor patient for respiratory depression. May produce hypotension in conscious sedation.

■ Milk of Magnesia

See **Magnesium Hydroxide**.

■ Mineral Oil

Indications: Constipation.

Actions: Emollient laxative.

Dosage: 15–30 mL PO prn.

Supplied: Liquid.

■ Minocycline (Minocin)

Indications: Infections caused by susceptible strains of many gram-positive and gram-negative bacteria, *Rickettsiae, Mycoplasma pneumoniae, Chlamydia,* syphilis, gonorrhea.

Actions: Bacteristatic; interferes with protein synthesis.

Dosage: 50 mg PO QID or 100 mg PO/IV BID.

Supplied: Capsules and tablets 50 mg, 100 mg; suspension 50 mg/5 mL; injections 100 mg.

Notes: A tetracycline antibiotic.

■ Minoxidil (Loniten, Rogaine)

Indications: Severe hypertension; treatment of male pattern baldness.

Actions: Peripheral vasodilator; stimulates vertex hair growth.

Dosage: *Oral*: 2.5–10 mg PO BID–QID.
Topical: Apply twice daily.

Supplied: Tablets 2.5 mg, 10 mg; topical solution 2%.

Notes: Pericardial effusion and volume overload may occur; hypertrichosis after chronic use.

■ Misoprostol (Cytotec)

Indications: Prevention of NSAID-induced gastric ulcers.

Actions: Synthetic prostaglandin with both antisecretory and mucosal protective properties.

Dosage: 200 μg PO QID.

Supplied: Tablets 200 μg.

Notes: DO NOT take if pregnant; can cause miscarriage with potentially dangerous bleeding. GI side effects are most common.

■ Molindone (Moban)

Indications: Management of psychotic disorders.

Actions: Piperazine phenothiazine.

Dosage: 5–100 mg PO TID–QID.

Supplied: Tablets 5 mg, 10 mg, 25 mg, 50 mg, 100 mg; concentrate 20 mg/mL.

■ Morphine Sulfate [C]

Indications: Relief of severe pain.

Actions: Narcotic analgesic.

Dosage: *Oral*: 10–30 mg every 4 hours prn; sustained-release tablets 30–60 mg every 8–12 hours.
Intramuscular: 5–20 mg every 4 hours prn.
Intravenous: 2.5–15 mg every 4 hours prn.
Epidural: by experienced anestheologist.

Supplied: Tablets 10 mg, 15 mg, 30 mg; sustained-release tablets 15 mg, 30 mg, 60 mg; solution 10 mg/5 mL, 20 mg/5 mL, 100 mg/5 mL; suppositories 5 mg, 10 mg, 20 mg; injection 2 mg/mL, 4 mg/mL, 5 mg/mL, 8 mg/mL, 10 mg/mL, 15 mg/mL; preservative-free injection 0.5 mg/mL, 1 mg/mL.

Notes: Large number of narcotic side effects. May require scheduled dosing to relieve severe chronic pain.

■ Moxalactam (Moxam)

See Table 7–8C, pp 494–495.

■ Nabilone (Cesamet) [C]

Indications: Nausea and vomiting associated with cancer chemotherapy.

Actions: Antiemetic.

Dosage: 1–2 mg PO BID.

Supplied: Capsules 1 mg.

Notes: Principal psychoactive substance in marijuana. Many CNS side effects.

■ Nadolol (Corgard)

See Table 7–7, p 492.

■ Nafcillin (Nafcil, Unipen)

See Table 7–5, p 489.

■ Nalbuphine (Nubain)

Indications: Moderate to severe pain.

Actions: Narcotic agonist-antagonist.

Dosage: 10–20 mg IM, IV every 4–6 hours prn.

Supplied: Injection 10 mg/mL, 20 mg/mL.

Notes: Causes CNS depression and drowsiness.

■ Nalidixic Acid (NegGram)

Indications: Urinary tract infections caused by susceptible strains of *Proteus, Klebsiella, Enterobacter,* and *E. coli.*

Actions: Interferes with DNA polymerization.

Dosage: 1 g PO QID for 7–14 days.

Supplied: Tablets 250 mg, 500 mg, 1 g; suspension 250 mg/5 mL.

Notes: Resistance emerges within 48 hours in significant percentage of trials. May enhance effect of oral anticoagulants. May cause CNS adverse effects that reverse on discontinuation of the drug.

■ Naloxone (Narcan)

Indications: Complete or partial reversal of narcotic depression.

Actions: Narcotic antagonist.

Dosage: 0.4–2.0 mg IV, IM, or SC every 5 minutes, maximum total dose of 10 mg.

Supplied: Injection 0.4 mg/mL, 1.0 mg/mL.

Notes: May precipitate acute withdrawal in addicts. If no response after 10 mg, suspect a nonnarcotic cause.

■ Naproxen (Naprosyn, Anaprox)

See Table 7–9, p 496.

■ Neomycin-Polymyxin Bladder Irrigant (Neosporin G.U. Irrigant)

Indications: Continuous irrigant for prophylaxis against bacteriuria and gram-negative bacteremia associated with indwelling catheter use.

Actions: Bactericidal.

Dosage: 1 mL irrigant added to 1 L 0.9% NaCl; continuous irrigation of the bladder with 1–2 L of solution per day.

Supplied: Ampules 1 mL, 20 mL.

Notes: Potential for bacterial or fungal superinfection. Possibility for neomycin-induced ototoxicity or nephrotoxicity.

■ Neomycin Sulfate

Indications: Hepatic coma.

Actions: Suppresses GI bacterial flora.

Dosage: 1–4 g PO QID.

Supplied: Tablets 500 mg; oral solution 125 mg/5 mL.

■ Niacin (Nicobid)

Indications: Adjunctive therapy in patients with significant hyperlipidemia who do not respond adequately to diet and weight loss.

Actions: Inhibits lipolysis, decreases esterification of triglyceride, increases lipoprotein lipase activity.

Dosage: 1–2 g TID with meals; up to 8 g per day.

Supplied: Sustained-release capsules 125 mg, 250 mg, 300 mg, 400 mg, 500 mg; tablets 20 mg, 25 mg, 50 mg, 100 mg, 500 mg; elixir 50 mg/5 mL.

Notes: Upper body facial flushing and warmth after dose. May cause GI upset.

■ Nicardipine (Cardene)

Indications: Chronic stable angina, hypertension.

Actions: Calcium channel–blocking agent.

Dosage: 20–40 mg PO TID.

Supplied: Capsules 20 mg, 40 mg.

■ Nifedipine (Procardia, Adalat)

Indications: Vasospastic or chronic stable angina; hypertensive crisis.

Actions: Calcium channel blocking agent.

Dosage: 10–30 mg PO q8h; maximum dose of 180 mg/d; SR 30–90 mg once daily.

Supplied: Capsules 10 mg, 20 mg; tablets SR 30 mg, 60 mg, 90 mg.

Notes: Headaches common on initial treatment; reflex tachycardia may occur.

■ Nitrofurantoin (Macrodantin, Furadantin)

Indications: Urinary tract infections.

Actions: Bacteriostatic; interferes with carbohydrate metabolism.

Dosage: *Suppression*: 50–100 mg PO QD.
Usual dose: 50–100 mg PO QID.

Supplied: Capsules and tablets 50 mg, 100 mg; suspension 25 mg/5 mL.

Notes: GI side effects are common. Should be taken with food, milk, or antacid. Macrocrystals (Macrodantin) cause less nausea than other forms of drug.

■ Nitroglycerin (Tridil, Nitrolingual, Nitro-Bid Ointment, Nitrobid, Nitrodisc, Transderm-Nitro, Others)

Indications: Angina pectoris; acute and prophylactic therapy; congestive heart failure; blood pressure control.

Actions: Relaxation of vascular smooth muscle.

Dosage: *Sublingual*: 1 tablet sublingually every 5 minutes prn × 3 doses.
Translingual: 1–2 metered doses sprayed onto oral mucosa.
Oral: 2.5–9.0 mg TID.
Intravenous: 5–20 μg/min titrated to effect.
Topical: 1–2 in. ointment to chest wall every 6 hours, then wipe off at night.
Transdermal: 5- to 20-cm patch QD.

Supplied: Sublingual tablets 0.15 mg, 0.3 mg, 0.4 mg, 0.6 mg; translingual spray 0.4 mg/dose; sustained-release capsules 2.5 mg, 6.5 mg, 9 mg; sustained-release tablets 2.6 mg, 6.5 mg, 9.0 mg; injection 0.5 mg/mL, 0.8 mg/mL, 5 mg/mL, 10 mg/mL; ointment 2%; transdermal patches delivering 2.5, 5, 7.5, 10, or 15 mg/24 h.

Notes: Tolerance to nitrates will develop with chronic use after 1–2 weeks; this can be avoided by providing a nitrate-free period each day. Shorter-acting nitrates should be used on a TID basis and long-acting patches and ointment should be removed before bedtime to prevent the development of tolerance.

■ Nitroprusside (Nipride)

Indications: Hypertensive emergency; aortic dissection; pulmonary edema.

Actions: Reduces systemic vascular resistance.

Dosage: 0.5–10 μg/kg/min IV infusion titrated to desired effect.

Supplied: Injection 50 mg/vial.

Notes: Thiocyanate, the metabolite, is excreted by the kidney. Thiocyanate toxicity occurs at plasma levels of 5–10 mg/dL. If used to treat aortic dissection, a beta blocker must be used concomitantly.

■ Nizatidine (Axid)

Indications: Treatment of duodenal ulcers.

Actions: H2 antagonists.

Dosage: *Active ulcer*: 150 mg PO BID or 300 mg PO QHS.
Maintenance: 150 mg PO QHS.

Supplied: Capsules 150 mg, 300 mg.

■ Norepinephrine (Levophed)

Indications: Acute hypotensive states.

Actions: Peripheral vasoconstrictor acting on both the arterial and venous beds.

Dosage: Initially 8–12 μg/min, titrate to response.

Supplied: Injection 1 mg/mL.

Notes: Correct blood volume depletion as much as possible prior to initiation of vasopressor therapy. Drug interaction with tricyclic antidepressants leading to severe, prolonged hypertension. Infuse into large vein to avoid extravasation. Phentolamine 5–10 mg/10 mL normal saline solution injected locally as antidote to extravasation.

■ Norfloxacin (Noroxin)

Indications: Treatment of complicated and uncomplicated urinary tract infections caused by a wide variety of pathogens including *E. coli, Enterobacter cloacae, Proteus mirabilis,* indole-positive *Proteus* species, *Pseudomonas aeruginosa, Staph. aureus*, and *Staph. epidermidis.*

Actions: Inhibits DNA gyrase.

Dosage: 400 mg PO BID.

Supplied: Tablets 400 mg.

Notes: NOT for use in pregnancy. To be taken 1 hour before or 2 hours after meals. Do not take with antacids.

■ Nortriptyline (Aventyl, Pamelor)

Indications: Endogenous depression.

Actions: Tricyclic antidepressant.

Dosage: 25 mg PO TID–QID, maximum of 150 mg/d.

Supplied: Capsules 10 mg, 25 mg, 75 mg; solution 10 mg/5 mL.

Notes: Many anticholinergic side effects including blurred vision, urinary retention, and dry mouth.

■ Nystatin (Mycostatin, Nilstat)

Indications: Treatment of *Candida* infections (thrush, vaginitis).

Actions: Alters membrane permeability.

Dosage: *Oral*: 400,000–600,000 U PO 4 or 5 times daily.
Vaginal: 1 tablet per vagina daily.
Topical: Apply 2 or 3 times daily.

Supplied: Oral suspension 100,000 U/mL; oral tablets 500,000 U; troches 200,000 U; vaginal tablets 100,000 U; topical cream, ointment, and powder 100,000 U/g.

Notes: Not absorbed orally, therefore not effective for systemic infections.

■ Omperazole (Prilosec)

Indications: Treatment of duodenal ulcers.

Actions: Proton-pump inhibitor.

Dosage: 20–40 mg QD.

Supplied: Capsules 20 mg.

■ Opium, Camphorated Tincture of (Paregoric) [C]

Indications: Diarrhea; relief of severe pain in place of morphine; sedative-hypnotic.

Actions: Antispasmodic, narcotic analgesic.

Dosage: 5–10 mL up to 4 times a day.

Supplied: Liquid.

Notes: CNS depressant activity results from morphine content (2 mg/ 5 mL).

■ Opium, Tincture [C]

Indications: Diarrhea; relief of severe pain in place of morphine; sedative-hypnotic.

Actions: Antispasmodic, narcotic analgesic.

Dosage: 0.6 mL 4 times a day.

Supplied: Liquid 10% opium.

Notes: CNS depressant activity results from morphine content (0.6 mL = 6 mg).

■ Oxacillin (Bactocil, Prostaphlin)

See Table 7–5, p 489.

■ Oxazepam (Serax) [C]

Indications: Anxiety; acute alcohol withdrawal.

Actions: Benzodiazepine.

Dosage: *Anxiety*: 10–15 mg PO TID–QID.
Alcohol withdrawal: 15–30 mg PO TID–QID.

Supplied: Capsules 10 mg, 15 mg, 30 mg; tablets 15 mg.

■ Oxtriphylline (Choledyl)

Indications: Asthma, bronchospasm.

Actions: Relaxes the smooth muscle of the bronchi and pulmonary blood vessels.

Dosage: 200 mg PO QID; sustained-release tablets 400–600 mg every 12 hours.

Supplied: Tablets 100 mg, 200 mg; sustained-release tablets 400 mg, 600 mg; syrup pediatric 50 mg/5 mL; elixir 100 mg/5 mL.

Notes: Contains 64% theophylline.

■ Oxybutynin (Ditropan)

Indications: Symptoms associated with neurogenic or reflex neurogenic bladder.

Actions: Antispasmodic.

Dosage: 5 mg PO BID–QID.

Supplied: Tablets 5 mg; syrup 5 mg/5 mL.

Notes: Anticholinergic side effects.

■ Oxycodone (Percocet, Percodan, Tylox) [C]

Indications: Moderate to moderately severe pain.

Actions: Narcotic analgesic.

Dosage: 1 or 2 tablets/capsules PO every 4–6 hours prn.

Supplied: Percocet tab—5 mg oxycodone, 325 mg acetaminophen; Percodan tab—4.5 mg oxycodone, 325 mg aspirin; Tylox capsule—5 mg oxycodone, 500 mg acetaminophen.

■ Pancreatin, Pancrealipase (Pancrease, Cotazyme)

Indications: For patients deficient in pancreatic exocrine enzymes (cystic fibrosis, chronic pancreatitis, other pancreatic insufficiency, and for steatorrhea of malabsorption syndrome).

Actions: Supplementation of pancreatic enzymes.

Dosage: 1–3 tablets PO after meals.

Supplied: Tablets.

Notes: Avoid antacids. May cause nausea, abdominal cramps, or diarrhea.

■ Pancuronium (Pavulon)

Indications: Aid in management of patient on mechanical ventilator.

Actions: Nondepolarizing muscle relaxant.

Dosage: 2–4 mg IV every 2–4 hours prn.

Supplied: Injection 1 mg/mL, 2 mg/mL.

Notes: Patient must be intubated and on controlled ventilation. Use adequate amount of sedation or analgesia (morphine, etc).

■ Penbutolol (Levatol)

See Table 7–7, p 492.

■ Penicillin G (Potassium or Sodium) Aqueous (Pfizerpen, Pentids)

Indications: Most gram-positive infections (except penicillin-resistant staphylococci), including streptococci, clostridia, corynebacteria, and some coliforms, and others. Also syphilis.

Actions: Interferes with cell wall synthesis.

Dosage: *Oral*: 400,000–800,000 U PO QID.
Intravenous: Doses vary greatly depending on indications, range from 1.2–2.4 million units per day.

Supplied: Tablets 200,000 U, 250,000 U, 400,000 U, 500,000 U, 800,000 U; powder for oral suspension 200,000 U/5 mL, 400,000 U/5 mL; powder for injection.

Notes: Beware of hypersensitivity reactions. Drug of choice for group A streptococcal, pneumococcal, and syphilis infections.

■ Penicillin G Benzathine (Bicillin)

Indications: Useful as a single-dose treatment regimen for streptococcal pharyngitis, rheumatic fever and glomerulonephritis prophylaxis, and syphilis.

Actions: Interferes with cell wall synthesis.

Dosage: 1.2–2.4 million units deep IM injection.

Supplied: Injection 300,000 U/mL, 600,000 U/mL.

Notes: Sustained action with detectable levels up to 4 weeks. Considered drug of choice for treatment of noncongenital syphilis. Bicillin L-A contains the benzathine salt only. Bicillin C-R contains a combination of the benzathine and procaine salts and is used for most acute strep infections (300,000 U procaine with 300,000 U benzathine/mL or 900,000 U benzathine with 300,000 U procaine/2 mL).

■ Penicillin G Procaine (Wycillin, Others)

Indications: Moderately severe infection caused by penicillin-sensitive organisms that respond to low persistent serum levels (syphilis and uncomplicated pneumococcal pneumonia).

Actions: Interferes with cell wall synthesis.

Dosage: 2.4–4.8 million units IM with 1 g of probenecid PO.

Supplied: Injection 300,000 U/mL, 500,000 U/mL, 600,000 U/mL.

Notes: A long-acting parenteral penicillin. Blood levels up to 15 hours. Give probenecid at least 30 minutes prior to administration of penicillin to prolong action.

■ Penicillin V (Pen-Vee K, V-Cillin K, Others)

Indications: Most gram-positive infections (except penicillin-resistant staphylococci), including streptococci, clostridia, corynebacteria, and some coliforms, and others. Also *N. meningitidis* and syphilis.

Actions: Interferes with cell wall synthesis.

Dosage: 250–500 mg PO QID.

Supplied: Tablets 125 mg, 250 mg, 500 mg; powder for oral suspension 125 mg/5 mL, 250 mg/5 mL.

Notes: A well-tolerated oral penicillin (250 mg = 400,000 U Pen G).

■ Pentamadine Isethionate (Pentam 300, NebuPent)

Indications: Treatment and prevention of *Pneumocystis carinii* pneumonia.

Actions: Inhibits the synthesis of DNA, RNA, phospholipids, and protein.

Dosage: *Intravenous*: 4 mg/kg IV or deep IM injection daily.
Inhalation: 300 mg once every 4 weeks, administered via Respirgard II nebulizer.

Supplied: Injection 300 mg/vial; aersol 300 mg.

Notes: Monitor patient for severe hypotension after IV/IM dosing. Associated with pancreatic islet cell necrosis leading to hyperglycemia or hypoglycemia. Monitor hematology labs for leukopenia and thrombocytopenia. IM dosing may result in sterile abscess formation.

■ Pentazocine (Talwin) [C]

Indications: Moderate to severe pain.

Actions: Narcotic agonist-antagonist.

Dosage: 30 mg IM or IV; 50–100 mg PO every 3–4 hours prn.

Supplied: Tablets 50 mg (with naloxone 0.5 mg); injection 30 mg/mL.

Notes: 30–60 mg IM equianalgesic to 10 mg morphine IM. Associated with considerable dysphoria.

■ Pentobarbital (Nembutal, Others) [C]

Indications: Insomnia; convulsions; induction of coma after severe head injury.

Actions: Barbiturate.

Dosage: *Sedative*: 20–40 mg PO every 6–12 hours.
Hypnotic: 100–200 mg PO QHS.
Induced coma: load 3–5 mg/kg IV × 1, then maintenance 2–3.5 mg/kg/dose hourly prn to keep level at 25–40 μg/mL.

Supplied: Capsules 50 mg, 100 mg; elixir 20 mg/5 mL; suppositories 30 mg, 60 mg, 120 mg, 200 mg; injection 50 mg/mL.

Notes: Can cause respiratory depression. May produce profound hypotension when given rapidly to induce coma. Tolerance to sedative-hypnotic effect acquired within 1–2 weeks.

■ Pentoxifylline (Trental)

Indications: Intermittent claudication.

Actions: Lowers blood viscosity by restoring erythrocyte flexibility.

Dosage: 400 mg PO TID with meals.

Supplied: Tablets 400 mg.

Notes: Treat for at least 8 weeks to see full effect.

■ Perphenazine (Trilafon)

Indications: Psychotic disorders; intractable hiccups; severe nausea.

Actions: Phenothiazine, antipsychotic, antiemetic.

Dosage: *Antipsychotic*: 4–8 mg PO TID, maximum 64 mg/d. *Hiccups*: 5 mg IM every 6 hours prn or 1 mg IV at not less than 1–2 mg/min intervals up to 5 mg.

Supplied: Tablets 2 mg, 4 mg, 8 mg, 16 mg; repetabs 8 mg; oral concentrate 16 mg/5 mL; injection 5 mg/mL.

■ Phenazopyridine (Pyridium, Others)

Indications: Symptomatic relief of discomfort from lower urinary tract irritation.

Actions: Local anesthetic on urinary tract mucosa.

Dosage: 200 mg PO TID.

Supplied: Tablets 100 mg, 200 mg.

Notes: GI disturbances. Causes red-orange urine color which can stain clothing. Can also stain contacts.

■ Phenobarbital [C]

Indications: Seizure disorders; insomnia; anxiety.

Actions: Barbiturate.

Dosage: *Sedative-hypnotic*: 30–120 mg PO or IM QD prn.
Anticonvulsant: Loading dose of 10–12 mg/kg in 3 divided doses, then 1–3 mg/kg/24 h PO/IV.

Supplied: Tablets 8 mg, 16 mg, 32 mg, 65 mg, 100 mg; elixir 20 mg/5 mL; injection 30 mg/mL, 60 mg/mL, 65 mg/mL, 130 mg/mL.

Notes: Tolerance develops to sedation. Long half-life allows single daily dosing. See Table 7–11, p 498.

■ Phenylephrine (Neo-Synephrine)

Indications: Treatment of vascular failure in shock, anaphylaxis, or drug-induced hypotension; nasal congestion; mydriatic.

Actions: Postsynaptic alpha-receptor stimulant.

Dosage: *Mild to moderate hypotension*: 2–5 mg IM or SC elevates BP for 2 hours; 0.1–0.5 mg IV elevates BP for 15 minutes.
Severe hypotension or shock: initiate continuous infusion at 100–180 μg/min; after BP is stabilized, maintenance rate of 40–60 μg/min.
Intranasal: 1 or 2 sprays in each nostril.

Supplied: Injection 10 mg/mL; nasal solution 0.125%, 0.16%, 0.2%, 0.25%, 0.5%, 1%; ophthalmic solution 0.12%, 2.5%, 10%.

Notes: Promptly restore blood volume if loss has occurred. Use with extreme caution in patients with hyperthyroidism, bradycardia, partial heart block, myocardial disease, or severe arteriosclerosis. Use large veins for infusion to avoid extravasation; phentolamine 10 mg in 10–15 mL normal saline solution for local injection as antidote for extravasation. Activity potentiated by oxytocin, monoamine oxidase inhibitors, and tricyclic antidepressants.

■ Phenytoin (Dilantin)

Indications: Tonic-clonic and partial seizures.

Actions: Inhibits seizure spread in motor cortex.

Dosage: *Load*: 15–20 mg/kg IV at a maximum infusion rate of 25 mg/min OR orally in 400-mg doses at 4-hour intervals.
Maintenance: 200 mg PO or IV BID or 300 mg QHS initially, then follow plasma concentrations.

Supplied: Capsules 30 mg, 100 mg; chewable tablets 50 mg; oral suspension 30 mg/5 mL, 125 mg/5 mL; injection 50 mg/mL.

Notes: Caution with cardiac depressant side effects, especially with IV administration. Follow levels as needed (see Table 7–11, p 498.). Nystagmus and ataxia are early signs of toxicity. Gum hyperplasia occurs with long-term use. Avoid use of oral suspension if possible because of erratic absorption. Avoid use in pregnancy.

■ Physostigmine (Antilirium)

Indications: Antidote for tricyclic antidepressant, atropine, and scopolamine overdose.

Actions: Reversible cholinesterase inhibitor.

Dosage: 2 mg IV/IM every 15 minutes.

Supplied: Injection 1 mg/mL.

Notes: Rapid IV administration associated with convulsions. Cholinergic side effects. May cause asystole.

■ Phytonadione (Vitamin K) (Aquamephyton, Others)

Indications: Coagulation disorders caused by faulty formation of factors II, VII, IX, and X; hyperalimentation.

Actions: Supplementation; needed for the production of factors II, VII, IX, and X.

Dosage: *Anticoagulant-induced prothrombin deficiency*: 2.5 to 10.0 mg PO or IV SLOWLY.
Hyperalimentation: 10 mg IM or IV every week.

Supplied: Tablets 5 mg; injection 2 mg/mL, 10 mg/mL.

Notes: With parenteral treatment, usually see first change in prothrombin in 12–24 hours. Anaphylaxis can result from IV dosage. Should be administered slowly IV.

■ Pindolol (Visken)

See Table 7–7, p 492.

■ Piperacillin (Pipracil)

See Table 7–6, p 490.

■ Piroxicam (Feldene)

See Table 7–9, p 496.

■ Plasma Protein Fraction (Plasmanate, Others)

Indications: Shock and hypotension.

Actions: Plasma volume expansion.

Dosage: 250 to 500 mL IV initially (not >10 mL/min); subsequent infusions should depend on clinical response.

Supplied: Injection 5%.

Notes: Hypotension associated with rapid infusion. 130–160 mEq sodium per liter.

■ Pneumococcal Vaccine, Polyvalent (Pneumovax)

Indications: Immunization against pneumococcal infections in patients predisposed to or at high risk of acquiring these infections (elderly, sickle cell disease, anatomic or functional asplenia, immunosupression, chronic obstructive pulmonary disease, diabetes mellitus, chronic renal disease).

Actions: Active immunization.

Dosage: 0.5 mL IM.

Supplied: Injection, 25 μg of polysaccharide isolates per 0.5-mL dose.

Notes: Revaccination of adults can increase the severity of adverse reactions. Do not vaccinate during immunosupressive therapy.

■ Polyethylene Glycol-Electrolyte Solution (Go-LYTLEY, Colyte)

Indications: Bowel cleansing prior to examination.

Actions: Osmotic cathartic.

Dosage: After 3- to 4-hour fast, drink 240 mL of solution every 10 minutes until 4 L consumed.

Supplied: Powder for reconstitution to 4 L in container.

Notes: First bowel movement should occur in approximately 1 hour. May cause some cramping or nausea.

■ Potassium Supplements

Indications: Prevention or treatment of hypokalemia.

Actions: Supplementation of potassium.

TABLE 7–3. ORAL POTASSIUM SUPPLEMENTS

Brand name	Salt	Form	Potassium (mEq/dosing unit)
Kaochlor 10%	KCl	Liquid	20 mEq/15 mL
Koachlor S-F 10% (sugar-free)	KCl	Liquid	20 mEq/15 mL
Kaon Elixir	K+ gluconate	Liquid	20 mEq/15 mL
Kaon	K+ gluconate	Tablets	5 mEq/tablet
Kaon-Cl	KCl	Tablet, SR	6.67 mEq/tablet
Kaon-Cl 20%	KCl	Liquid	40 mEq/15 mL
KayCiel	KCl	Liquid	20 mEq/15 mL
K-Lor	KCl	Powder	15 or 20 mEq/packet
Klorvess	KCl	Liquid	20 mEq/15 mL
Klotrix	KCl	Tablet, SR	10 mEq/tablet
K-Lyte	K+ bicarbonate	Effervescent tablet	25 mEq/tablet
K-Tab	KCl	Tablet, SR	10 mEq/tablet
Micro-K	KCl	Capsules	8 mEq/capsule
Slow-K	KCl	Tablet, SR	8 mEq/tablet

SR = sustained-release.
From Gomella LG, ed. Clinician's Pocket Reference. *6th ed. Norwalk, Conn: Appleton & Lange; 1989. Used with permission.*

Dosage: 16–24 mEq/d, divided QD–BID.

Supplied: See Table 7–3.

Notes: Can cause GI irritation. Powder and liquids must be mixed with beverage (unsalted tomato juice very palatable). Use cautiously in renal insufficiency, and along with NSAIDs and angiotensin-converting enzyme inhibitors.

■ Prazepam (Centrax) [C]

Indications: Anxiety disorders.

Actions: Benzodiazepine.

Dosage: 5–10 mg PO three or four times a day, or 20–50 mg PO as single bedtime dose to minimize daytime drowsiness.

Supplied: Capsules 5 mg, 10 mg, 20 mg; tablets 10 mg.

■ Prazosin (Minipres)

Indications: Hypertension.

Actions: Peripherally acting alpha-adrenergic blocker.

Dosage: 1 mg PO TID; can increase to a total daily dose of 5 mg QID.

Supplied: Capsules 1 mg, 2 mg, 5 mg.

Notes: Can cause orthostatic hypotension; therefore, patient should take first dose at bedtime. Tolerance develops to this effect. Tachyphylaxis may result.

■ Prednisone

See Table 7–4, p 476.

■ Prednisolone

See Table 7–4, p 476.

■ Probenecid (Benemid, Others)

Indications: Gout; maintenance of serum levels of penicillins or cephalosporins.

Actions: Renal tubular-blocking agent.

Dosage: *Gout*: 0.25 gm BID for 1 week; then 0.5 g PO BID.
Antibiotic effect: 1–2 g PO 30 minutes prior to dose of antibiotic.

Supplied: Tablets 500 mg.

■ Probucol (Lorelco)

Indications: Adjunctive therapy for reduction of serum cholesterol.

Actions: Lowers serum cholesterol.

Dosage: 500 mg PO BID with morning and evening meals.

Supplied: Tablets 250 mg, 500 mg.

Notes: May note prolongation of QT interval on ECG. Diarrhea or loose stools are common. May also lower high-density lipoprotein cholesterol.

■ Procainamide (Pronestyl, Procan)

Indications: Treatment of supraventricular and ventricular arrhythmias.

Actions: Class 1A antiarrhythmic.

Dosage: *Emergency cardiac care*: 100–200 mg/dose IV every 5 minutes until dysrhythmia resolves, hypotension ensues, or dose totals 1 g; then maintenance of 1–4 mg/min IV infusion.
Chronic dosing: 50 mg/kg/d PO in divided doses every 4–6 hours.

Supplied: Tablets and capsules 250 mg, 375 mg, 500 mg; sustained-release tablets 250 mg, 500 mg, 750 mg, 1000 mg; injection 100 mg/mL, 500 mg/mL.

Notes: Can cause hypotension and a lupuslike syndrome. Dosage adjustment required with renal impairment. See Table 7–11, p 498.

■ Prochlorperazine (Compazine)

Indications: Nausea; vomiting; agitation; psychotic disorders.

Actions: Phenothiazine antiemetic and antipsychotic.

Dosage: *Antiemetic*: 5–10 mg PO TID–QID OR 25 mg rectally BID OR 5–10 mg deep IM every 4–6 hours.
Antipsychotic: 10–20 mg IM acutely OR 5–10 mg PO TID–QID for maintenance.

Supplied: Tablets 5 mg, 10 mg, 25 mg; sustained-release capsules 10 mg, 15 mg, 30 mg; syrup 5 mg/5 mL; suppositories 2.5 mg, 5 mg, 25 mg; injection 5 mg/mL.

Notes: Much larger dose may be required for antipsychotic effect. Extrapyramidal side effects are common. Treat acute extrapyramidal reactions with diphenhydramine.

■ Promethazine (Phenergan)

Indications: Nausea; vomiting; motion sickness.

Actions: Phenothiazine antihistamine; antiemetic.

Dosage: 12.5–50 mg PO rectally, or IM BID–QID prn.

Supplied: Tablets 12.5 mg, 25 mg, 50 mg; syrup 6.25 mg/mL, 25 mg/mL; suppositories 12.5 mg, 25 mg, 50 mg; injection 25 mg/mL, 50 mg/mL.

Notes: High incidence of drowsiness.

■ Propantheline (Pro-Banthine)

Indications: Symptomatic treatment of small intestine hypermotility, spastic colon, ureteral spasm, bladder spasm, pylorospasm.

Actions: Antimuscarinic agent.

Dosage: 15 mg PO ac and 30 mg PO HS.

Supplied: Tablets 7.5 mg, 15 mg.

Notes: Anticholinergic side effects such as dry mouth and blurred vision are common.

■ Propoxyphene (Darvon, Darvocet) [C]

Indications: Mild to moderate pain.

Actions: Narcotic analgesic.

Dosage: 32–65 mg PO every 4 hours prn.

Supplied: Darvon (propoxyphene HCl) 32 mg, 65 mg; Darvon-N (propoxyphene napsylate), 100 mg = 65 mg of propoxyphene HCl; Darvocet-N (propoxyphene napsylate/acetaminophen); Darvon compound (propoxyphene HCl/aspirin/caffeine).

Notes: Intentional overdose can be lethal.

■ Propranolol (Inderal)

See Table 7–7, p 492.

■ Propranolol IV (Inderal)

Indications: Ventricular arrhythmias; supraventricular tachycardia.

Dosage: 1–3 mg IV; dose may be repeated 1 time after 2 minutes; no more propranolol should be given for 4 hours.

Supplied: Injection 1 mg/mL.

Notes: Administration rate 1 mg/min. Monitor blood pressure, heart rate, and electrocardiogram carefully.

■ Propylthiouracil (PTU)

Indications: Hyperthyroidism.

Actions: Inhibits production of T3 and T4, and conversion of T4 to T3.

Dosage: Begin at 100 mg PO every 8 hours (may need up to 1200 mg/d for control); after patient is euthyroid (6–8 weeks), taper dose by one-third every 4–6 weeks to a maintenance dose of 50–150 mg/24 h; treatment is usually able to be discontinued in 2–3 years.

Supplied: Tablets 50 mg.

Notes: Follow patient clinically. Monitor thyroid function tests.

■ Protamine Sulfate

Indications: Reversal of heparin effect.

Actions: Neutralizes heparin.

Dosage: Based on amount of heparin reversal desired; given slow IV, 1 mg will reverse approximately 100 U of heparin given in the preceding 3–4 hours to maximum dose of 50 mg.

Supplied: Injection 10 mg/mL.

Notes: Follow coagulation studies. May have anticoagulant effect if given without heparin.

■ Protriptyline (Vivactil)

Indications: Endogenous depression.

Actions: Tricyclic antidepressant.

Dosage: 5–10 mg PO TID–QID.

Supplied: Tablets 5 mg, 10 mg.

Notes: Monitor elderly patients for cardiovascular side effects. Anticholinergic effects.

■ Pseudoephedrine (Sudafed, Novafed, Afrinol, Others)

Indications: Decongestant.

Actions: Sympathomimetic.

Dosage: 30–60 mg PO every 6–8 hours; sustained-release capsules 120 mg PO every 12 hours.

Supplied: Tablets 30 mg, 60 mg; sustained-release capsules 120 mg; liquid 15 mg/5 mL; syrup 30 mg/5 mL.

Notes: Contraindicated in patients with hypertension or coronary artery disease and patients taking monoamine oxidase inhibitors. An ingredient in many cough and cold preparations.

■ Psyllium (Metamucil, Serutan, Effer-Syllium)

Indications: Constipation; diverticular disease of the colon.

Actions: Bulk laxative.

Dosage: 1 teaspoon (7 g) in a glass of water QD–TID.

Supplied: Granules 4 g/tsp, 2.5 g/tsp; powder 3.5 g/packet.

Notes: Do not use if bowel obstruction is suspected. One of the safest laxatives. Psyllium in effervescent (Effer-Syllium) form usually contains potassium and should be used with caution in patients with renal failure.

■ Pyridoxine

Indications: Treatment and prevention of vitamin B_6 deficiency.

Actions: Supplementation of vitamin B_6.

Dosage: *Deficiency*: 2.5–10.0 mg PO QD.
Drug-induced neuritis: 50 mg PO QD.

Supplied: Tablets 10 mg, 25 mg, 50 mg, 100 mg, 200 mg, 250 mg, 500 mg; injection 100 mg/mL.

■ Quinidine (Quinidex, Quinaglute)

Indications: Prevention of tachydysrhythmias.

Actions: Class 1A antiarrhythmic.

Dosage: *Premature atrial and ventricular contractions*: 200–300 mg PO TID–QID.
Conversion of atrial fibrillation or flutter: use after digitalization, 200 mg every 2–3 hours for 8 doses; then increase daily dose to maximum of 3–4 g or until normal rhythm.

Supplied: *Sulfate*: tablets 100 mg, 200 mg, 300 mg; capsules 200 mg, 300 mg; sustained-release tablets 300 mg; injection 200 mg/mL.
Gluconate: sustained-release tablets 324 mg, 330 mg; injection 80 mg/mL.

Notes: Contraindicated in digitalis toxicity and atrioventricular block. Follow serum levels if available (see Table 7–11, p 498). Extreme hypotension seen with IV administration. Sulfate salt contains 83% quinidine. Gluconate salt contains 62% quinidine.

■ Ranitidine (Zantac)

Indications: Duodenal ulcer; active benign ulcers; hypersecretory conditions; gastroesophageal reflux.

Actions: H2 receptor antagonist.

Dosage: *Ulcer*: 150 mg PO BID, 300 mg PO QHS, or 50 mg IV every 6–8 hours.
Maintenance: 150 mg PO QHS.
Hypersecretion: 150 mg PO BID.

Supplied: Tablets 150 mg, 300 mg; syrup 15 mg/mL; injection 25 mg/mL.

Notes: Reduce dose with renal failure. Give with antacids prn. Note oral and parenteral doses are different.

■ Rifampin (Rifadin)

Indications: Tuberculosis; treatment and prophylaxis of *N. meningitidis, H. influenzae*, or *Staph. aureus* carriers.

Actions: Inhibits DNA-dependent RNA polymerase activity.

Dosage: *N. meningitidis and H. influenzae carrier*: 600 mg PO QD × 4 days.
Tuberculosis: 600 mg PO or IV QD OR twice weekly with combination therapy regimen.

Supplied: Capsules 150 mg, 300 mg; injection 600 mg/vial.

Notes: Multiple side effects. Causes orange-red discoloration of bodily secretions including tears and can stain contacts. Never used as a single agent to treat active tuberculosis infections.

■ Secobarbital (Seconal) [C]

Indications: Insomnia.

Actions: Rapidly acting barbiturate.

Dosage: 100 mg PO, IM, QHS, PRN.

Supplied: Capsules 50 mg, 100 mg; tablets 100 mg; injection 50 mg/mL.

Notes: Beware of respiratory depression. Tolerance acquired within 1–2 weeks.

■ Silver Sulfadiazine (Silvadene)

Indications: Prevention of sepsis in second-degree and third-degree burns.

Actions: Bactericidal.

Dosage: Aseptically cover affected area with $\frac{1}{16}$-in. coating BID.

Supplied: Cream 1%.

Notes: Can have systemic absorption with extensive application.

■ Simethicone (Mylicon)

Indications: Symptomatic treatment of flatulence.

Actions: Defoaming action.

Dosage: 40–125 mg PO pc and HS prn.

Supplied: Tablets 40 mg, 80 mg, 125 mg; capsules 125 mg; drops 40 mg/0.6 mL.

■ Sodium Bicarbonate

Indications: Alkalinization of urine; treatment of metabolic acidosis.

Dosage: Titrate to effect based on blood gases or urine pH.

Supplied: Injection 0.5 mEq/mL, 1 mEq/mL; tablets 325 mg, 650 mg.

Notes: 1 g neutralizes 12 mEq of acid.

■ Sodium Polystyrene Sulfonate (Kayexalate)

Indications: Treatment of hyperkalemia.

Actions: Sodium and potassium ion-exchange resin.

Dosage: 15–60 g PO or 30–60 g PR every 6 hours based on serum potassium.

Supplied: Powder, suspension 15 g/60 mL sorbitol.

Notes: Can cause hypernatremia. Given with agent such as sorbitol to promote movement through bowel.

■ Sorbitol

Indications: Constipation.

Actions: Laxative.

Dosage: 30–60 mL of a 20–70% solution prn.

Supplied: Liquid 70%.

■ Spironolactone (Aldactone)

Indications: Treatment of hyperaldosteronism; essential hypertension; edematous states (congestive heart failure, cirrhosis).

Actions: Aldosterone antagonist, potassium-sparing diuretic.

Dosage: 25–100 mg PO QID.

Supplied: Tablets 25 mg, 50 mg, 100 mg.

Notes: Can cause hyperkalemia and gynecomastia. Avoid prolonged use. Diuretic of choice for cirrhotic edema and ascites.

■ SSKI

Indications: As an expectorant to help thin tenacious mucus in various chronic pulmonary conditions; thyroid storm.

Actions: Enhances the secretion of respiratory fluids, thus decreasing the viscosity of the mucus; iodine supplementation.

Dosage: 0.3–0.6 mL (300–600 mg) 3 or 4 times a day diluted in water; maximum dose is 6 mL (6 g) per day.

Supplied: Solution 1000 mg/mL.

Notes: Not for use during pregnancy as it may lead to fetal goiter. Drug interaction with lithium and antithyroid agents to enhance hypothyroid effects. Thyroid function tests may be altered. Watch for chronic iodine poisoning.

■ Steroids

The following relates only to the commonly used systemic glucocorticoids.

Indications: Endocrine disorders (adrenal insufficiency); rheumatoid disorders; collagen-vascular diseases; dermatologic diseases; allergic states, edematous states (cerebral, nephrotic syndrome); immunosuppression for transplantation; hypercalcemia; malignancies (breast, lymphomas).

TABLE 7–4. COMPARISON OF GLUCOCORTICOIDS

Drug	Equivalent Dose (mg)	Relative Mineralcorticoid Activity	Duration (h)	Route
Cortisone (Cortone)	25.00	2	8–12	PO, IM
Hydrocortisone (Solu-Cortef)	20.00	2	8–12	PO, IM, IV
Prednisone (Deltasone)	5.00	1	12–36	PO
Prednisolone (Delta-Cortef)	5.00	1	12–36	PO, IM, IV
Methylprednisolone (Depo-Medrol, Solu-Medrol)	4.00	0	36–72	PO, IM, IV
Dexamethasone (Decadron)	0.75	0	36–72	PO, IV

From Gomella LG, ed. Clinician's Pocket Reference. *6th ed. Norwalk, Conn: Appleton & Lange; 1989. Used with permission.*

Dosage: Varies with indications and institutional protocols; some commonly used dosages are listed here:
Acute adrenal insufficiency (Addisonian crisis): hydrocortisone 100 mg IV every 6 hours.
Chronic adrenal insufficiency: hydrocortisone 20 mg PO QAM, 10 mg PO QPM; may need mineralocorticoid supplementation such as desoxycorticosterone acetate.
Hypercalcemia of malignancy: hydrocrotisone 250–500 mg PO/IV initially; then prednisone 10–30 mg PO QD.
Cerebral edema: dexamethasone 10 mg IV; then 4–6 mg IV every 4–6 hours.

Notes: See Table 7–4. All steroids can cause hyperglycemia and adrenal suppression. Never acutely stop steroids, especially if chronic treatment. Taper dose.

■ Streptokinase (Streptase, Kabikinase)

Indications: Coronary artery thrombosis; acute massive pulmonary embolism; deep vein thrombosis.

Actions: Activates plasminogen to plasmin that degrades fibrin.

Dosage: *Pulmonary embolus*: loading dose of 250,000 IU IV through a peripheral vein over 30 minutes, then 100,000 IU/h IV for 24–72 hours.
Transmural MI: 1,500,000 IU IV over 60 minutes.

Supplied: Powder for injection.

Notes: If maintenance infusion is not adequate to maintain thrombin clotting time two to five times control, refer to package insert, PDR, or American Hospital Formulary Service for adjustments. Heparinization is required after streptokinase administration.

■ Streptomycin

Indications: Tuberculosis; bacterial endocarditis.

Actions: Aminoglycoside antibiotic; interferes with protein synthesis.

Dosage: 1–4 g/d IM in 2–4 divided doses.

Supplied: Injection 400 mg/mL; powder for injection 1 g, 5 g.

Notes: Nephrotoxic and ototoxic. Decrease dose in renal impairment.

■ Sucralfate (Carafate)

Indications: Treatment of duodenal ulcers; gastric ulcers.

Actions: Forms ulcer-adherent complex that protects it against acid, pepsin, and bile salts.

Dosage: 1 g PO QID.

Supplied: Tablets 1 g.

Notes: Administer 1 hour prior to meals and HS. Antacids may also be used if taken one-half hour after sucralfate. Treatment should be continued for 4–8 weeks unless healing is demonstrated by x-ray or endoscopy. Constipation is most frequent side effect.

■ Sulfamethoxazole

See **Trimethoprim-Sulfamethoxazole.**

■ Sulfasalazine (Azulfidine)

Indications: Ulcerative colitis.

Actions: Sulfonamide antibiotic.

Dosage: 500 mg–1 g PO BID–QID.

Supplied: Tablets 500 mg; enteric-coated tablets 500 mg; oral suspension 250 mg/5 mL.

Notes: Can cause severe GI upset. Discolors urine.

■ Sulfinpyrazone (Anturane)

Indications: Chronic gouty arthritis.

Actions: Inhibits renal tubular absorption of uric acid.

Dosage: 100–200 mg PO BID.

Supplied: Tablets 100 mg; capsules 200 mg.

■ Sulfisoxazole (Gantrisin, Others)

Indications: Acute uncomplicated urinary tract infections.

Actions: Sulfonamide antibiotic.

Dosage: 500 mg–1 g PO QID.

Supplied: Tablets 500 mg; oral suspension 500 mg/5 mL; syrup 500 mg/5 mL.

Notes: Avoid use in last half of pregnancy (causes fetal hyperbilirubinemia).

■ Sulindac (Clinoril)

See Table 7–9, p 496.

■ Temazepam (Restoril) [C]

Indications: Insomnia.

Actions: Benzodiazepine.

Dosage: 15–30 mg PO QHS prn.

Supplied: Capsules 15 mg, 30 mg.

Notes: Reduce dose in elderly.

■ Terazosin (Hytrin)

Indications: Hypertension.

Actions: Peripherally acting antiadrenergic agent.

Dosage: Initially 1 mg PO HS; titrate up to maximum of 5 mg PO QHS.

Supplied: Tablets 1 mg, 2 mg, 5 mg.

Notes: Hypotension and syncope following first dose; dizziness, weakness, nasal congestion, peripheral edema common; must be used with thiazide diuretic.

■ Terbutaline (Brethine, Bricanyl)

Indications: Reversible bronchospasm (asthma, chronic obstructive pulmonary disease).

Actions: Sympathomimetic bronchodilator.

Dosage: 2.5–5 mg PO TID; 0.25 mg SC, may repeat in 15 minutes (maximum 0.5 mg in 4 hours); metered dose inhaler, 2 inhalations every 4–6 hours.

Supplied: Tablets 2.5 mg, 5 mg; injection 1 mg/mL; metered dose inhaler 0.2 mg/dose or 200 μg/dose.

Notes: Use with caution in diabetes, hypertension, and hyperthyroidism. High doses may precipitate beta-1-adrenergic effects.

■ Terfenadine (Seldane)

Indications: Seasonal allergic rhinitis.

Actions: Relatively nonsedating antihistamine.

Dosage: 60 mg PO BID.

Supplied: Tablets 60 mg.

■ Tetanus Immune Globulin

Indications: Passive immunization against tetanus for any person with a suspect contaminated wound and unknown immunization status or if less than 3 doses of tetanus toxoid have been given in the past.

Actions: Passive immunization.

Dosage: 250–500 U IM (higher doses if delay in initiation of therapy).

Supplied: Injection 250-U vial or syringe.

Notes: May begin active immunization series at different injection site if required.

■ Tetanus Toxoid

Indications: Protection against tetanus.

Actions: Active immunization.

Dosage: 0.5 mL as tetanus/diphtheria toxoid for tetanus and diphtheria prophylaxis.

Supplied: Injection: tetanus toxoid, fluid 4–5 Lf U/0.5 mL; tetanus toxoid, adsorbed 5 Lf U/0.5 mL, 10 Lf U/0.5 mL.

■ Tetracycline (Achromycin V, Sumycin)

Indications: Broad-spectrum antibiotic active against *Staphylococcus, Streptococcus, Chlamydia, Rickettsia,* and *Mycoplasma.*

Actions: Interferes with protein synthesis.

Dosage: 250–500 mg PO QID.

Supplied: Capsules 100 mg, 250 mg, 500 mg; tablets 250 mg, 500 mg; oral suspension 250 mg/5 mL; injection 250 mg/mL, 500 mg/mL.

Notes: IM and IV routes are not recommended. Use with caution in pregnancy. Do not use if impaired renal function (see **Doxycycline**).

■ Theophylline (Theolair, Theodur, Somophyllin, Others)

Indications: Asthma; bronchospasm.

Actions: Relaxes smooth muscle of the bronchi and pulmonary blood vessels.

Dosage: 24 mg/kg/24 h PO divided every 6 hours; sustained-release products may be divided every 8–12 hours.

Supplied: Elixir 80 mg/15 mL, 150 mg/15 mL; liquid 80 mg/15 mL, 160 mg/15 mL; capsules 100 mg, 200 mg, 250 mg; tablets 100 mg, 125 mg, 200 mg, 225 mg, 250 mg, 300 mg; sustained-release capsules 50 mg, 75 mg, 100 mg, 125 mg, 200 mg, 250 mg, 260 mg, 300 mg; sustained-release tablets 100 mg, 200 mg, 250 mg, 300 mg, 400 mg, 500 mg.

Notes: See Table 7–11, p 498.

■ Thiamine (Vitamin B_1)

Indications: Thiamine deficiency (beriberi); alcholic neuritis; Wernicke's encephalopathy.

Actions: Dietary supplementation.

Dosage: *Deficiency*: 100 mg IM QD for 2 weeks, then 5–10 mg PO QD for 1 month.

Wernicke's encephalopathy: 100 mg IV × 1 dose, then 100 mg IM QD for 2 weeks.

Supplied: Tablets 5 mg, 10 mg, 25 mg, 50 mg, 100 mg, 500 mg; injection 100 mg/mL, 200 mg/mL.

Notes: IV thiamine administration associated with anaphylactic reaction. Must be given slowly IV.

■ Thioridazine (Mellaril)

Indications: Psychotic disorders; short-term treatment of depression; agitation; organic brain syndrome.

Actions: Phenothiazine antipsychotic.

Dosage: Initially 50–100 mg PO TID; maintenance 10–50 mg PO BID–QID.

Supplied: Tablets 10 mg, 15 mg, 25 mg, 50 mg, 100 mg, 150 mg, 200 mg; oral concentrate 30 mg/mL; oral suspension 25 mg/5 mL, 100 mg/5 mL.

Notes: Low incidence of extrapyramidal effects.

■ Thiothixene (Navane)

Indications: Psychotic disorders.

Actions: Antipsychotic.

Dosage: *Mild to moderate psychosis*: 2 mg PO TID.
Severe psychosis: 5 mg PO BID; increase to maximum dose of 30 mg TID.
IM use: 2 mg 2–5 times per day; maximum 30 mg/d.

Supplied: Capsules 1 mg, 2 mg, 5 mg, 10 mg, 20 mg; oral concentrate 5 mg/mL; injection 2 mg/mL, 5 mg/mL.

Notes: Drowsiness and extrapyramidal side effects are most common.

■ Ticarcillin (Ticar)

See Table 7–6, p 490.

■ Ticarcillin/Potassium Clavulanate (Timentin)

See Table 7–6, p 490.

■ Timolol (Timoptic, Blocadren)

(See also Table 7–7, p 492.)

Indications: Glaucoma; hypertension; reduction in risk of reinfarction or cardiovascular mortality immediately after an acute myocardial infarction.

Actions: Beta-adrenergic blocking agent.

Dosage: *Glaucoma*: 1 gtt of 0.25% to 0.50% solution in each eye BID (Timoptic).
Hypertension and reinfarction: See Timolol (Blocadren) in Table 7–7, p 492.

Supplied: Tablets 5 mg, 10 mg, 20 mg; ophthalmic solution 0.25%, 0.5%.

■ Tobramycin (Nebcin)

Indications: Serious gram-negative infections, especially *Pseudomonas*.

Actions: Aminoglycoside antibiotic; interferes with protein synthesis.

Dosage: Based on renal function; refer to Tables 7–13 and 7–14, p 499.

Supplied: Injection 10 mg/mL, 40 mg/mL.

Notes: Nephrotoxic and ototoxic. Decrease dose with renal insufficiency. Monitor creatinine clearance and serum concentration for dosage adjustments. See Table 7–12, p 498.

■ Tocainide (Tonocard)

Indications: Suppression of ventricular arrhythmias including premature ventricular contractions and ventricular tachycardia.

Actions: Class 1B antiarrhythmic.

Dosage: 400–600 mg PO every 8 hours.

Supplied: Tablets 400 mg, 600 mg.

Notes: Properties similar to those of lidocaine. Reduce dose in renal failure. CNS and GI side effects are common.

■ Tolazamide (Tolinase, Ronase, Others)

See Table 7–10, p 497.

■ Tolbutamide (Orinase)

See Table 7–10, p 497.

■ Tolmetin (Tolectin)

See Table 7–9, p 496.

■ Trazodone (Desyrel)

Indications: Major depression.

Actions: Antidepressant.

Dosage: 50–150 mg PO QD–QID; maximum 600 mg/d.

Supplied: Tablets 50 mg, 100 mg, 150 mg.

Notes: May take 1–2 weeks for symptomatic improvement. Anticholinergic side effects.

■ Triamterene (Dyrenium)

Indications: Edema associated with congestive heart failure; cirrhosis.

Actions: Potassium-sparing diuretic.

Dosage: 50–100 mg PO QD–BID.

Supplied: Capsules 50 mg, 100 mg.

Notes: Can cause hyperkalemia, blood dyscrasias, liver damage, and other reactions.

■ Triazolam (Halcion) [C]

Indications: Insomnia.

Actions: Benzodiazepine.

Dosage: 0.125–0.5 mg PO HS prn.

Supplied: Tablets 0.125 mg, 0.25 mg, 0.5 mg.

Notes: Additive CNS depression with alcohol and other CNS depressants.

■ Trifluoperazine (Stelazine)

Indications: Psychotic disorders.

Actions: Phenothiazine antipsychotic.

Dosage: 2–5 mg PO BID.

Supplied: Tablets 1 mg, 2 mg, 5 mg, 10 mg; oral concentrate 10 mg/mL; injection 2 mg/mL.

Notes: Decrease dosage in elderly and debilitated patients. Oral concentrate must be diluted to 60 mL or more prior to administration.

■ Trihexyphenidyl (Artane)

Indications: Parkinsonism; drug-induced extrapyramidal disorders.

Actions: Anticholinergic.

Dosage: 2–5 mg PO QD–QID.

Supplied: Tablets 2 mg, 5 mg; sustained-release capsules 5 mg; elixir 2 mg/5 mL.

Notes: Contraindicated in narrow-angle glaucoma.

■ Trimeprazine (Temaril)

Indications: Pruritis associated with allergic and nonallergic conditions.

Actions: Phenothiazine antihistamine.

Dosage: 2.5 mg PO QID prn OR 5 mg PO every 12 hours sustained-release.

Supplied: Tablets 2.5 mg; sustained-release capsules 5 mg; syrup 2.5 mg/5 mL.

Notes: Extrapyramidal reactions may occur in elderly.

■ Trimethaphan (Arfonad)

Indications: Treatment of hypertensive crisis; treatment of pulmonary edema with pulmonary hypertension associated with systemic hypertension.

Actions: Ganglionic blocking agent.

Dosage: 0.3–6 mg/min IV infusion titrated to effect.

Supplied: Injection 50 mg/mL.

Notes: Additive effect with other antihypertensive agents. Vasopressors may be used to reverse hypotension if required. Phenylephrine is vasopressor of choice for reversal of effects.

■ Trimethobenzamide (Tigan)

Indications: Nausea and vomiting.

Actions: Anticholinergic antiemetic.

Dosage: 250 mg PO or 200 mg rectally or IM TID–QID prn.

Supplied: Capsules 100 mg, 250 mg; suppositories 100 mg, 200 mg; injection 100 mg/mL.

Notes: In the presence of viral infections, may contribute to Reye's syndrome. May cause Parkinsonian-like syndrome.

■ Trimethoprim (Trimpex, Proloprim)

Indications: Urinary tract infections caused by susceptible gram-positive and gram-negative organisms.

Actions: Inhibits dihydrofolate reductase.

Dosage: 100 mg PO BID OR 200 mg PO QD.

Supplied: Tablets 100 mg, 200 mg.

Notes: Reduce dose in renal failure. If creatinine clearance 15–30 mL/min, give half dose; <15 mL/min is not well studied.

■ Trimethoprim-Sulfamethoxazole (Bactrim, Septra)

Indications: Urinary tract infections; otitis media; sinusitis; bronchitis; traveler's diarrhea; *Shigella*; *Pneumocystis carinii*; *Nocardia*.

Actions: Combined actions of sulfonamide and trimethoprim.

Dosage: 1 DS tablet PO BID or 10 mg/kg/24 h (based on trimethoprim component) IV in 3 or 4 divided doses.
Pneumocystis carinii: 20 mg/kg/d (trimethoprim component) in 3 or 4 divided doses.

Supplied: Tablets—regular 80 mg TMP and 400 mg SMX, DS 160 mg TMP and 800 mg SMX; oral suspension 40 mg TMP and 200 mg SMX per 5 mL; injection 80 mg TMP and 400 mg SMX per 5 mL.

Notes: Reduce dosage in renal failure. If creatinine clearance 15–30 mL/min, use half dose. Contraindicated if clearance <15 mL/min.

■ Triprolidine-Pseudoephedrine (Actifed)

Indications: Symptomatic relief of allergic and vasomotor rhinitis.

Actions: Antihistamine and decongestant combination.

Dosage: 1 tablet PO TID–QID or 2 tsp (10 mL) TID–QID.

Supplied: Tablets—triprolidine 2.5 mg + pseudoephedrine 60 mg; syrup—triprolidine 1.25 mg + pseudoephedrine 30 mg per 5 mL.

■ Urokinase (Abbokinase)

Indications: Pulmonary embolism; coronary artery thrombosis; restoration of patency to IV catheters.

Actions: Converts plasminogen to plasmin that causes clot lysis.

Dosage: *Systemic effect*: 4400 IU/kg IV over 10 minutes, followed by 4400 IU/kg/h for 12 hours.
Restoration of catheter patency: inject 5000 IU into catheter and gently aspirate.

Supplied: Powder for injection 5000 IU/mL, 250,000 IU/5-mL vial.

Notes: Do not use systemically within 10 days of surgery, delivery, or organ biopsy.

■ Valproic Acid and Divalproex (Depakene and Depakote)

Indications: Absence seizures; in combination for tonic/clonic seizures.

Actions: Anticonvulsant.

Dosage: 15–60 mg/kg/24 h, divided every 8 hours.

Supplied: Valproic Acid—capsules 250 mg; syrup 250 mg/5 mL. Divalproex—enteric-coated tablets 125 mg, 250 mg, 500 mg.

Notes: Monitor liver functions and follow serum levels (see Table 7–11, p 498). Concurrent use of phenobarbital and phenytoin may alter serum levels of these agents.

■ Vancomycin (Vancocin, Vancoled)

Indications: Serious infections caused by penicillin-resistant staphylococci and in enterococcal endocarditis in combination with aminoglycosides in penicillin-allergic patients; oral treatment of *C. difficile* pseudomembranous colitis.

Actions: Interferes with protein synthesis.

Dosage: *Intravenous*: 1 g every 12 hours OR 500 mg every 6 hours.
Oral: 250–500 mg PO every 6 hours.

Supplied: Capsules 125 mg, 250 mg; powder for oral solution; powder for injection 500 mg, 1000 mg per vial.

Notes: Ototoxic and nephrotoxic. Not absorbed orally, provides local effect in gut only. Give IV dose slowly over 1 hour to prevent "red-man syndrome." Adjust dose in renal failure. Follow levels. See Table 7–12, p 498.

■ Vasopressin (Antidiuretic Hormone) (Pitressin)

Indications: Treatment of diabetes insipidus; relief of gaseous GI tract distension; severe GI bleeding.

Actions: Posterior pituitary hormone; potent GI vasoconstrictor.

Dosage: *Diabetes insipidus*: 5–10 U SC or IM TID–QID or 1.5–5.0 U IM every 1–3 days of the Pitressin tannate in oil.
GI bleeding: 0.2–0.4 U/min.

Supplied: Injection 20 U/mL.

Notes: Should be used with caution with any vascular disease.

■ Vecuronium (Norcuron)

Indications: Skeletal muscle relaxation used in conjunction with mechanical ventilation.

Actions: Nondepolarizing neuromuscular blocker.

Dosage: 0.08–0.1 mg/kg IV bolus; maintenance of 0.010–0.015 mg/kg after 25–40 minutes followed with additional doses every 12–15 minutes.

Supplied: Powder for injection 10 mg.

Notes: Drug interactions leading to increased effect of vecuronium include aminoglycosides, tetracycline, and succinylcholine. Less cardiac effects than with pancuronium.

■ Verapamil (Calan, Isoptin)

Indications: Supraventricular tachyarrhythmias (paroxysmal atrial tachycardia, atrial flutter, or fibrillation); vasospastic (Prinzmetal's) and unstable (crescendo, preinfarction) angina; chronic stable angina (classic effort-associated); hypertension.

Actions: Calcium channel blocker.

Dosage: *Tachyarrhythmias*: 5–10 mg IV over 2 minutes (may repeat in 30 minutes).
Angina: 240–480 mg/24 h divided in 3 or 4 doses.
Hypertension: 80–180 mg PO TID or sustained-release tablet 180–240 mg PO QD.

Supplied: Tablets 40 mg, 80 mg, 120 mg; sustained-release tablets 180 mg, 240 mg; injection 5 mg/2 mL.

Notes: Use with caution in elderly patients. Reduce dose in renal failure. Constipation is a common side effect.

■ Vidarabine (Vira-A)

Indications: Treatment of herpes simplex encephalitis.

Actions: Antiviral agent.

Dosage: 15 mg/kg/24 h by slow IV infusion over 12–24 hours.

Supplied: Injection 200 mg/mL.

Notes: Early diagnosis and treatment are essential to success of therapy. Treat only patients with positive herpes simplex virus cell culture. May suppress RBC and platelet counts. Avoid administration of allopurinol with vidarabine. Acyclovir is the drug of choice for herpes simplex encephalitis.

■ Vitamin B_{12}

See **Cyanocobalamin.**

■ Vitamin K

See **Phytonadione.**

■ Warfarin Sodium (Coumadin)

Indications: Prophylaxis and treatment of pulmonary embolism and venous thrombosis; atrial fibrillation with embolization.

Actions: Inhibits hepatic production of vitamin K–dependent clotting factors in this order: VII–IX–X–II.

Dosage: Need to individualize dosage to keep prothrombin time (PT) at 1.12–2.0 times control, depending on the indication for use; initially 10–15 mg PO, IM, or IV QD for 1–3 days; then maintenance, 2–10 mg PO, IV, or IM QD; follow daily PT during initial phase to guide dosage.

Supplied: Tablets 2 mg, 2.5 mg, 5 mg, 7.5 mg, 10 mg; powder for injection 50 mg/vial.

Notes: PT needs to be checked periodically while on maintenance dose. Beware of bleeding caused by overanticoagulation (PT >3 times control). Caution patient on effects of taking coumadin with other medications, especially aspirin. To correct overcoumadinization rapidly, use vitamin K, fresh-frozen plasma, or both. Highly teratogenic; do not use in pregnancy.

■ Zidovudine (Retrovir)

Indications: Management of patients with HIV infections.

Actions: Antiviral agent.

Dosage: *Symptomatic HIV infection*: 200 mg every 4 hours for 1 month, then 100 mg PO every 4 hours.
Asymptomatic HIV infection: 100 mg PO every 4 hours.
Intravenous: 1–2 mg/kg every 4 hours.

Supplied: Capsules 100 mg; syrup 50 mg/5 mL; injection.

Notes: Not a cure for HIV infections.

TABLE 7–5. ANTISTAPHYLOCOCCAL PENICILLINS

Drug (Brand Name)	Daily Dosage Range, Adult (g)	Usual Dosing Interval (h)	Supplied	Notes
Methicillin (Staphcillin)	4–18	4–6	Injection	1. Interstitial nephritis can occur with high doses 2. Reduce dose in renal failure
Oxacillin (Prostaphlin)	4–12	4–6	Injection Oral	1. Poorly absorbed orally, cloxacillin or dicloxacillin better for oral use 2. Interstitial nephritis can occur with high doses 3. Reduce dose in renal failure
Nafcillin (Unipen)	4–18	4–6	Injection Oral	1. Poorly absorbed orally, cloxacillin or dicloxacillin better for oral use 2. Injectable highest activity against *Staph. aureus*
Cloxacillin (Tegopen, Cloxapen)	1–2	6	Oral	Administer on an empty stomach at least 1 hour ac or 2 hours pc
Dicloxacillin (Dynapen)	0.5–1	6	Oral	See *Cloxacillin*

Note. These agents should be used only for infections caused by penicillinase-producing *Staphylococcus aureus* and *Staphylococcus epidermidis*. Other bacteria (*Streptococcus, Clostridia*, etc.) normally sensitive to penicillin are less sensitive to the antistaphylococcal penicillins and treatment failures can result. The methicillin or oxacillin disk is the class disk for all the antistaphylococcal penicillins, and sensitivity results apply to all drugs in this class. Hospital strains of methicillin-resistant *Staph. aureus* (MRSA) and *Staph. epidermidis* are becoming more frequent. Vancomycin is the drug of choice for MRSA. Antistaphylococcal penicillins should not be used in penicillin-allergic patients.
Modified from Gomella LG, ed. Clinician's Pocket Reference. *6th ed. Norwalk, Conn: Appleton & Lange; 1989. Used with permission.*

TABLE 7–6. ANTIPSEUDOMONAL PENICILLINS

Drug (Brand Name)	Daily Dosage Range, Adult (g)	Usual Dosing Interval (h)	Na+ (mEq/g)	Supplied	Notes
Carbenicillin (Geopen, Pyopen)	8–40[a]	4	4.7	Injection Oral[b]	1. When used alone, resistant gram-negative bacteria may occur 2. Hypokalemia and bleeding may occur with high doses 3. Na^+ content may cause congestive heart failure
Ticarcillin (Ticar)	2–24[a]	4–6	5.4	Injection	1. See Note 1 for *Carbenicillin* 2. Hypokalemia, bleeding, and less sodium than carbenicillin
Ticarcillin-potassium clavulanate (Timentin)	9–12	4–6	5.4	Injection	Clavulanate protects ticarcillin from degradation by β-lactamases
Mezlocillin (Mezlin)	2–24[a]	4–6	1.85	Injection	1. More active than ticarcillin against Enterobacteriacae, same activity against *Pseudomonas aeruginosa*

(*continued*)

TABLE 7–6. (*Continued*)

Drug (Brand Name)	Daily Dosage Range Adult (g)	Usual Dosing Interval (h)	Na+ (mEq/g)	Supplied	Notes
					2. Good anaerobic activity against *Bacillus fragilis*
Azlocillin (Azlin)	2–24[a]	4–6	1.85	Injection	1. More active than ticarcillin against *P. aeruginosa* 2. Same activity as ticarcillin against Enterobacteriacae
Piperacillin (Pipracil)	2–24[a]	4–6	1.85	Injection	Good activity against *P. aeruginosa*, Enterobacteriacae, and anaerobes (*B. fragilis*)

Note. These antibiotics were developed for the treatment of serious systemic *Pseudomonas aeruginosa* infections. These are usually treated in combination with an aminoglycoside because the combination is synergistic against *Pseudomonas aeruginosa*. Like penicillin and ampicillin, mezlocillin, piperacillin and azlocillin show synergism against *enterococci* (Group D strep) where carbenicillin and ticarcillin do not. For carbenicillin and ticarcillin, the class disk (carbenicillin) determines the sensitivity for both drugs. For mezlocillin, piperacillin and azlocillin sensitivities must be obtained for each drug. These drugs should not be used in penicillin-allergic patients.

[a]Reduce dose in renal failure.

[b]The oral form of this drug is to be used only for simple urinary tract infections, never for serious infections of any type.

Modified from Gomella LG, ed. Clinician's Pocket Reference, *6th ed. Norwalk, Conn: Appleton & Lange; 1989. Used with permission.*

TABLE 7–7. BETA-ADRENERGIC BLOCKING AGENTS

Drug (Brand Name)	Receptor Activity	Half-Life (h)	Excretion	Dosing Range and Frequency[a]	
				Angina Pectoris	*Hypertension*
Acebutolol* (Sectral)	β_1	3–4	Hepatic, renal	N.A.	200 mg PO BID 400 mg PO QD
Atenelol (Tenormin)	β_1	6–9	Renal	50–100 mg PO QD[b]	50–100 mg PO QD[b]
Carteolol (Cartrol)	β_1, β_2	6	Renal	N.A.	2.5–10 mg PO QD
Labetalol (Normodyne, Trandate)	β_1, β_2, α	6–8	Hepatic	N.A.	100–400 mg PO BID
Metoprolol (Lopressor)	β_1	3–7	Hepatic, renal	50–100 mg PO BID	50–100 mg PO BID–TID
Nadolol (Corgard)	β_1, β_2	20–40	Renal	40–240 mg PO QD[b]	40–320 mg PO QD[b]
Penbutolol (Levatol)	β_1, β_2	5	Hepatic, renal	N.A.	20–40 mg PO QD
Pindolol* (Visken)	β_1, β_2	3–4	Hepatic, renal	N.A.	10–40 mg PO BID
Propranolol[c] (Inderal)	β_1, β_2	3–5	Hepatic	80–240 mg PO BID–TID	80–480 mg PO BID–TID
Timolol (Blocadren)	β_1, β_2	4	Hepatic, renal	10–40 mg PO BID	N.A.

[a]Other uses of beta blockers include post myocardial infarction to reduce mortality, pheochromocytoma, and hypertrophic subaortic stenosis.
[b]Reduce dose in renal failure.
[c]For arrhythmias, adult: 80–120 mg PO divided TID–QID. For migraine prophylaxis: 80–240 mg PO divided BID–TID.
*Intrinsic Sympathetic Activity (ISA)
Modified from Gomella LG, ed. Clinician's Pocket Reference. *6th ed. Norwalk, Conn: Appleton & Lange; 1989. Used with permission.*

TABLE 7–8. CEPHALOSPORINS

Drug (Brand Name)	Daily Dosing, Adult	Usual Interval (h)	Half-Life	Supplied	Notes
■ FIRST-GENERATION CEPHALOSPORINS					
Cefadroxil (Duricef, Ultracef)	1–2 g PO	12	1.5 h	Caps Tablets	
Cephalothin (Keflin)	2–12 g[a]	4–6	30–45 min	Injection	IV use causes phlebitis; IM use is painful
Cephapirin (Cefadyl)	2–12 g[a]	4–6	30–45 min	Injection	Possibly less phlebitis; IM use less painful than Keflin
Cefaclor (Ceclor)	1–4 g[a]	4–6	45 min	Oral	High-level activity against *Hemophilus influenzae*
Cephalexin (Keflex)	1–4 g[a]	4–6	45 min	Oral	
Cephradine (Velocef, Anspor)	1–4 g PO 2–8 g IV	4–6	45 min	Oral Injection	Less active than cephalothin against *Staph. aureus*
Cefazolin (Ancef, Kefzol)	1.5–12 g[a]	8	2 h	Injection	1. Best first-generation for surgical prophylaxis 2. IM dose fairly well tolerated

(*continued*)

TABLE 7–8. (*Continued*)

Drug (Brand Name)	Daily Dosing, Adult	Usual Interval (h)	Half-Life	Supplied	Notes
■ SECOND-GENERATION CEPHALOSPORINS					
Cefamandole (Mandol)	3–12 g[a]	4–6	40 min	Injection	1. High level of activity against *Hemophilus influenzae* 2. Disulfiram reaction with alcohol use 3. Monitor prothrombin time closely with long-term use 4. Does not cross blood-brain barrier
Cefotetan (Cefotan)	2–4 g	12	4 h	Injection	1. Activity against *B. fragilis* 2. May cause hypoprothrombinemia
Cefoxitin (Mefoxin)	2–12 g[a]	4–6	45 min	Injection	Best cephalosporin against *B. fragilis;* good for mixed aerobic/anaerobic infections in obstetrics/gynecology, surgery
Cefuroxime (Zinacef, Ceftin, Axetil)	2.25–9 g IV[a] 500 mg–1 g PO	8	1.5 h	Injection Oral	Crosses blood-brain barrier; can be used for some organisms in meningitis at higher doses
Ceforanide (Precef)	1–4 g[a]	12	2.2 h	Injection	Less effective against *Staph. aureus*
Cefonicid (Monocid)	1–4 g[a]	24	4 h	Injection	Less effective against *Staph. aureus*
Cefmetazole (Zefazone)	2–8 g[a]	6–12	1.2 h	Injection	Active against anaerobic bacteria
■ THIRD-GENERATION CEPHALOSPORINS					
Cefotaxime (Claforan)	2–12 g[a]	4–8	1 h	Injection	1. Crosses blood-brain barrier 2. Give half dose if creatinine clearance < 20

Moxalactam (Moxam)	2–12 g[a]	8	2.5 h	Injection	1. Crosses blood-brain barrier 2. Serious bleeding can occur from hypoprothrombinemia and thrombocytopenia; minimize by prophylactic vitamin K and dose of <4 g/d
Cefoperazone (Cefobid)	2–12 g	8–12	2.5 h	Injection	1. Hepatic/renal excretion allows normal dosing in renal failure 2. Disulfiram reactions and hypoprothrombinemia can occur 3. Do not use alone with *Pseudomonas*
Ceftizoxime (Ceftizox)	2–12 g[a]	8–12	2.5 h	Injection	1. Spectrum similar to that of cefotaxime 2. Less activity against *B. fragilis*
Ceftazidime (Fortraz, Tazidime, Tazicef)	2–12 g[a]	8–12	2.5 h	Injection	1. Best third-generation against *Pseudomonas* 2. No activity against *B. fragilis* 3. Crosses blood-brain barrier
Ceftriaxone (Rocephin)	1–4 g	24	8 h	Injection	1. Long half-life allows once-a-day dose 2. Home therapy possible 3. No change in renal failure to 2 g/d 4. Crosses blood-brain barrier
Cefixime (Suprax)	400 mg	12–24	3.5 h	Oral	May cause GI irritation

Note. Cephalosporins are most commonly divided into groups on the basis of their activity against gram-negative bacteria. The use of the terms *first-*, *second-*, and *third-generation cephalosporin* reflects the gram-negative activity, with the third-generation having the greatest and the first-generation the least. The resistance or sensitivity pattern to cephalothin applies to all the first-generation cephalosporins. For the second- and third-generation cephalosporins sensitivity to the individual agents must be determined. In patients showing severe allergic reactions to penicillins, cephalosporins must be used cautiously as cross-sensitivity can exist.

[a]Reduce dose in renal failure.

Modified from Gomella LG, ed. Clinician's Pocket Reference. *6th ed. Norwalk, Conn: Appleton & Lange; 1989. Used with permission.*

TABLE 7–9. NONSTEROIDAL ANTI-INFLAMMATORY AGENTS

Drug (Trade Name)	Maximum Daily Doses (MG)	Dosing Frequency	Notes
■ **PROPIONIC ACIDS**			
Fenoprofen (Nalfon)	3200	TID, QID	Approval for arthritis and analgesia
Flurbiprofen (Ansaid)	300	BID, TID, QID	Approval for arthritis
Ibuprofen (Motrin, Rufen, Advil, Nuprin)	3200	BID, TID, QID	1. Approval for arthritis, analgesia, and dysmenorrhea 2. Many generic products are available
Ketoprofen (Orudis)	300	TID, QID	Approval for arthritis and analgesia
Naproxen (Naprosyn, Anaprox)	1500	BID	1. Approval for arthritis and analgesia 2. Very GI irritating
■ **INDOLES**			
Indomethacin (Indocin)	200	QD, BID, TID	1. Approval for arthritis 2. Sustained-release product available
Sulindac (Clinoril)	400	BID	1. Approval for arthritis 2. Less renal toxicity
■ **HETEROPHENYL ACETIC ACIDS**			
Tolmetin (Tolectin)	2000	TID, QID	Approval for arthritis
■ **OXICAMS**			
Piroxicam (Feldene)	20	BID	1. Approval for arthritis 2. Very GI irritating
■ **PHENYLACETIC ACIDS**			
Diclofenac (Voltaren)	200	BID, TID	Approval for arthritis
■ **SALICYLIC ACIDS**			
Aspirin	3000–6000	QID, six times per day	Approval for arthritis and analgesia
Diflunisal (Dolobid)	1500	BID	1. Approval for arthritis and analgesia 2. May prolong prothrombin time

TABLE 7–10. SULFONYLUREAS

Drug (Trade Name)	Duration of Activity (h)	Equivalent Dose (mg)	Maximum Daily Dose (mg)
■ **FIRST GENERATION**			
Acetohexamide (Dymelor)	12–18	500	1500
Chlorpropamide (Diabinese)	36–72	250	500
Tolazamide (Tolinase)	24	250	1000
Tolbutamide (Orinase)	6–8	1000	3000
■ **SECOND GENERATION**			
Glyburide (DiaBeta, Micronase)	24	5	20
Glipizide (Glucotrol)	12–24	10	40

TABLE 7–11. DRUG LEVELS

Drug	Therapeutic Level	Toxic Level
Carbamazepine	8.0–12.0 μg/mL	>15.0 μg/mL
Digoxin	0.8–2.0 ng/mL	>2.4 ng/mL
Ethanol		100–200 mg/100 mL (legally drunk, labile behavior) 150–300 mg/ 100 mL (confusion) 250–400 mg/100 mL (stupor) 350–500 mg/100 mL (coma) >450 mg/100 mL (death)
Ethosuximide	40.0–100.0 μg/mL	>150.0 μg/mL
Lidocaine	1.5–6.5 μg/mL	>6.0–8.0 μg/mL
Lithium	0.6–1.2 mmol/L	>2.0 mmol/L
Phenobarbital	15.0–40.0 μg/mL	>45.0 μg/mL
Phenytoin	10.0–20.0 μg/mL	>25.0 μg/mL
Procainamide *N*-acetylprocainamide (NAPA-active metabolite of procainamide)	4.0–10.0 μg/mL	>16.0 μg/mL
Quinidine	3.0–7.0 μg/mL	>7 μg/mL
Salicylate	20–30 μg/mL	40–50 μg/dL
Theophylline	10.0–20.0 μg/mL	>20.0 μg/mL
Valproic acid	50–100 μg/mL	>150 μg/mL

Note. Each lab may have its own set of values that may vary slightly from those given.
Modified from Gomella LG, ed. Clinician's Pocket Reference. *6th ed. Norwalk, Conn: Appleton & Lange; 1989. Used with permission.*

TABLE 7–12. DRUG LEVELS: ANTIBIOTICS

Antibiotic	Trough (μg/mL) (maintain below upper limit)	Peak (μg/mL
Amikacin	5.0–7.5	25–35
Gentamicin	1.5–2.0	5–8
Tobramycin	1.5–2.0	5–8
Netilmicin	0.5–2.0	6–10
Vancomycin	5.0–10.0	20–40

Modified from Gomella LG, ed. Clinician's Pocket Reference. *6th ed. Norwalk, Conn: Appleton & Lange; 1989. Used with permission.*

TABLE 7–13. AMINOGLYCOSIDE DOSING IN ADULTS

1. Select the loading dose:

Gentamicin	1.5–2.0 mg/kg
Tobramycin	1.5–2.0 mg/kg
Amikacin	5.0–7.5 mg/kg

2. Calculate the estimated creatinine clearance (CrCl) based on serum creatinine (SCr), age, and weight (kg) OR a formal creatinine clearance can also be ordered, if time permits.

   $$\text{CrCl for male} = \frac{(140 - \text{age}) \times (\text{weight in kg})}{(\text{ScCr}) \times (72)}$$

   $$\text{CrCl for female} = 0.85 \times (\text{CrCl male})$$

3. By using Table 7–14 you can now select the maintenance dose (as a percentage of the chosen loading dose) most appropriate for the renal function of the patient based on CrCl and dosing interval. Shaded areas are the suggested percentages and intervals for any given creatinine clearance.
4. This is only an empirical dose to begin therapy. Serum levels should be monitored routinely for optimal therapy. Use Table 7–12.

Note. See Table 7–12 for the trough and peak levels of the aminoglycosides gentamicin, tobramycin, and amikacin. Peak levels should be drawn 30 minutes after the dose is completely infused; trough levels should be drawn 30 minutes prior to the dose. As a general rule, draw the peak and trough around the fourth maintenance dose. Therapy can be initiated with the recommended guidelines. THESE CALCULATIONS ARE NOT VALID FOR NETILMICIN.

From Gomella LG, ed. Clinician's Pocket Reference. *6th ed. Norwalk, Conn: Appleton & Lange; 1989. Used with permission.*

TABLE 7–14. PERCENTAGE OF LOADING DOSE REQUIRED FOR DOSAGE INTERVAL SELECTED

Creatinine Clearance (mL/min)	Dosing Interval		
	8 hours	*12 hours*	*24 hours*
90	90%	—	—
90	88	—	—
70	84	—	—
60	79	91%	—
50	74	87	—
40	66	80	—
30	57	72	92%
25	51	66	88
20	45	59	83
15	37	50	75
10	29	40	64
7	24	33	55
5	20	28	48
2	14	20	35
0	9	13	25

Note. Shaded areas indicate suggested dosage intervals.

From Hull JH, Sarubbi FA. Gentamicin serum concentrations: Pharmacokinetic predictions. Ann Intern Med *1976; 85:183–189. Used with permission.*

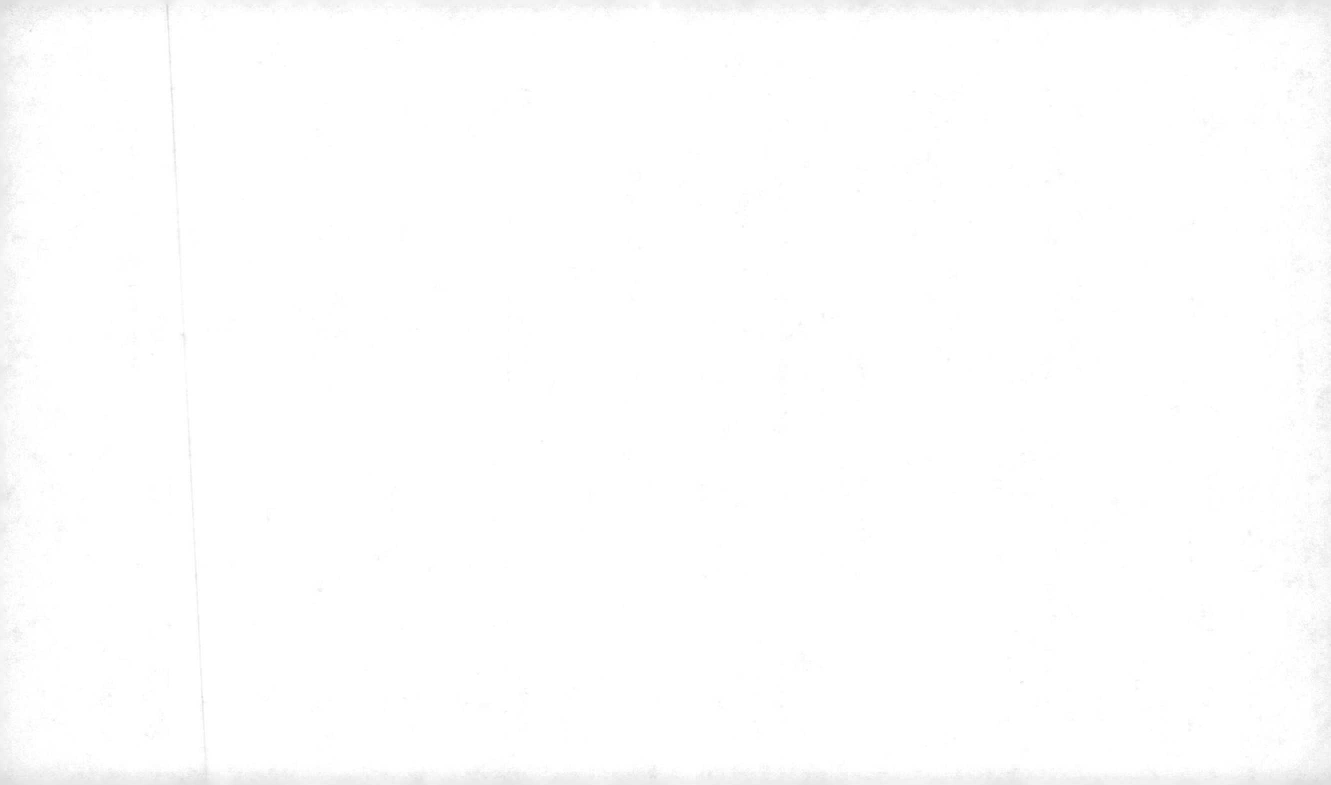

Appendix

TABLE A–1. TEMPERATURE CONVERSION

°F	°C	°C	°F
0	−17.7	0	32.0
95.0	35.0	35.0	95.0
96.0	35.5	35.5	95.9
97.0	36.1	36.0	96.8
98.0	36.6	36.5	97.7
98.6	37.0	37.0	98.6
99.0	37.2	37.5	99.5
100.0	37.7	38.0	100.4
101.0	38.3	38.5	101.3
102.0	38.8	39.0	102.2
103.0	39.4	39.5	103.1
104.0	40.0	40.0	104.0
105.0	40.5	40.5	104.9
106.0	41.1	41.0	105.8
°C = (°F − 32) × 5/9		°F = (°C × 9/5) + 32	

From Gomella LG, ed. Clinician's Pocket Reference. *6th ed. Norwalk, Conn: Appleton & Lange; 1989. Used with permission.*

TABLE A–2. WEIGHT CONVERSION

lb	kg	kg	lb
1	0.5	1	2.2
2	0.9	2	4.4
4	1.8	3	6.6
6	2.7	4	8.8
8	3.6	5	11.0
10	4.5	6	13.2
20	9.1	8	17.6
30	13.6	10	22.0
40	18.2	20	44.0
50	22.7	30	66.0
60	27.3	40	88.0
70	31.8	50	110.0
80	36.4	60	132.0
90	40.9	70	154.0
100	45.4	80	176.0
150	68.2	90	198.0
200	90.8	100	220.0
kg = lb × 0.454		lb = kg × 2.2	

From Gomella LG, ed. Clinician's Pocket Reference. *Norwalk, Conn: Appleton & Lange; 1989. Used with permission.*

TABLE A–3. GLASGOW COMA SCALE

Parameter		Response	Score
Eyes	Open	Spontaneously	4
		To verbal command	3
		To pain	2
		No response	1
Best motor response	To verbal command	Obeys	6
	To painful stimuls	Localizes pain	5
		Flexion-withdrawal	4
		Decorticate (flex)	3
		Decerebrate (extent)	2
		No response	1
Best verbal response		Oriented, converses	5
		Disoriented, converses	4
		Inappropriate responses	3
		Incomprehensible sounds	2
		No response	1

Note. The Glasgow Coma Scale (EMV Scale) is a fairly reliable, objective way to monitor changes in levels of consciousness. It is based on eye opening, motor responses, and verbal responses (EMV). A person's EMV score is based on the total of the three different responses. The score ranges from 3 (lowest) to 15 (highest).

From Gomella LG, ed. Clinician's Pocket Reference. *6th ed. Norwalk, Conn: Appleton & Lange; 1989. Used with permission.*

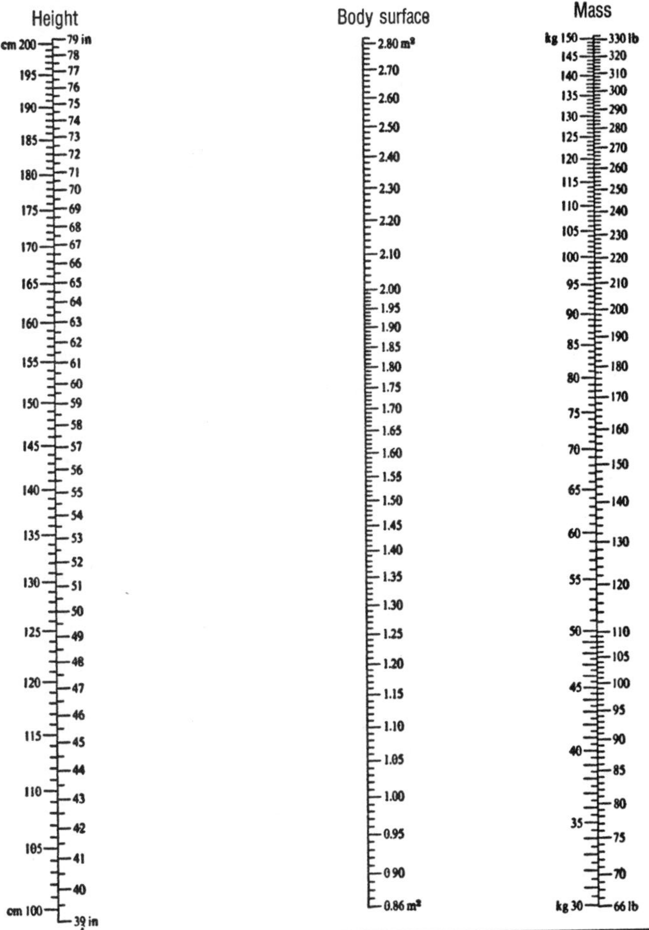

Figure A–1. Body surface area. To determine the body surface of an adult, use a straight-edge to connect height and mass. The point of intersection in the body surface line gives the body surface area in meters squared (m^2). *(From Lentner C, ed.* Geigy Scientific Tables. *8th ed. Basel: CIBA Geigy; 1981:vol 1, p 227.)*

TABLE A-4. ENDOCARDITIS PROPHYLAXIS

	Dosage for Adults	Dosage for Children[a]
DENTAL AND UPPER RESPIRATORY PROCEDURES[b]		
Oral[c]		
Amoxicillin[d]	3 g 1 h before procedure and 1.5 g 6 h later	50 mg/kg 1 h before procedure and 25 mg/kg 6 h later
Penicillin allergy: Erythromycin	1 g 2 h before procedure and 500 mg 6 h later	20 mg/kg 2 h before procedure and 10 mg/kg 6 h later
Parenteral[c,e]		
Ampicillin	2 g IM or IV 30 min before procedure	50 mg/kg IM or IV 30 min before procedure
plus		
Gentamicin	1.5 mg/kg IM or IV 30 min before procedure	2 mg/kg IM or IV 30 min before procedure
Penicillin allergy: Vancomycin	1 g IV infused *slowly over 1 h* beginning 1 h before procedure	20 mg/kg IV infused *slowly over 1 h* beginning 1 h before procedure

■ **GASTROINTESTINAL AND GENITOURINARY PROCEDURES**[b]

Oral[e]		
Amoxicillin[d]	3 g 1 h before procedure and 1.5 g 6 h later	50 mg/kg 1 h before procedure and 25 mg/kg 6 h later
Parenteral[c,e]		
Ampicillin	2 g IM or IV 30 min before procedure	50 mg/kg IM or IV 30 min before procedure
plus		
Gentamicin	1.5 mg/kg IM or IV 30 min before procedure	2 mg/kg IM or IV 30 min before procedure
Penicillin allergy: Vancomycin	1 g IV infused *slowly over 1 h* beginning 1 h before procedure	20 mg/kg IV infused *slowly over 1 h* beginning 1 h before procedure
plus		
Gentamicin	1.5 mg/kg IM or IV 30 min before procedure	2 mg/kg IM or IV 30 min before procedure

Note. For patients with previous endocarditis, valvular heart disease, prosthetic heart valves, most forms of congenital heart disease (but not uncomplicated secundum atrial septal defect), idiopathic hypertrophic subaortic stenosis, and mitral valve prolapse with regurgitation. Viridans streptococci are the most common cause of endocarditis after dental or upper respiratory procedures; enterococci are the most common cause of endocarditis after gastrointestinal or genitourinary procedures.

[a]Should not exceed adult doses.

[b]For a review of the risk of bacteremia and endocarditis with various procedures, see Durack D in Mandell GL et al, eds. *Principles and Practice of Infectious Disease.* 3rd ed. New York: Churchill Livingstone; 1990:716.

[c]Oral regimens are more convenient and safer. Parenteral regimens are more likely to be effective; they are recommended especially for patients with prosthetic heart valves, those who have had endocarditis previously, or those taking continuous oral penicillin for rheumatic fever prophylaxis.

[d]Amoxicillin is recommended because of its excellent bioavailability and good activity against streptococci and enterococci.

[e]A single dose of parenteral drugs is probably adequate, because bacteremia after most dental and diagnostic procedures is of short duration. An additional dose may be given 8 hours later in patients judged to be at higher risk.

From Med Lett *1989; 31:112. Used with permission.*

TABLE A–5. SPECIMEN TUBES FOR VENIPUNCTURE

Tube Color	Additives	General Use
Red	None	Clot tube to collect serum for chemistry, cross-matching, serology
Red and black (hot pink)	Silicone gel for rapid clot	As above, but not for osmolality or blood bank work
Blue	Sodium citrate (binds calcium)	Coagulation studies (best kept on ice, not for fibrin split products)
Blue/yellow label		Fibrin split products
Royal blue		Heavy metals, arsenic
Purple	Disodium EDTA (binds calcium)	Hematology, not for lipid profiles
Green	Sodium heparin	Ammonia, cortisol, ionized calcium (best kept on ice)
Green/glass beads		LE prep
Gray	Sodium fluoride	Lactic acid
Yellow	Transport medium	Blood cultures

Note. Individual labs may vary slightly from these listings.
From Gomella LG, Lefor AT: Surgery On Call. *Norwalk, Conn, Appleton & Lange, 1990, p 411. Used with permission.*

Index